REVISED EDITION

UNDERSTANDING CANADIAN PRESCRIPTION DRUGS

A

Consumer's

Guide

to

Correct

Use

DOROTHY L. SMITH
PHARM. D.

KEY PORTER BOOKS

Canadian Cataloguing in Publication Data

Smith, Dorothy L.
 Understanding Canadian prescription drugs

Rev. ed.
ISBN 1-55013-316-0

1. Drugs — Popular works. 2. Drugs — Canada —
Popular works. I. Title.

RS51.S55 1992   615'.1   C92-093657-1

Key Porter Books Limited
70 The Esplanade
Toronto, Ontario
M5E 1R2

This logo is the trademark of the Canadian Pharmaceutical Association – the national professional association of pharmacists.

Jacket photo: Greg Eligh
Typesetting: Computer Composition of Canada, Inc.

Printed and Bound in Canada

 93 94 95 96 6 5 4 3

To Trevor, Shannon and Jennifer

As you grow up, may you always remember
that one of our purposes in life is to use our talents
— whatever they may be — to help other people.

CONTENTS

CONTENTS

FOREWORD

The Canadian Pharmaceutical Association is the national voluntary association for pharmacists. Pharmacists have an extensive knowledge of medicines and can help patients identify and solve problems they may have with their medications.

Because the human body is complex and modern medicines are potent, it is important to have an understanding of both the benefits and the risks of our medication usage. Medicines may act differently on different individuals or even affect the same person differently at different times. Medicines may interact when taken together, with increased or reduced effects. Consequently, those of us who use medications may feel a need for additional information to help us respond to our particular situations. This book will be an aid in answering many of your questions.

We encourage you to ask your pharmacist about any additional information you may need on the medicines you take. Pharmacists are well trained and are accessible. I recommend that you take advantage of this by taking your specific questions on medications to your pharmacist.

Leroy Fevang
Executive Director
Canadian Pharmaceutical Association

ACKNOWLEDGEMENTS

I often wonder whether the preparation of a book is a "labor of love" or a "love of labor." Regardless, it has been a true pleasure to prepare the second edition of this Canadian home reference book on prescription drugs. When Phyllis Bruce, Editor-in-Chief of Key Porter Books, asked me to prepare a second edition, we knew there would be thousands of hours of work ahead of us. However, we felt that Canadians taking prescription drugs need a home reference source that applies to *Canadian* medications.

A very special thank you is extended to the Canadian Pharmaceutical Association for its continued endorsement of the book. As Leroy Fevang, Executive Director of the Canadian Pharmaceutical Association, states in the Foreword, the Canadian Pharmaceutical Association strongly encourages patients to ask pharmacists any questions they may have about their prescription drugs.

I am especially grateful to Dr. Linda Hensman for her dedication and assistance in the preparation of this second edition. The development of books can be very tedious, and I am thankful that our friendship has managed to survive yet another updating process!

I am also indebted to the distinguished Canadian pharmacists and physicians who took time from their busy schedules to serve as members of the Professional Advisory Board. The members of the Advisory Board represent almost every area of medical and pharmacy practice in Canada and I would like to thank them for their excellent recommendations.

I would also like to thank two future pharmacists, Cindy Smith and Carrie Renehan, who worked as summer assistants in the preparation of this second edition. I hope that you will take the background you have learned in this project and apply it to your practices once you become graduate pharmacists. You will have to continuously improve your patient counselling skills and stay up-to-date on the new information that is released every day.

ACKNOWLEDGEMENTS

It was a real pleasure to work with Lisa Bloomfield and Kathleen Crawford, and I would like to thank them for the painstaking efforts they took to ensure the accuracy of the word processing and the final printout.

Gratitude is also expressed to Carmen Krogh, Editor-in-Chief and Director of Publications, and Patricia Carruthers-Czyzewski, CPS Resource/Program Development of the Canadian Pharmaceutical Association. Whenever I had a question or special request, they were always cooperative and responded so quickly.

A very special thank you goes to Dr. Eleanor Vogt, who once again helped me during the final review stage of the Advisory Board comments. Ellie's contribution to the book was invaluable and demonstrated her commitment to helping consumers better understand their medications.

I would also like to thank my mother, Mrs. Edna Smith, for initially recognizing the need for this book. Thank you also for still being willing to come for a visit, even though the galleys always seem to arrive at the same time and we all end up proofreading. You have justly earned an honorary degree in drug information!

It has been a great experience working with you in the preparation of the second edition. I am deeply indebted to all of you. Thank you for being so willing to invest your time, knowledge and expertise.

Dr. Dorothy L. Smith
April 1992

CANADIAN ADVISORY BOARD

PATIENT EDUCATION CONSULTANT

Linda R. Hensman, B.Sc.(Pharm), Pharm.D.
Assistant Executive Director
St. Clare's Mercy Hospital
St. John's, Newfoundland
and
Adjunct Assistant Professor of Clinical Pharmacy
School of Pharmacy
Memorial University of Newfoundland
St. John's, Newfoundland

PROFESSIONAL ADVISORY BOARD

J. Dennis Andrews, Pharm.D.
Clinical Pharmacist
Department of Pharmacy
St. Helena Hospital & Health Center
Deer Park, California

Dean H. Ast, B.S.P.
Community Pharmacist/Owner
Hill Avenue Drugs Ltd.
Regina, Saskatchewan

Helena A. Bardos, B.Sc.(Pharm)
Pharmacist/Manager
Ambulatory Care Pharmacy
Shaughnessy Hospital
and
Clinical Instructor
Faculty of Pharmaceutical Sciences
University of British Columbia
Vancouver, British Columbia

B. Marie Berry, B.A., B.Sc.(Pharm)
Community Pharmacist
Vimy Park Pharmacy
Winnipeg, Manitoba

Graeme H. Bethune, B.Sc., M.D.,
C.C.F.P.
Family Physician
Halifax, Nova Scotia
and
Lecturer
Department of Family Medicine
Dalhousie University
Halifax, Nova Scotia

Sharon E. Bettess, B.Sc.Pharm.,
M.Sc.
Instructor, Pharmacy Technician
Program
Robertson Career College
Winnipeg, Manitoba

James L. Blackburn, B.S.P., M.S.,
Pharm.D.
Professor and Dean
College of Pharmacy
University of Saskatchewan
Saskatoon, Saskatchewan

Michel P. Leveille, M.D.
Nephrologist and
Assistant Professor of Medicine
Department of Medicine
University of Montreal
Montreal, Quebec

Joanne A. Logie, B.S.P.
Dispensing Pharmacist
Safeway #14 Pharmacy
Delta, British Columbia

Stuart Maddin, B.A., M.D.C.M.,
   F.R.C.P.(C)
Clinical Professor of Dermatology
Division of Dermatology
Department of Medicine
Director of the Dermatopharmacology
   Unit
University of British Columbia
Vancouver, British Columbia

Barbara L. Madej, B.S.P.
Chief Pharmacist
Community Clinic Pharmacy
Saskatoon, Saskatchewan

Claude Mailhot, B. Pharm., D.P.H.,
   Pharm.D.
Associate Professor of Clinical Pharmacy
Faculty of Pharmacy
University of Montreal
   and
Adjunct Researcher
Research Centre
Sacre-Coeur Hospital
Montreal, Quebec

Janine J. Matte, B.Sc.Pharm.,
   M.Sc.Pharm.
Clinical Pharmacist
J. Matte L.Petit Pharmacists
Quebec City, Quebec
   and
Chief Pharmacist
Foyer Lac Etchemin
Lac Etchemin, Quebec
   and
Director
Info-Medicaments
Quebec City, Quebec

Louise Matte, B.Sc.(Biology), B.Pharm.,
   M.A. (Health Science Education)
Biologist & Pharmacist Consultant
   and
President
Concept Info — Sante Globale
   and
Coordinator of the Community
   Pharmacy
Clinical Training Program
School of Pharmacy
Laval University
Sainte-Foy, Quebec

Brenda J. McBean Cochran, B.S.P.,
   M.Sc.(Clin.Pharm.)
President
BMC Health Associates
Halifax, Nova Scotia

James P. McCormack, Pharm.D.
Assistant Professor
Faculty of Pharmaceutical Sciences
University of British Columbia
Vancouver, British Columbia

David J. McCutcheon, M.D., M.B.A.,
   C.H.E.
Vice-President, Medical Services
Victoria General Hospital
Halifax, Nova Scotia

Janet McGillivray, B.S.P.
Director, Continuing Education
Manitoba Pharmaceutical Association
Winnipeg, Manitoba

Elaine H. MacPhail, B.Sc.Pharm.,
   M.H.P.(Hospital Pharmacy)
Pharmacist, Providence Centre
Scarborough, Ontario

Adi E. Mehta, M.D., F.R.C.P.(C)
Associate Professor of Internal Medicine
   and Endocrinology
Faculty of Medicine
University of Manitoba
   and
Director
Diabetes Education Centre
Health Sciences Centre
Winnipeg, Manitoba

Linda G. Suveges, B.S.P., M.Sc., Ph.D.
Associate Professor and Head
Pharmacy Practice Section
College of Pharmacy
University of Saskatchewan
Saskatoon, Saskatchewan

Terry W. Talbot, M.D., F.R.C.P.(C)
  (Gastroenterology) & F.F.C.P.(C)
  (Internal Medicine)
Gastroenterologist
Private Practice
Edmonton, Alberta

Patricia A. Thomson, B.S.P.
Pharmacy Department Head
Pinders Drugs — Grosvenor
Saskatoon, Saskatchewan

Jacques Trottier, B.Sc.Phm.
Community Pharmacist/Owner
Victoria Pharmacy
Ottawa, Ontario
  and
President
PROVIPHARM Inc.
Ottawa, Ontario

Louyse I. Trottier, B.Sc.Phm.
Community Pharmacist/Owner
Victoria Pharmacy
Ottawa, Ontario

Lynn R. Trottier, B.Sc.(Pharm)
Acting Coordinator, Clinical
Pharmacy Programs and Research
University Hospital, UBC Site
  and
Assistant Clinical Professor
Division of Clinical Pharmacy
Faculty of Pharmaceutical Sciences
University of British Columbia
Vancouver, British Columbia

C. Brian Tuttle, B.Sc.(Pharm),
  M.Sc.Phm.
Director, Drug Information Services
Regional Drug Information Service
Camp Hill Medical Centre
  and
Honorary Special Lecturer
College of Pharmacy
Dalhousie University
Halifax, Nova Scotia

Ronald H. Waller, B.Sc.(Pharm),
  M.Sc.(Pharm)
Community Pharmacist/Co-Owner
Lakeside Clinical Pharmacy Ltd.
  and
Fellow
American Society of Consultant
  Pharmacists
Kelowna, British Columbia

Dennis E. Walter, M.B.B.S.(London)
General Practitioner
Private Practice
Regina, Saskatchewan

Trevor M. Watson, B.A., B.Sc.(Pharm)
Pharmacy Practitioner
Derma Apothecary Shop Ltd.
Vancouver, British Columbia
  and
Chairman
Canadian Drug Advisory Committee
  (1988-1991)

Nancy Winslade, Pharm.D.
Assistant to the Dean
Faculty of Pharmacy
  and
Pharmacist
Sunnybrook Health Science Centre
University of Toronto
Toronto, Ontario

Donna M. Woloschuk, B.S.P., Pharm.D.
Clinical Pharmacist
Oncology/Bone Marrow Transplantation
Department of Pharmaceutical Services
Health Sciences Centre
Winnipeg, Manitoba

D. Wayne Wurtz, B.S.P.
Field Officer
Saskatchewan Pharmaceutical
  Association
Regina, Saskatchewan

Marguerite M. Yee, B.Sc.(Pharm)
Senior Instructor
Division of Pharmaceutics, Clinical
  Pharmacy
Faculty of Pharmaceutical Sciences
University of British Columbia
Vancouver, British Columbia

ADVISORY BOARD

TAKING PRESCRIPTION DRUGS CORRECTLY

It is difficult to believe, but research has shown that one of every two prescription drugs is not being taken correctly. It has been estimated that:

✓ 50% of patients (including children) are not taking their prescription drugs correctly.

✓ 30% of prescription drugs are being misused in a manner that poses a serious threat to the patient's health.

✓ 60% of patients cannot identify their medicines.

✓ 40% of patients receive drugs prescribed by two or more doctors.

✓ 10% of patients over age 65 share prescription medicines with others.

✓ 3-30% of hospital admissions are due to incorrect use of drugs by patients at home.

✓ One of every two patients with high blood pressure will stop taking the prescribed medications and never tell their physicians. Of the patients who continue taking the medications, only two-thirds will take enough to control their blood pressure. The result can be life-threatening medical complications such as a heart attack, stroke or congestive heart failure.

Modern medicines can be very effective in curing and preventing diseases and relieving the symptoms of many medical conditions. They can save days previously lost from work and help a person return to work earlier. However, in order for prescription drugs to be effective, they must be:

Properly PRESCRIBED by the PHYSICIAN
▽
Properly DISPENSED by the PHARMACIST
▽
AND
▽
Properly ADMINISTERED by the PATIENT

The responsibility of the patient in the drug therapy is just as important as that of the physician and pharmacist.

Studies have shown that patients forget 50% of the prescription instructions given to them by physicians by the time they arrive at the pharmacy. It has also been shown that the directions on a prescription label do not provide enough information for people who are responsible for treating themselves or family members. "Take 1 capsule every 6 hours" and "Take as directed" are inadequate instructions. Patients need more information.

Before people can take a drug correctly, they have to know the *exact times* to take the medicine, *how* to administer it and *how long* to take it. Before they can avoid drug interactions with food, alcohol, nonprescription drugs or other prescription drugs, they must first know *what* these interactions are. Before they can *manage* or handle a harmless but annoying side effect, they must know what the symptoms of the side effect are. Finally, since every drug carries a risk, people must know which symptoms of an adverse drug reaction should prompt them to call their doctors.

In addition to the need for more information about prescription drugs, people need information that is PRACTICAL and CONCISE and that they can UNDERSTAND. It is the intent of this book to provide the patient with a translation of complicated medical terminology into easy-to-understand language.

This book contains general information on the most commonly prescribed drugs in Canada. Many people in Canada are still using instructions from books that have been published in the United States and apply only to American medications. This is a dangerous practice since Canadian medications are different from American medications in many ways. For example, a Canadian medication may have exactly the same brand name as an American medication but contain different ingredients, have different uses, different storage requirements and even different times and methods of administration!

The medication instructions in this book have been carefully prepared in cooperation with a review board of distinguished Canadian physicians and pharmacists. The content of the instructions was based on the recommendations of these physicians and pharmacists, the official pharmaceutical manufacturers' literature, the *Compendium of Pharmaceuticals and Specialties 1990,* and the medical literature. It cannot be emphasized too greatly that the medication instructions are general in nature and are to be used only under the direction and guidance of a health care professional. The instructions are not intended to take the place of the patient's doctor or pharmacist. Every patient is special because of his or her medical condition, age, weight, other medications that have been prescribed and daily activities. It is often necessary to adjust the drug therapy depending upon these factors. The author and publisher cannot be responsible for errors in publication or any consequences arising from the use of the information contained in this book.

The next time you receive a prescription, it is important that you understand how to take the medication correctly. If you have any questions at all about your medications, do not hesitate to ask your doctor or pharmacist. It is the hope of everyone involved in the preparation of this book that you will find the information helpful and that you will have a speedy recovery.

HOW TO USE THIS BOOK

I. READ THE PRESCRIPTION LABEL

Determine the name of the medicine on the prescription label. If you have difficulty with the spelling of the drug name, check with your pharmacist.

II. INDEX

Turn to the index at the back of the book to find the medicine you are interested in and the number of the page in this book that discusses the drug and how to take it. Then turn to that page.

III. SPECIFIC DRUG INSTRUCTIONS

GENERIC NAMES

All of the medicines included in the book are arranged alphabetically under the generic name for each drug.

All drugs have a generic name. The generic name is the standard drug name that is recognized by health professionals and scientific organizations.

BRAND NAMES

The most commonly prescribed brand names (or trade names) are listed in alphabetical order.

The brand name is the name that the pharmaceutical manufacturer gives to its brand of the drug. If a drug is still protected by the patent granted to the original manufacturer, only one brand name will appear. However, if the patent protection has expired, other companies can manufacture that generic drug and give each of their products a different name. Some manufacturers prefer to sell their products under the generic name. Other manufacturers prefer to market their drug

4

products under a trade name that is unique to their company. This is why there is sometimes only one brand name for a generic drug and at other times there are several brand names.

This is the only consumer book that provides general information on the most commonly prescribed generic drugs as well as additional information on the specific brand you are taking. With many drug products, the specific brand instructions are extremely important.

Special instructions for brand names are indicated throughout the book. For example, in the monograph for "ERYTHROMYCIN," some brands of this antibiotic have special administration instructions. Whenever some brands of medicine have special instructions, the names of those brands will be indicated in the following way:

If you were prescribed APO-ERYTHRO BASE, APO-ERYTHRO E-C, E-MYCIN, ERYC, ERYTHROMID, NOVORYTHRO BASE, PCE:

It is very important to know which brand of medicine you are taking. If you have any questions, ask your pharmacist.

Purpose
The drug monographs contain a description of the usual purpose(s) of each medicine.

Before a person takes a prescription drug, it is important to understand the reason the drug has been prescribed. Only approved uses of the drugs are included. Investigational or experimental uses of a drug are not included. If you do not understand why a particular medicine has been prescribed for you, ask your doctor.

Allergies/Warnings
The drug monographs contain the most common allergy warnings. If you have ever had an allergic reaction to any of the drugs listed in the warning, do not take the medicine. Call your doctor or pharmacist.

It is important to tell your physician and pharmacist if you are allergic to any medicines, foods or color dyes (for example, tartrazine). This will help prevent you from receiving a prescription for a drug to which you may be allergic. Some medicines are closely related to each other in chemical structure, and you could experience an allergic reaction if you were allergic to one of the medicines and later received the other similar medicine. Some medicines are flavored or colored with ingredients to which some people are allergic.

The drug monographs also contain selected warnings for medical conditions in which the drug may be contraindicated or which may require special dosage calculations and/or special monitoring by the physician.

Some people have a history of medical conditions that could make them more susceptible to developing adverse effects with certain drugs. For example, a person who has an ulcer should not receive a prescription for a drug that can irritate the ulcer. If you have any of the medical conditions listed, be sure that your doctor knows before you take any of the medicine. As a general rule, be sure to tell *every* physician treating you the names of any drugs you are allergic to, all drugs you are taking and the medical conditions for which you are being or have been treated. Complete the Medicine Card in this book and carry it in your wallet next to your driver's license. Consider joining Canadian Medic-Alert (293 Eglinton Avenue East, Toronto, Ontario M4P 2Z8, or phone (416) 481-5171) and wearing one of the Medic-Alert necklaces or bracelets that will contain your medical and drug history. Ask your physician or pharmacist for the Medic-Alert application form.

How to Use This Medicine

Time of Administration
Each drug monograph provides recommendations regarding the time(s) that the specific drug should be taken.

Ask your pharmacist to suggest exact times that will fit in with your daily meals and work schedule. Try to follow these times as closely as possible. For example, if you are prescribed a medicine that is to be taken "three times a day," the day (24 hours) should be divided into three equal time periods. The doses should be spaced 8 hours apart (24 hours/day divided by 3 doses/day = 8 hours apart). Then, determine the exact times *you* should take the medicine so that it interferes the least amount possible with your daily activities. For example, one person may be able to take the medicine at 7 A.M.-3 P.M.-10 P.M. and another person may find a 9 A.M.-5 P.M.-12 midnight schedule to be better. The times you take the medicine can be flexible, but ask your pharmacist for advice because some medicines should not be taken at meals and others must be taken with food.

Many parents ask if they must wake their child up during the middle of the night to give a dose of the medicine. This depends on the specific medicine and the child's illness. Many times, a convenient schedule can be planned that does not interfere with the child's sleep.

Some drugs must be taken on an empty stomach (1 hour before or 2 hours after eating food) in order to be absorbed completely. In contrast, other drugs that are irritating to the stomach should be taken immediately after eating some food to help prevent stomach upset.

In special circumstances, these times may have to be changed by your doctor or pharmacist, depending on your medical condition or other drugs you are taking. People who have liver or kidney problems metabolize and excrete some medicines differently, and it may be necessary for the doctor to alter the dosage schedule of some of their medicines. Some people may be taking another prescription medicine that will make it necessary to change the normal times of administration of these drugs so that they are not taken at the same time and will not interact with each other.

How to Administer
Instructions for the correct method of administering a drug are included whenever necessary.

In addition, the section "How to Administer Medications" contains instructions for:

- Oral Liquid Medicines
- Oral Liquid Syringes
- Medicine Droppers
- Medicine Spoons
- Buccal Tablets
- Sublingual Tablets
- Eye Drops
- Eye Ointments
- Ear Drops
- Nose Drops
- Nasal Sprays
- Metered-Dose Inhalers
- Dry Powder Diskhalers
- Creams, Ointments, Gels, Solutions and Lotions
- Aerosol Sprays
- Transdermal Patches
- Rectal Suppositories
- Rectal Enemas
- Rectal Creams
- Vaginal Creams, Ointments and Gels
- Vaginal Suppositories
- Vaginal Tablets, Ovules and Inserts

Special Instructions

Length of Therapy

It is important to know how long you should take the prescribed medicine.

Many people make the mistake of stopping a medicine before the treatment is completed. This can prevent the medicine from providing the full benefit and may result in unnecessary adverse complications.

Pregnancy/Breastfeeding

Warnings regarding the use of each medicine during pregnancy and breastfeeding are included. Women who are pregnant or breastfeeding should not take any medicines or home remedies without consulting their doctor or pharmacist.

Drug Interactions

Warnings regarding the use of the prescribed medicine with certain foods and/or nonprescription drugs are included.

Some foods (including milk and fruit juices) can interfere with the absorption of some drugs into the blood and decrease their effectiveness. For example, the antibiotic tetracycline should not be taken with milk or dairy products because the antibiotic will bind with the calcium in these dairy products and prevent the body from absorbing some of the antibiotic. As a result, the antibiotic will be less effective. Many of these interactions can be avoided by simply avoiding those specific foods during the time (usually 2 or 3 hours) the drug is being absorbed or, in some cases, by avoiding the foods during the entire drug treatment.

Many people make a mistake in thinking that medicines they can buy without a prescription aren't "drugs." All over-the-counter products contain drugs and many are capable of interacting with prescription medicines. A person taking a prescription medicine should never self-medicate with any nonprescription drug without first checking with his or her doctor or pharmacist.

This book does not contain information on prescription drug interactions with other prescription drugs. It is the responsibility of the physician (before prescribing the drug) and the pharmacist (before dispensing the drug) to review the individual drug therapy of each patient. There are too many other factors to consider, such as the medical condition of the patient, to even attempt to cover this area in a comprehensive, safe and accurate manner. If you are taking any other medications, consult with your pharmacist or doctor regarding the safety of the combination.

Alcohol
Warnings are included regarding the dangers of drinking alcoholic beverages while taking certain prescription drugs.

It is generally not a good idea to drink alcoholic beverages while taking any drug. However, alcoholic beverages are definitely contraindicated with some medicines because they can interact with the drug and cause potentially serious side effects.

Special Precautions
This book contains information on how to manage commonly occurring side effects and provides advice on when to consult your doctor or pharmacist. Special attention has been given to translating the technical medical names of these symptoms into easy-to-understand language.

Every medicine can cause side effects. People should know which side effects a drug commonly causes and what precautionary measures they can take to either avoid or manage the side effect if it occurs. For example, if a medicine commonly causes drowsiness, dizziness or blurred vision, people should be careful driving an automobile, flying an airplane or operating electrical equipment until they know how they respond to the drug.

When to Call Your Doctor
Selected warning signs that should prompt the patient to call the doctor are included for each drug.

Patients should always call their doctor or pharmacist if they feel that the drug is not "agreeing" with them or if they develop some symptoms that they have never experienced before and that they feel may be due to the drug.

In addition, there are warning signs with some medicines that should prompt a person to seek medical advice. This can help ensure that the person continues to receive the maximum benefit from the treatment. It may be necessary for the doctor to adjust the dose of the medicine or to prescribe another drug that does not cause the same problem.

Allergic Reactions
Always call your doctor or go to the nearest hospital emergency department if you think you are allergic to a medicine. The more common signs of an allergic reaction are a skin rash, hives, itching, swelling of the face or difficulty in breathing.

9

Refills
Dangerous side effects can develop with some medicines if they are stopped suddenly. This book contains reminders with these drugs to call the pharmacist for a refill 2 or 3 days before the medicine will be used up.

Storage
Special storage instructions are included.

In general, a cool, dry place is the best storage place for most medicines. It is important not to store prescription drugs in the bathroom medicine cabinet. The bathroom often becomes hot and steamy and the heat and humidity can destroy some drugs or make them less effective.

Some medicines must be stored in the refrigerator while others should be stored at room temperature. If a person takes a medicine that has deteriorated because of improper storage, the drug could become less effective and, in some cases, dangerous.

Never take a medicine that is outdated. The expiration date will appear on the prescription label if the medicine is expected to become outdated in a short time period. If you have any questions about the expiration date of a prescription drug, call your pharmacist.

Miscellaneous
These prescription drug instructions are general in nature and may have to be altered by your doctor or pharmacist because of your medical condition or other drugs you may be taking. The instructions are selective and do not cover all possible uses, actions, precautions, side effects or interactions.

If you have *any* questions about the medicine you are taking, ask your doctor or pharmacist. Sometimes, a question that you may think is very unimportant can be very important to your health.

IV. MEDICINE CARDS

Four Medicine Cards are included in this book and it is recommended that you or anyone in your family taking prescription drugs complete one of the cards and carry it in the wallet or purse. The Medicine Card could help save your life if you were ever in an accident. The doctors treating you would know immediately what allergies you have, which drugs you have been taking and the phone numbers of your doctors and pharmacist.

V. APPENDICES

APPENDIX A contains a listing of foods that are high in potassium. This is important for some patients taking diuretics (water pills).

APPENDIX B contains general instructions for diabetics on diet, foot care and treatment of hypoglycemia and hyperglycemia.

APPENDIX C contains tips to detect tampering of medicines that can be purchased without a prescription.

APPENDIX D contains a list of foods that have been reported to trigger migraine headaches.

APPENDIX E contains helpful ways to reduce nausea and vomiting from chemotherapy.

APPENDIX F contains first aid procedures to take when someone is having an epileptic seizure.

APPENDIX G contains a listing of the names, addresses and phone numbers of the Poison Control Centers in Canada.

APPENDIX H contains a listing of the Canadian Drug Information Centers, which can be contacted for information on prescription drugs.

Canadian and U.S. Medications Differ by 30%

Prescription drugs available in Canada are frequently different from those available in the United States, even though they may be manufactured by the same pharmaceutical company and sold under the same brand name.

During the preparation of the manuscript for this book, it became evident that more than 30% of the medication instructions differed between the two countries. There are three common reasons for this:

1. There are many cases of a Canadian product requiring different administration instructions from the American product because of differences in formulation of the product between the two countries.

2. Even the types of medical problems for which the federal governments have approved the drug to be safe and effective often differ between the two countries.

3. There are some Canadian medications that have exactly the same name as the American product but have different ingredients or different strengths. As a result, the contraindications, warnings and side effects can vary between the two products.

It is very important for Canadians to follow the medication instructions for Canadian products and not to use American reference sources.

GENERIC DRUGS

• *Generic and brand name drugs are simply two ways of naming pharmaceutical products.*

When a drug is first discovered, it is known by its chemical name or generic name, also called the "active ingredient." The pharmaceutical company that discovered the drug then gives the drug a special brand name or trade name. This brand name medicine will be the only product available in Canada until the patent expires. After the patent has expired, the drug can be copied and marketed by other pharmaceutical companies. The copies of the original product are usually marketed under the generic name or a new brand name. Therefore, after a patent has expired, the medicine may be available under both the original brand name and several generic names.

• *Generic and brand name drugs are similar but NOT exactly the same.*

Generic and brand name products must be alike only as far as the ACTIVE ingredients (the actual drug) are concerned. This can represent as little as 10% of a tablet or capsule.

The remaining 90% is composed of INACTIVE INGREDIENTS — such as starch, lactose, sugar, lubricants, preservatives, dyes and flavoring agents. These ingredients are needed to bind the drug particles together so that a tablet or capsule will disintegrate (break apart) after it is swallowed, and subsequently dissolve in the blood. They also make the product large enough so that a person can easily pick it up. Inactive ingredients are generally considered to be "trade secrets" and the various manufacturers must select their own inactive ingredients and manufacturing processes.

If a person is allergic to an inactive ingredient, it is important to avoid taking medicines that contain these chemicals. The Canadian Health Protection Branch is currently recommending that all pharmaceutical manufacturers list all inactive ingredients in their medicines. Until this information appears on product labels, patients can ask their pharmacist or doctor to check the content of specific medicines.

- *More than one company often manufactures the same generic drug.*

Some provincial governments cover the costs of prescription drugs under the terms of a provincial drug plan. The provincial formulary or list of covered drugs may contain several products with the same active ingredient(s) but made by different manufacturers. Provincial laws vary, but in most provinces, the pharmacist may legally substitute a generic or the least expensive product with the same active ingredient(s) for the prescribed medication *unless* the physician or patient specifically requests otherwise. This means that a patient could receive a different company's product if the provincial drug list changed and the pharmacy adjusted its stock accordingly.

- *There is no question that all drugs — brand name as well as generic — are of high quality.*

All drugs must be approved by the federal government before they can be marketed. However, differences may exist, not only between the brand name drug and a generic, but from generic to generic, because of the different inactive ingredients and the manufacturing processes used by each company. Differences can also exist between brand name drug products.

There have been isolated reports that when some patients were switched between different manufacturers' products of the SAME DRUG (generic or brand name drugs) at refills, they experienced a change in the incidence of side effects and/or in the effectiveness of the drug products in controlling their symptoms. These reports have sparked a call for well-designed research studies.

- *A very complex issue*

Generic drugs are safe and effective and may save the patient money as long as they are used wisely. For most conditions (i.e., colds, infections, pain, etc.), problems will probably not arise when one product is substituted for another. However, repeated substitution of different manufacturers' products may be inadvisable for:

- *chronically ill patients with life-threatening conditions such as high blood pressure, blood clots, heart disease, thyroid disease and asthma;*

14

- *patients receiving medications with doses that must be kept within a narrow therapeutic range. Examples include:*

> Medicines for seizures (anticonvulsants)
> Heart medicines
> Thyroid medicines
> Insulins
> Blood thinners (anticoagulants)
> Birth control pills
> Long-acting or sustained release products

A patient should probably stay on the SAME MANUFACTURER'S PRODUCT (regardless of whether it is a brand name medicine or a generic product) for any of these chronic conditions or medications. This is a very complex medical and scientific issue, and until the questions are all answered, it would be wise to discuss any questions you have with your doctor and pharmacist. Depending on your medical condition and the drugs you are being prescribed, they may recommend the same manufacturer's product for each refill.

Provincial laws vary but several provinces require the pharmacist to type the name of the drug and its manufacturer on the prescription label. This is a valuable law since it assures that a person will know the name of the medicine and will be able to request the same manufacturer's product each time the prescription medicine is refilled. If the name of the manufacturer does not appear on the label, just ask the pharmacist.

- *Ask Questions.*

Ask your doctor or pharmacist if you are being prescribed a medication for which it would be wise to stay on the same manufacturer's product at each refill. Ask how much your prescription will cost if you purchase the brand name product or one of the generic products. Remember, you have the right to request a particular manufacturer's product, but you may have to pay the difference in price between the two products.

The cost of the medicine you purchase is only one factor. It is also important to consider your need for the wide range of monitoring and counselling services that pharmacists can offer. Have all your prescriptions dispensed at the same pharmacy so that the pharmacist can keep accurate medication records for you and provide you with the professional advice you need in order to take your medicines correctly.

What Is in a Tablet Other Than the Drug?

In addition to the medicine, tablets may contain the following ingredients:

Diluents (such as lactose, starch or dextrose) to add bulk and make the tablet large enough to be handled and to ensure a consistent size.

Disintegrants (such as starch) to speed up the rate at which the tablet will break down and dissolve in the body.

Coatings to protect the tablet from light, air and moisture, to disguise an unpleasant taste and to add color. Some coatings contain tartrazine (a yellow dye) and people who are hypersensitive to tartrazine should tell their doctor so that another medicine can be prescribed.

Some coatings are specially designed to protect the tablet from dissolving in the stomach fluids or to pass through the stomach and into the small intestine intact. These are called enteric coatings. Tablets with enteric coatings should not be chewed or given with milk or antacids because this may remove the protective coating on the tablet.

Long-acting tablets and capsules are formulated to provide two or three doses over a long period of time. This eliminates the need for the person to take a medicine so often. However, if these medicines are crushed or chewed, all of the medicine will be released at one time and the person will receive too much of the medicine at that time. Side effects or toxicity could result.

This book gives special instructions for medicines that have enteric coatings or are long-acting.

HOW TO ADMINISTER MEDICATIONS

ORAL LIQUID MEDICINES

The best way to administer liquid medicines is by using an *oral liquid syringe, medicine dropper* or *medicine spoon*.

If your doctor has prescribed liquid medicine for you, follow the instructions for using the oral liquid syringe, medicine spoon, or medicine dropper.

Do not use household teaspoons or tablespoons because they are not accurate enough.

When a prescription indicates that "1 teaspoon" of a medicine should be administered, this means a teaspoon that is equal to 5 mL of liquid. However, household teaspoons range in size from 2.5 mL to 9.7 mL. Studies have also shown that the volume of liquid measured using the *same* teaspoon varies greatly depending upon the person using the spoon.

Do not use the same syringe or medicine spoon to administer medicine to another person. Germs could be transferred to the other person.

If the instructions tell you to shake the bottle first, be sure to do so; otherwise, if the ingredients have separated or settled, you may receive an incorrect dose.

Oral Liquid Syringe
- Measure the correct amount of medicine either using a plastic adapter or measuring directly from a medicine cup.

ORAL LIQUID SYRINGE WITH ADAPTER
- Wet the plastic bottle adapter with warm water. Press the adapter into the mouth of the medicine bottle.
  - Remove the cap from the tip of the oral liquid syringe.
  - Fit the tip of the syringe into the adapter.
  - Turn the markings on the syringe toward you so that you will be able to read them.

Medicine

Adapter

Barrel

Oral
Liquid
Syringe

Plunger

Oral liquid syringe with adapter

- The plunger rod should be pushed down completely into the syringe barrel.
- Turn the bottle (with the adapter and syringe connected) upside down.
- The barrel of the syringe is calibrated. Slowly pull down the plunger to the correct dosage mark on the barrel of the syringe.
- Overfill the syringe a small amount (approximately 1 mL). This will help remove any bubbles and ensure that an accurate dose is being measured.
- Pull the plunger back until the line on the plunger is level with the correct dosage amount indicated on the outside of the oral liquid syringe.
- Remove the syringe from the adapter.

ORAL LIQUID SYRINGE WITHOUT ADAPTER
- Pour a small amount of the liquid medicine into a clear container (a cup or a small glass).
- Remove the cap from the tip of the syringe.

Oral liquid syringe without adapter

- Turn the markings on the syringe toward you so that you will be able to read them.
- The plunger rod should be pushed down completely into the syringe barrel.
- Place the tip of the syringe into the medicine.
- The barrel of the syringe is calibrated. Slowly pull the plunger up to the correct dosage mark of the barrel of the syringe.
- Overfill the syringe a small amount (approximately 1 mL). This will help remove any bubbles and ensure that an accurate dose is being measured.
- Pull the plunger up until the line on the plunger is level with the correct dosage amount indicated on the outside of the oral liquid syringe. You may wish to mark this line with a piece of tape.
- Remove the syringe from the liquid.

For an infant:
- If the medicine is being given to an infant, the infant's head should be well supported with one hand while the infant is

held in the lap. Be sure the infant's head and shoulders are raised.
- Gently press down on the chin with your thumb in order to open the infant's mouth.
- Point the tip of the oral liquid syringe to the inside cheek or the back side of the mouth. This will help prevent choking or drooling.
- SLOWLY push the plunger to release the medicine. You may find it helpful to divide the dose into small amounts so that the child will be able to swallow the medicine more easily. Allow the infant to swallow naturally.

Administering medicine to an
infant using an oral liquid syringe

For a child or adult:
- Have the person sit upright and point the tip of the oral liquid syringe to the inside cheek or the back side of the mouth. This will help prevent choking or drooling.
- SLOWLY push the plunger rod to release the medicine. Allow the person to swallow naturally.
- Ask your pharmacist if drinking some water after taking the medicine is okay.

General Instructions
- Rinse the oral liquid syringe with warm water. The plunger rod may be removed. Dry the plunger rod thoroughly.

- Replace the storage cap on the syringe. Keep the storage cap away from children since they could swallow the cap. Store the oral liquid syringe in a cool, dry place.

Medicine Dropper

- Withdraw the correct amount of medicine from the bottle by squeezing the bulb of the dropper. If the dropper is calibrated, check that you have the correct dose by holding the dropper upright and looking at it at eye level.
- Hold the infant so that his head and shoulders are slightly elevated.
- Press down gently on the infant's chin with your thumb to open the infant's mouth. If the infant will not open his mouth, try stroking the side of his cheek.
- Drop the prescribed number of drops into the infant's mouth. If you are using a calibrated dropper, place the dropper between the infant's cheek and gum to help prevent him from spitting out the medicine. Allow the child to swallow naturally.

Using a medicine dropper

- Ask your pharmacist if giving the child some water to drink after taking the medicine is okay.
- Rinse the medicine dropper with warm water after each use and shake gently to remove any drops of water.

Medicine Spoon

- Pour the liquid medicine into the medicine spoon to the correct dosage line.
- Have the child or adult sit upright and *slowly* tip the spoon forward to release the liquid medicine. Allow the person to swallow naturally.

Using a calibrated medicine spoon

- Encourage the child or adult to suck all the medicine from the spoon so that the entire dose is administered.
- Ask your pharmacist if giving the child some water to drink after taking the medicine is okay.
- Rinse the medicine spoon with warm water after each use.

BUCCAL TABLETS

- Place a tablet *in the pouch* between the cheek and the teeth. Close your mouth and let the tablet dissolve completely. *Do not swallow or chew* the tablet since this type of tablet works faster when it is absorbed through the lining of the mouth.

Buccal tablet dissolving in pouch of cheek

- Try not to swallow until the tablet is dissolved and do not rinse your mouth for a few minutes. Do not eat, drink or smoke while the tablet is dissolving.

SUBLINGUAL TABLETS

- Place a tablet *under your tongue* and let it dissolve completely. *Do not swallow or chew* the tablet since this type of tablet works faster when it is absorbed through the lining of the mouth.

Sublingual tablet dissolving
under the tongue

- Try not to swallow until the tablet is dissolved and do not rinse your mouth for a few minutes afterwards. Do not eat, drink or smoke while the tablet is dissolving.

EYE DROPS

- The person administering the eye drops should wash his or her hands with soap and water before administering the eye drops.
- The eye drops must be kept clean. Do not touch the dropper against the face or anything else.

Instilling eye drops in pouch of eyelid

- Lie down or tilt your head backward and look up at the ceiling.
- Rest your hand on your cheek and gently pull down the lower lid of your eye to form a pouch.
- Hold the dropper in your other hand and approach the eye from the side. Place the dropper as close to the eye as possible without touching it. Resting your hand against the forehead or nose may help steady your hand.
- Place the prescribed number of drops into the *pouch* of the eye.
- Close your eyes for 1 to 2 minutes. Do not rub them.
- Apply gentle pressure for a minute with your fingers to the bridge of the nose and the inner corner of the eye to prevent the eye drops from being drained from the eye.

- Try not to blink more often than usual and do not close the eyes tightly after you have instilled the drops. This can remove the medicine from the place on the eye where you want the medicine to work.
- Blot the excess solution around the eye with a tissue.

Alternative (Closed-Eyes) Method

If you have difficulty instilling eye drops with your eyes open, check with your doctor or pharmacist to see if you can use the following method:

- Lie down on your back and close your eyes.
- Place the prescribed number of drops on the eyelid in the corner of the eye nearest the nose. (This is called the inner canthus.)
- Then blink your eyes and the drops will fall naturally into the eyes as the eyelids are opened. You may wish to tilt the head slightly to the outside to help the drops run in.
- Wipe off any remaining drops on the eyelids with a clean tissue.

Instilling eye drops using
the closed eyes method

NOTE: The CLOSED-EYES METHOD may be particularly helpful in administering eye drops to children.

General Instructions

If necessary, have someone else administer the eye drops for you.

If you are using more than one kind of eye drop, wait at least 5 minutes before instilling the second kind.

Some eye drops may blur the vision for a few minutes. Do not drive a car or operate dangerous machinery or do jobs that require you to be alert until your vision has cleared.

Call your doctor if the condition for which the eye drops are being used persists or becomes worse or if the drops cause itching or burning for more than just a few minutes after use. Many eye drops sting for a short time after use.

Keep the eye drop bottle tightly closed when not in use. Do not use the eye drops if they change in color or in any other way after being purchased. Do not use outdated eye drops as they could be contaminated or ineffective.

EYE OINTMENTS

- The person administering the eye ointment should wash his or her hands with soap and water before administering the eye ointment.
- If the top of the tube is sealed when the cap is removed, invert the cap and pierce a hole in the seal. This will allow the medicine to be squeezed from the tube.
- The tip of the ointment tube must be kept clean. Do not touch the tip of the tube against the face or anything else.
- Stand in front of a mirror and tilt your head forward slightly.
- Rest your hand on your cheek and gently pull down the lower lid of your eye to form a pouch.
- Hold the tube in your other hand and place the tube as close to the eye as possible without touching it. Resting your hand against the forehead or nose may help steady your hand.
- Place the prescribed amount of ointment (usually ½ inch) along the pouch (inside surface of lower lid) of the eye.
- Close your eyes for 1 to 2 minutes. Do not rub your eyes.
- Wipe off any excess ointment around the eye with a tissue.
- Clean the tip of the ointment tube with a tissue.

General Instructions

If necessary, have someone else administer the eye ointment for you. Vision may be blurred for a few minutes after the ointment is applied. Do not drive a car or operate dangerous machinery or do jobs that require you to be alert until your vision has cleared.

Call your doctor if the condition for which the eye ointment is being used persists or becomes worse or if the ointment causes itching or burning for more than just a few minutes after use. Some eye ointments sting for a short time immediately after use.

Keep the eye ointment tube tightly closed when not in use. Do not use outdated eye ointments as they could be contaminated or ineffective.

Placing prescribed dose of eye
ointment in pouch of lower eyelid

EAR DROPS

- Warm the ear drops to body temperature by holding the bottle in your hands for a few minutes. Do *not* heat the drops in hot water because this could cause pain and dizziness.
- The person administering the ear drops should wash his or her hands with soap and water.
- The ear drops must be kept clean. Do not touch the dropper against the ear or anything else that could contaminate it.
- Shake the bottle before use if necessary.
- Tilt your head or lie on your side so that the ear you are treating is facing up.

In *adults and children over 3 years:*
• Gently pull the top of the ear *up and back.*

In *children under 3 years:*
• Gently pull the top of the ear *down and back.*

Child: Pull Ear
Down and Back

Adult: Pull Ear
Up and Back

Administering ear drops

NOTE: Pulling the top of the ear will help to straighten the ear canal so that the ear drops can reach the eardrum.

• Place the prescribed number of drops into the ear. Do not insert the dropper into the ear canal as it may cause injury.
• Remain in the same position for a short time (5 to 10 minutes) after you have administered the drops. This will allow the ear drops to run down into the ear canal.
• Dry the ear lobe if there are any ear drops on it.

General Instructions

If you must administer drops in both ears, wait about 5 to 10 minutes before placing the drops in the second ear. This will help keep the medicine in the ear canal of the first ear for at least 5 to 10 minutes before you have to tilt your head to put drops in the other ear. It is generally not recommended that cotton be placed in the ear after the ear drops have been instilled because the cotton can soak up the drug.

Do not use the ear drops more frequently or in larger quantities than prescribed by your doctor.

Do not use the ear drops if they change in color or change in any way after being purchased.

Call your doctor if the condition for which these ear drops are being used persists or becomes worse or if the ear drops cause itching or burning for more than just a few minutes after use.

Do not use this medicine at the same time as any other ear medicine without the approval of your doctor. Some medicines cannot be mixed.

These instructions may be altered by your doctor or pharmacist because of your medical condition or the specific medicine in the ear drops.

NOSE DROPS

- Blow your nose gently to clean the nostrils.
- Sit in a chair and tilt your head backward or lie down on a bed with your head extending over the edge of the bed or lie down and place a pillow under your shoulders so that your head is tipped backward.

For *children*:
- Let the head hang over the edge of a table, bed or parent's lap and follow the same procedure.

For *infants*:
- While holding the child on your lap, tilt the child's head slightly backward and use your hand to support the child's head.

Administering nose drops

- Insert the dropper into the nostril about 1/3 inch and drop the prescribed number of drops into the nose.
- Try not to touch the inside of the nose with the dropper as it will probably make you sneeze and will contaminate the dropper.
- Immediately bend your head forward toward your knees. Stay in this position for a few seconds and then sit upright. The drops will then trickle down the back of the throat.
- Repeat for the other nostril if necessary.
- Remain in the same position for at least 5 minutes.

General Instructions

Clean the plastic nasal piece with warm water after each use. Dry well.

NASAL SPRAYS

- Blow your nose gently to clean the nostrils.
- Sit upright with your head slightly forward.
- Shake the container.
- Insert the spray tip firmly into the nostril. The spray tip should be pointed at the *back* and *outer side* of the nose to obtain the best results. Close the other nostril by pressing your finger on the side of it.

Using a nasal spray

- With your mouth closed, sniff gently and squeeze the bottle to release a firm, quick spray.
- Remove the spray tip from your nostril. Bend your head forward for a few seconds to allow the spray to spread over the nasal membranes. Then tilt the head upright or backward and the spray will trickle down the back of the throat.
- Hold your breath a few seconds and then breathe out through your mouth.
- Repeat for the other nostril if necessary.

General Instructions

Clean the plastic nasal piece with warm water after each use. Dry well.

METERED-DOSE INHALERS

When medicine is inhaled correctly,
it reaches the tiny air passages in the lungs.

If troubled with mucous or phlegm in the lungs, try to clear your chest as completely as possible before using this medicine. This will help the drug to reach more deeply into your lungs.

Hold the inhaler according to the specific instructions for that drug contained on the label or in the package.

Shake the container well each time before use.

There are 2 basic methods of using medicine in inhalers. Follow whichever method has been recommended by your doctor.

Method I. Closed-Mouth Instructions

- Breathe out fully and place the lips tightly around the mouthpiece. The mouthpiece should be over the tongue and well into the mouth.
- Tilt the head slightly back.
- Start to breathe in slowly and deeply through the mouth. At the middle of a deep breath in, press down the top of the inhaler as far as it will go to release a "puff." By starting to breathe in before inhaling the medicine, you will help to prevent the medicine from staying in the mouth and you will get more of the medicine into the lungs.
- Keep your tongue down to avoid blocking the mist.
- Take the inhaler out of your mouth and close your mouth.
- Hold your breath for a few seconds (10 to 15 seconds). This helps the medicine to reach the tiny air passages in the lungs where its action is needed. Breathe out through your nose slowly.
- Check your technique in front of a mirror. If you see a white mist escaping into the air, you may not be breathing in correctly or your lips may not be sealed around the mouthpiece.

Closed-Mouth Method: The angle
at which the inhaler must be held depends on
the specific product

Closed-Mouth Method Using an Inhaler Aid

General Instructions

For people who have difficulty coordinating their breathing and inhaling the medicine, inhaler aids are now available. One example is the Aerochamber. The inhaler aid (also called an Extender Device or Spacer) is designed to be attached to the inhaler and has a chamber in which the spray from the inhaler is deposited. The person then breathes through the inhaler aid rather than directly from the inhaler. Because of the new additional space between the mouth and the inhaler, the patient has a few more seconds to inhale the medication after it has been released into the device. This makes it possible for the patient to inhale the medication more slowly and thus help the drug reach more deeply into the lungs.

Inhaler aids also allow time for the propellants in the spray to evaporate. This makes the particles of medication travel more slowly and there is less chance the medication will be deposited on the back of the throat.

Each brand of inhaler aid is slightly different. Be sure you understand how to correctly use the brand you have purchased. It is also important to select a device that will fit the specific inhaler you are using. Not all inhaler aids will fit all inhalers.

Inhaler

Chamber of the
Inhaler Aid

Using an inhaler aid attached
to the inhaler

Method II. Open-Mouth Instructions
- Open your mouth.
- Place the tip of the pressurized inhaler approximately 1 inch in front of your opened mouth.
- Breathe out through your mouth as completely as possible.

Open-Mouth Method

- Start to breathe in slowly and deeply through your mouth. In the middle of a deep breath in, press down the top of the inhaler as far as it will go to release a "puff." By starting to breathe in before you release a "puff," you will help to prevent the medicine from staying in the mouth and will get it to the lungs.
- Keep your tongue down to avoid blocking the mist.
- Close your mouth.
- Hold your breath for approximately 10 to 15 seconds. This helps the medicine to reach the tiny air passages in the lungs where its action is needed. Then breathe out through your nose slowly.

General Instructions for Both Methods

If your doctor has prescribed 2 "puffs," wait at least 30 seconds between "puffs" so that the valve pressure in the inhaler can build up.

Rinse your mouth with warm water after you have inhaled the medicine. This will help prevent your mouth and throat from becoming dry.

The mouthpiece of the inhaler should be kept clean and dry.

Failure to follow these instructions carefully can cause your medicine not to work properly or completely.

These instructions may be altered by your doctor or pharmacist because of your medical condition or the specific medicine in the inhaler.

Store the inhaler at room temperature. Do not place it in hot water or near radiators, stoves or other sources of heat. Do not puncture, burn or incinerate the container (even when it is empty).

DRY POWDER DISKHALERS

- Assemble the diskhaler according to the package instructions. Each foil "blister" in the diskhaler contains one dose of medicine in the form of a fine, dry powder.
- Just before you are ready to inhale a dose, pierce one "blister" according to the package instructions.
- Breathe out slowly and as completely as possible.
- Place the mouthpiece of the diskhaler between your teeth and lips. Tilt your head back. Keep the diskhaler level. Be sure that your fingers or lips do not cover the air inlet holes on the sides of the mouthpiece.

- Breathe in through your mouth as quickly and as deeply as you can.
- Hold your breath briefly as you remove the diskhaler from your mouth. Breathe out slowly.
- If your doctor has prescribed 2 "puffs," repeat the above steps but remember the following:
  - Do not puncture the foil "blister" until *immediately* before use.
  - If you are using several different types of medications, ask your doctor or pharmacist about the order in which they should be used. It can make a big difference in how well your medicines will work.

General Instructions

Do not use the dry powder diskhaler more often than your doctor has prescribed. If your breathing is not helped by the prescribed dose, contact your doctor immediately or go to the nearest emergency room.

CREAMS, OINTMENTS, GELS, SOLUTIONS AND LOTIONS

- Each time you apply the medicine, wash your hands, and gently cleanse the skin area well with water unless otherwise directed by your doctor. Do not allow the skin to dry completely. Pat with a clean towel until almost dry.

Applying an ointment

- If you were prescribed a lotion, shake the bottle well before using.
- If you were prescribed a cream, ointment or gel and if the top of the tube is sealed, invert the cap and pierce a hole in the seal. This will allow the medicine to be squeezed from the tube.
- Apply a small amount of the drug to the affected area and spread lightly. Only the medicine that is actually touching the skin will work. A thick layer is not more effective than a thin layer. Do not cover the area with a bandage unless directed by your doctor.
- Wash your hands immediately after applying the medicine so that you do not accidentally get any medicine in your eyes or mouth.

AEROSOL SPRAYS

- Shake the container well each time before using.
- Cleanse the affected area well with water unless otherwise directed by your doctor. Do not allow the skin to dry completely. Pat with a clean towel until slightly damp.

- Hold the container straight up and about 15 to 20 cm (6 to 8 inches) away from the skin.
- Spray the affected area for 1 to 3 seconds.
- Shake the container well between sprays.

Using an aerosol spray

General Instructions
- Do not spray into the eyes, nose or mouth, and try to avoid inhaling the vapors.
- Do not smoke while using the spray and do not use near an open flame, fire or heat.
- Do not place the aerosol container in hot water or near radiators, stoves or other sources of heat. Do not puncture or incinerate the container (even when it is empty). Do not store at temperatures greater than 50° C or 120° F.
- Do not use the spray near food.

TRANSDERMAL PATCHES

- Apply the patch at the same time(s) every day so that the level of the medicine in your body is constant.
- Apply to a non-hairy area of the body. Some patches must be applied to certain parts of the body (e.g., behind the ear). Check with your pharmacist.

- Do not apply the patch over cuts, scrapes or areas with calluses or scars because this can change the absorption of the drug through the skin.
- Do not apply the patch on skin folds or wear under tight clothing since the patch may fall off.
- Do not use the same spot all the time but rotate to different areas. This will help prevent skin irritation.
- Wash your hands with soap and water before applying the patch. Dry hands completely.
- Cleanse the area chosen with soap and water. Rinse and wipe the area completely dry with a clean tissue.
- Do not apply a patch directly after showering, bathing or swimming. Wait until you are sure the skin is completely dry.
- Open the package and remove and throw away the protective backing. Do not touch the inside (sticky side) because the medicine is in this area. Do not cut the patches unless recommended by the manufacturer.

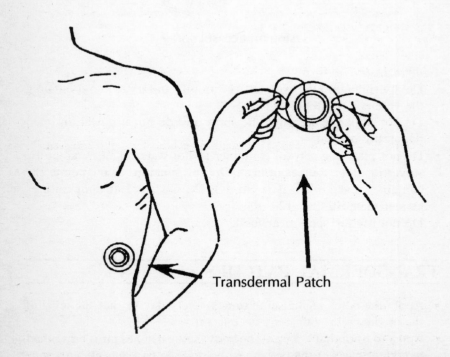

Transdermal Patch

Applying a transdermal patch

- Attach the patch to the skin and press firmly in place for 10 to 15 seconds. Run your finger along the outside edge of the patch to seal it.
- The medicine in the patch will be slowly released through the skin and directly into the bloodstream.
- Remove and throw away the patch after the specified time or before applying the next patch unless otherwise directed by your doctor.

Leaking Microwave Oven Causes Burn Under Transdermal Patch

The *New England Journal of Medicine* has reported that a leaking microwave oven was implicated in a case of a second-degree burn in a 51-year-old man with angina pectoris. The man had been using a transdermal patch containing nitroglycerin for several months without any ill effects. He had been applying the patches to his chest, and went to his doctor when he developed a burn on the chest which was of the size and shape of the patch containing the medication.

The man related that he had been sitting near a microwave oven that was in operation when he first began to feel warmth in the area of the patch. By the time he was able to pull the patch off, a second-degree burn had occurred.

The microwave was checked and found to have a leak. It was assumed that the microwave radiation heated the adhesive strip of aluminized (metallic) plastic in the transdermal patch and caused the burn.

Patients wearing transdermal patches that have metallic components should avoid sitting in front of operating microwave ovens that might be leaking.

RECTAL SUPPOSITORIES

- Remove the wrapper from the suppository. If the suppository is too soft, chill it *before* removing it from the foil wrapper by placing it under cold running water or in the refrigerator for a few minutes.

- Moisten the suppository with a little water by dipping it quickly into some cool water.
- Lie on your side and raise your knee to your chest.
- Insert the suppository into the rectum with the tapered (pointed) end first.
- Remain lying down for a few minutes so that the suppository will dissolve in the rectum. Wash your hands.
- Try to avoid having a bowel movement for at least 1 hour after administration, so that the drug will have time to work.

General Instructions

Rectal suppositories are more effective if they are used when the bowels are empty. If possible, try to insert the suppositories after a bowel movement. Check with your doctor or pharmacist if you have any questions about the best time(s) to use the suppositories.

Suppositories should generally be stored in a cool place. Do not store them in the refrigerator, however, unless directed by your pharmacist.

RECTAL ENEMAS

Procedure for Administering Medicated Enemas

Since the administration of the medication may make you want to have a bowel movement and for the medication to be most effective, it is recommended that the bowel be emptied prior to administration.

- Shake the bottle well if instructed to do so.
- Remove the plastic cap from the applicator tip. Hold the bottle at the neck so that you don't squeeze any of the medication out of the bottle.
- If you are going to administer the medication yourself:
  - Lie on your left side with the left leg straight out and the right leg flexed forward.

If you are going to have someone else administer the medication:
  - Kneel down and bend forward resting your arms on the bed or floor.

- Gently insert the lubricated tip into the rectum, pointed slightly toward the lower spine.
- Hold the bottle firmly and squeeze slowly to instill the medication. Do NOT release and squeeze the bottle, but apply constant pressure until the bottle is empty.

- After the medication has been administered, withdraw the tip and discard the bottle.
- Remain in position for 30 minutes. Try to retain the enema for as long as your doctor has prescribed.

Procedure for Administering Enemas Used for the Relief of Constipation

Shake the bottle well if instructed to do so.
- Remove the plastic cap from the applicator tip. Hold the bottle at the neck so that you don't squeeze any of the medication out of the bottle.
- If you are going to administer the medication yourself:
  - Lie on your left side with the left leg straight out and the right leg flexed forward.

If you are going to have someone else administer the medication:
  - Kneel down and bend forward resting your arms on the bed or floor.

- Gently insert the lubricated tip into the rectum, pointed slightly toward the lower spine.
- Hold the bottle firmly and squeeze slowly to instill the medication. Do NOT release and squeeze the bottle, but apply constant pressure until the bottle is empty.
- After the medication has been administered, withdraw the tip and discard the bottle.
- Go to the bathroom as soon as you feel the urge to have a bowel movement.

RECTAL CREAMS

Procedure for Applying to Rectal Skin Area
- Bathe and dry the rectal area.
- If the top of the tube is sealed when the cap is removed, invert the cap and pierce a hole in the sealed top. This will allow the medicine to be squeezed from the tube.
- Apply a small amount of the cream to the rectal area and spread lightly. Only the cream that is touching the skin will work. A thick layer of cream is not more effective than a thin layer of cream.

Procedure for Inserting Cream into Rectum
- Attach the plastic applicator to the opened tube of cream.
- A small amount of lubricant, such as petroleum jelly (e.g., Vaseline), or some of the cream, may be placed on the outside of the applicator.

- Lie on your side and raise your knee to your chest.
- Insert the applicator tip into the rectum and gently squeeze the tube to deliver the cream.
- Remove the applicator from the rectum and wash the applicator with warm, soapy water. Dry the plastic applicator.
- Replace the cap on the tube of cream.

VAGINAL CREAMS, OINTMENTS AND GELS

- Remove the cap from the tube of cream.
- If the top of the tube is sealed when the cap is removed, invert the cap and pierce a hole in the sealed top. This will allow the medicine to be squeezed from the tube.
- Screw the applicator to the tube.
- Squeeze the tube until the applicator plunger is fully extended. The applicator will now be filled with medicine. If your doctor has prescribed a smaller dose, fill it to the level indicated.
- Unscrew the applicator by the cylinder.
- Apply a small amount of cream to the outside of the applicator.
- Lie on your back with your knees drawn up and spread apart.
- Hold the filled applicator by the cylinder and gently insert it into the vagina as far as it will comfortably go without using force.
- While still holding the cylinder, push the plunger to deposit the cream into the vagina.
- While keeping the plunger depressed, remove the applicator from the vagina.

Insertion of vaginal cream
using an applicator

General Instructions

Discard the applicator if it is disposable. If the applicator is reusable, clean it thoroughly as follows:

- After each use, take the applicator apart by holding the cylinder and the top of the plunger and pulling to separate them. Generally, a "pop" is heard as they separate. Note: Some applicators have screw tops.
- Wash both sections of the applicator thoroughly with warm water and soap and rinse thoroughly. Sterilization of the applicator is unnecessary and extremely hot water should not be used on plastic applicators since it could soften them.
- Dry the applicator. Reassemble by dropping the plunger back into the cylinder as far as it will go.

VAGINAL TABLETS, OVULES AND INSERTS

- This is not an oral medicine and should not be swallowed.
- Remove the wrapper from the tablet. Quickly dip the tablet into some lukewarm water just to moisten it.
- Insert the wide end of the tablet high up into the vagina.

IF THERE IS AN APPLICATOR:

- Put the tablet into the applicator. Do not dip the tablet into water.
- Lie on your back with your knees drawn up and spread apart.
- Gently insert the applicator into the vagina as far as it will comfortably go and then depress the plunger to release the medication.
- Remove the applicator from the vagina.

Insertion of vaginal tablets
using an applicator

General Instructions

Discard the applicator if it is disposable. If the applicator is reusable, clean it thoroughly as follows:

- After each use, clean the applicator according to the instructions that came with your medicine. Extremely hot water should not be used on plastic applicators since it could soften them.
- Dry the applicator.

VAGINAL SUPPOSITORIES

- Remove the wrapper from the suppository.
- Lie on your back with your knees drawn up and spread apart.
- Insert the wide end of the suppository into the vagina.
- Remain lying down for a few minutes so that the suppository will melt.

General Instructions

Suppositories should generally be stored in a cool place. Do not store them in the refrigerator, however, unless directed by your pharmacist. If, for some reason, the suppositories become too soft to insert because of accidental storage in a warm place, they can be chilled in the refrigerator for a few minutes before use. Another method is to run cold water over the foil package *before* removing the suppository.

PRESCRIPTION DRUG INSTRUCTIONS

Disclaimer

These instructions are selective and do not cover all possible uses, actions, precautions, side effects or interactions of the medications included in this book. The information has been based on the official Canadian product labeling, the 1990 *Compendium of Pharmaceuticals and Specialties* and the recommendations of the distinguished physicians and pharmacists who reviewed the manuscript. The instructions may be altered by your doctor or pharmacist because of your medical condition or other drugs you may be taking.

The reader should not consult this book for decisions regarding the practice of medicine. This publication should be used for reference and information only. It should never take the place of your physician. You should not use this book to make medical decisions; rather, you should promptly consult your doctor whenever a medical question arises.

Allergic Reactions

Call your doctor immediately if you think you may be allergic to a medicine or if you develop a skin rash, hives, itching, swelling of the face or difficulty in breathing. If you cannot reach your doctor, phone a hospital emergency department or the closest emergency medical service.

Medications and Crossing the Canadian/U.S. Border

To prevent drug trafficking across the Canadian/U.S. border, customs officials have undertaken a strict policy of "zero tolerance" with respect to medicines, both prescription and nonprescription. All medications that are not properly labeled will be inspected and possibly confiscated.

So keep the following in mind when crossing the border:

- Keep all nonprescription medicines in the manufacturer's original package.
- Carry prescription medicines in the original dispensing package containing the prescription label. Do not mix them with other medicines or transfer them to an unlabeled container.
- If you have a chronic condition and require ongoing medications, carry them with a note from your doctor which certifies the medications, or with a copy of the prescription from the pharmacy.
- You may want to volunteer information about your medicines to the customs official before you are asked about them.

▶ **ACEBUTOLOL (ORAL)**
MONITAN, SECTRAL

ATENOLOL
APO-ATENOL, TENORMIN

ATENOLOL-CHLORTHALIDONE
TENORETIC

LABETALOL
TRANDATE

METOPROLOL
APO-METOPROLOL, BETALOC, BETALOC DURULES, LOPRESOR, LOPRESOR SR, NOVOMETOPROL

NADOLOL
APO-NADOL, CORGARD, SYN-NADOLOL

NADOLOL-BENDROFLUMETHIAZIDE
CORZIDE

OXPRENOLOL
SLOW-TRASICOR, TRASICOR

PINDOLOL
APO-PINDOL, SYN-PINDOLOL, VISKEN

PINDOLOL-HYDROCHLOROTHIAZIDE
VISKAZIDE

PROPRANOLOL
APO-PROPRANOLOL, DETENSOL, INDERAL, INDERAL LA,
NOVOPRANOL, PMS PROPRANOLOL

PROPRANOLOL-HYDROCHLOROTHIAZIDE
INDERIDE

SOTALOL
SOTACOR

TIMOLOL
APO-TIMOL, BLOCADREN

TIMOLOL-HYDROCHLOROTHIAZIDE
TIMOLIDE

Purpose
All of these medicines are beta-blockers and may be used to lower the blood pressure.

PROPRANOLOL is also used in other medical conditions to keep the heartbeat regular and steady and to treat certain types of tremors.

The following medicines are also used to help prevent future heart attacks in people who have already suffered from a heart attack: METOPROLOL, PROPRANOLOL and TIMOLOL.

The following medicines are also used to reduce chest pain (angina) by "calming" the heart so that it beats more slowly and less forcefully and requires less oxygen: ACEBUTOLOL, ATENOLOL, METOPROLOL, NADOLOL, PINDOLOL, PROPRANOLOL, SOTALOL and TIMOLOL.

PROPRANOLOL and TIMOLOL are also used in some patients to help prevent migraine attacks.

Allergies/Warnings

Be sure to tell your doctor and pharmacist if you are allergic to any medicine or if you have a history of allergies (such as hay fever) or have any type of respiratory disease such as asthma, emphysema or bronchitis.

If you were prescribed CORZIDE, INDERIDE, TENORETIC, TIMOLIDE or VISKAZIDE, be sure to tell your doctor and pharmacist if you are allergic to sulfa drugs, oral diabetes drugs, thiazide diuretics or any medicine.

Also tell your doctor if you burn easily when exposed to the sun.

How to Use This Medicine

Time of Administration

Try to take the medicine at the same time(s) every day so that you will have a constant level of the medicine in your body.

If you were prescribed CORZIDE, INDERIDE, TENORETIC, TIMOLIDE, *or* VISKAZIDE:

- When you first start taking this medicine, you will probably urinate (pass your water) more often and in larger amounts than usual. Therefore, if you are to take 1 dose each day, take it in the morning after breakfast. Do not initially take a dose at bedtime or you may have to get up during the night to go to the bathroom.
- If you are to take more than 1 dose each day, ask your doctor if you can take the last dose approximately 6 hours before bedtime so that you will not have to get up during the night to go to the bathroom. This effect will usually decrease after you have taken the drug for a while.

All of these medicines may be taken with food or on an empty stomach *except* TRANDATE, VISKAZIDE and VISKEN, which should be taken after food or meals.

How to Administer

Take this medicine with a full glass of water.

For BETALOC DURULES, INDERAL LA, LOPRESOR SR *or* SLOW-TRASICOR:

- Swallow the medicine whole. Do not crush or chew it or cut it.
- If you have trouble swallowing BETALOC DURULES, they may be cut in half.

Special Instructions

Length of Therapy

It may be necessary for you to take this medicine for a long time in spite of the fact that you may feel better. It is very important that you take the medicine as your doctor has prescribed and that you do not miss any doses. Otherwise, you cannot expect the drug to work for you.

Do not take any more of this medicine than your doctor has prescribed and *do not stop taking this medicine suddenly without the approval of your doctor.* It will be necessary for your doctor to reduce your dose slowly since your body will need time to adjust. It could be harmful and make your condition worse if you suddenly stopped taking the medicine.

Pregnancy/Breastfeeding

Women who are pregnant, breastfeeding or planning to become pregnant should tell their doctor before taking this medicine.

Drug Interactions

Some nonprescription drugs can aggravate your condition. Do not take any of the following without the approval of your doctor or pharmacist: cough, cold or sinus products; asthma, allergy or hay fever products; since they could increase your blood pressure. Read the label of the product to see if there is a warning. If there is, check with your doctor or pharmacist before using the product.

Do not smoke while you are on PROPRANOLOL because smoking can make the drug less effective.

Be sure to tell your doctor and pharmacist if you are taking any nonprescription drugs containing ASA or salicylates. They may decrease the effect of this medicine.

PROPRANOLOL may interfere with the glaucoma screening test.

Special Precautions

Ask your doctor how to check your pulse rate. Check your pulse regularly while you are taking this medicine. If your pulse becomes much slower than usual or if it is less than 50 beats per minute, check with your doctor about taking the drug that day. The dose of your medicine may have to be adjusted. A pulse rate that is too slow may cause circulation problems.

Follow any special diet your doctor may have ordered. If you have high blood pressure, he or she may want to limit the amount of salt in your diet. Check with your pharmacist before using a salt substitute because it may contain potassium.

In some people, this drug may cause dizziness or drowsiness. Do not drive a car, pilot an airplane, operate dangerous machinery or do jobs that require you to be alert if you are dizzy or drowsy. You should also be careful going up and down stairs, getting out of bed or out of chairs. Sit or lie down at the first sign of dizziness. Tell your doctor if the dizziness or drowsiness continues.

If you were prescribed LABETALOL, it is recommended that you lie down for 2 to 4 hours after taking the first dose or any increase in dose. This will help prevent fainting.

If your mouth becomes dry, drink water, suck ice chips or a hard, sour candy (sugarless) or chew gum (sugarless). Sugarless products are recommended in order to avoid dental problems. It is especially important to brush and floss your teeth regularly if you develop a dry mouth to help prevent gum problems.

If your eyes become dry, ask your pharmacist or doctor to recommend a lubricating/wetting solution or *artificial tears*. This side effect is more common in elderly people.

If you were prescribed SLOW-TRASICOR, do not become alarmed if you notice something that looks like a tablet in your stool. This medicine is contained in a wax core that has been designed to release the drug slowly in your body. The empty wax core is eliminated in the stool.

If you become more sensitive to the cold, dress warmly during cold weather and do not stay outside for long periods of time in cold weather. Call your doctor if you develop cold hands or feet or numbness or tingling in the fingers or toes.

It is recommended that patients receiving this drug stop smoking.

For patients with angina:
- Check with your doctor about the amount of exercise that is safe for you. This medicine can reduce chest pain resulting from too much exercise and make it difficult to tell when a person has exercised just the right amount.

For patients with diabetes:
- This medicine may cause a change in your blood sugar level. It may also mask or hide some of the signs of low blood sugar (such as blood pressure changes and faster pulse rate). Be alert for the other signs of low blood sugar that are not masked (such as sweating,

hunger or tiredness). If you think your blood sugar is lower than normal, call your doctor. It may be necessary to adjust the dose of your diabetes medications.

If you were prescribed CORZIDE, INDERIDE, TENORETIC, TIMOLIDE, *or* VISKAZIDE, *the following special instructions also apply:*

- This medicine normally causes your body to lose potassium. The body has warning signs to let you know if too much potassium is being lost. Call your doctor if you become unusually thirsty or if you develop leg cramps, unusual weakness, fatigue, vomiting, confusion or an irregular pulse. Since these symptoms may not be present in all patients, your doctor may wish to check your blood occasionally to see if it is low in potassium. Depending upon your dose, your doctor may prescribe some medicine to replace the potassium or he or she may recommend that you regularly eat foods that contain a lot of potassium (see Appendix A). *Do not change your diet unless your doctor tells you to.*
- This medicine may make some people more sensitive to sunlight and various tanning lamps. When you begin taking this medicine, try to avoid too much sun until you see how you are going to react. If your skin does become more sensitive to sunlight, tell your doctor and try not to stay in direct sunlight for extended periods of time. While in the sun, wear protective clothing and sunglasses. You may wish to ask your pharmacist about suitable sunscreen products. Call your doctor if you become sunburned.
- Tingling of the scalp is common when you first start taking TRANDATE. This is temporary and will usually disappear after you have taken the drug for a while.

When to Call Your Doctor

For all drugs EXCEPT TRANDATE:
- Most people experience few or no side effects from this drug. However, any medicine can sometimes cause unwanted effects. Call your doctor if you develop a skin rash, shortness of breath, wheezing, fever or sore throat, unusual bruising or bleeding, swelling of the legs or ankles, sudden weight gain of 5 pounds (2.5 kg) or more, impotence or decreased sexual ability, changes in vision, cold hands or feet or numbness or tingling of the fingers or toes, or if your pulse becomes slower than normal or is less than 50 beats per minute. Also call your doctor if you develop nightmares, depression, insomnia, unusual tiredness or headaches, or if you become confused.

If you were prescribed CORZIDE, INDERIDE, TENORETIC, TIMOLIDE, *or* VISKAZIDE:

- In addition to the previous symptoms, also call your doctor if you develop sharp stomach pain, persistent nausea, vomiting or diarrhea, sharp joint pain, a yellow color to the skin or eyes or dark-colored urine.

If you were prescribed TRANDATE:

- Unlike the other medicines, this drug rarely affects the heart rate.
- Call your doctor if you develop shortness of breath, difficulty breathing, difficulty urinating (passing your water), impotence or decreased sexual ability, a yellow color to the skin or eyes, dark-colored urine, unusual weakness or tiredness, unusual bruising or bleeding, changes in vision, muscle or joint pain, nasal stuffiness, unusual dizziness or fainting, unpleasant taste in the mouth, swelling of the legs or ankles, or sudden weight gain of 5 pounds (2.5 kg) or more.

Asthma Caused by a Pet's Drugs!

Two Canadian physicians recently reported that pet medications can trigger asthma attacks in sensitive people.

In one case, the pancreatic enzyme powder being mixed with a dog's food every evening entered the vent of a home's forced-air heating system and was circulated throughout the house. The air in the house became contaminated from the pancreatic enzyme powder. The owner of the pet was sensitive to the pet's medicine and suffered severe asthma attacks.

To help prevent the circulation of the medicine in the home, the following steps can be taken:

- Avoid shaking the powder.
- Use a spoon to measure a dose of the powder. Do not shake the medicine directly out of the container.
- Do not mix the powder and pet food in a drafty location.

Refills

Do not stop taking this medicine without your doctor's approval and do not go without medicine between prescription refills. Call your pharmacist for a refill 2 or 3 days before you will run out of the medicine.

Discuss with your pharmacist the implications of dispensing all your refills for this medicine with the same manufacturer's product. (*See* Generic Drugs, page 13.)

Miscellaneous

Carry an identification card in your wallet or wear a medical alert bracelet indicating that you are taking this medicine as well as the names and phone numbers of your doctors. If you do not already carry such a card, complete the Medicine Card in this book. Always tell your dentist, pharmacist and other doctors who are treating you that you are taking this medicine.

▶ ACETAMINOPHEN (ORAL)

ANACIN 3, ANACIN 3 EXTRA STRENGTH, APO-ACETAMINOPHEN, ATASOL, ATASOL FORTE, EXDOL, EXDOL STRONG, PANADOL, PANADOL CHEWABLE, ROBIGESIC, ROUNOX, TEMPRA, TEMPRA CHEWABLE, TEMPRA SYRUP, TYLENOL, TYLENOL CHEWABLE, TYLENOL EXTRA-STRENGTH, TYLENOL JUNIOR STRENGTH

ACETAMINOPHEN (RECTAL)

ABENOL SUPPOSITORIES, ACETAMINOPHEN SUPPOSITORIES

Purpose

This medicine is used to help reduce pain and/or fever.

Do not use for arthritic conditions without checking with your doctor because ACETAMINOPHEN does not treat the underlying cause (inflammation) of arthritic pain. ACETAMINOPHEN may relieve the pain but it will not relieve the inflammation (redness, swelling, stiffness) of arthritis.

Allergies/Warnings

If you have ever had an allergic reaction to ACETAMINOPHEN or any other medicine, tell your doctor and pharmacist before you take any of this medicine.

How to Use This Medicine

How to Administer

This medicine may be taken with food or a full glass of water.

For drops:
- If a dropper is used to measure the dose and you do not fully understand how to use it, *see* Medicine Dropper (page 21). Caution: Some drops are very concentrated. Be sure you know how much to use.

For syrups and elixirs:
- If a spoon is used to measure the dose, it is recommended that you use a medicine spoon or an oral liquid syringe, which you can obtain from your pharmacist. *See* Oral Liquid Syringe (page 17) and Medicine Spoon (page 22).

For chewable tablets (PANADOL CHEWABLE, TEMPRA CHEWABLE, TYLENOL CHEWABLE):
- This medicine must be chewed completely before swallowing.

For suppositories:
- *See* Rectal Suppositories (page 39).

Special Instructions

Length of Therapy
Children under 2 years of age should only be given this medicine with the approval of the doctor. Children under 12 years of age should not be given this medicine for more than 5 days in a row.

Pregnancy/Breastfeeding
Women who are pregnant, breastfeeding or planning to become pregnant should tell their doctor before taking this medicine.

Drug Interactions
Do not take any other medicine containing ACETAMINOPHEN without consulting your doctor or pharmacist while you are taking this medicine because you could take too much of this drug. Since many nonprescription drugs contain ACETAMINOPHEN, check the labels of any nonprescription drugs you may have and call your pharmacist if you have any questions about the contents.

Alcohol
Do not drink alcoholic beverages while taking this drug without the approval of your doctor. High doses of the drug taken for a long period in combination with large amounts of alcohol may cause liver damage.

What You Should Know About Your Medicines

Whenever you receive a medicine from a pharmacist, you should know the answer to these questions:

- What is the name of the medicine?
- Why has the medicine been prescribed for me?
- How will I know if the medicine is working correctly?
- How long will it take to have an effect?
- How should I administer the medicine?
- How much of the medicine should I take?
- At what exact time(s) during the day and night should I administer the drug?
- Does the drug have to be taken before, during or after eating some food or on an empty stomach?
- What does it mean to take a drug on an empty stomach?
- Are there any foods that should be avoided?
- Should alcoholic beverages be avoided while taking this medicine?
- Are there any nonprescription medicines that can interact with this prescription drug and should not be taken at the same time?
- What are the side effects that most commonly occur with this medicine? What should I do if I experience one of these side effects?
- What adverse effects should prompt me to call the doctor?
- How long should I take the medicine?
- Can the prescription be refilled, and how?
- How should the medicine be stored?

Remember: The more you know about your medicine, the better!

When to Call Your Doctor

Call your doctor if the medicine does not relieve your symptoms or if they get worse. If you are using the medicine to lower a fever and if the fever does not go away (for example, within 2 or 3 days), call your doctor.

Most people experience few or no side effects from this drug. However, any medicine can sometimes cause unwanted effects. Call your

doctor if you develop nausea or vomiting, stomach pain, diarrhea, unexplained sore throat or fever, unusual weakness or tiredness, unusual bruising or bleeding or a yellow color to the skin or eyes.

Get emergency help at once if you think that anyone has taken an overdose of this medicine. Overdoses can be very serious and treatment may need to be started even before the symptoms of an overdose appear, because the symptoms of liver damage may not appear until 4 to 6 days after the overdose has been taken. Overdose symptoms include nausea, vomiting, diarrhea, stomach cramps, swelling of abdomen, increased sweating, fever, loss of appetite or a yellow color to the skin or eyes.

Allergic Reactions
Call your doctor immediately if you think you may be allergic to the medicine or if you develop a skin rash, hives, itching, fever, swelling of the face or difficulty in breathing. If you cannot reach your doctor, phone a hospital emergency department.

Storage
For tablets and capsules:
• Store the medicine in a cool, dark place.

For suppositories:
• *See* Rectal Suppositories (page 39).

▶ ## ACETAMINOPHEN-CODEINE (ORAL)
EMPRACET-30, EMPRACET-60, EMTEC-30, LENOLTEC WITH CODEINE No. 4, ROUNOX + CODEINE, TYLENOL No. 4 WITH CODEINE, TYLENOL WITH CODEINE ELIXIR

ACETAMINOPHEN-CAFFEINE-CODEINE
ATASOL-8, ATASOL-15, ATASOL-30, EXDOL-8, EXDOL-15, EXDOL-30, LENOLTEC WITH CODEINE No. 1, No. 2 AND No. 3, NOVOGESIC C8, C15, AND C30, TRIATE C-8 AND C-30, TYLENOL No. 1, TYLENOL No. 1 FORTE, TYLENOL No. 2 WITH CODEINE, TYLENOL No. 3 WITH CODEINE

ACETAMINOPHEN-OXYCODONE
ENDOCET, OXYCOCET, PERCOCET, PERCOCET-DEMI

Purpose
This medicine is used to help relieve pain. Some products may also be used to reduce fever and coughing in some conditions.

Allergies/Warnings

If you have ever had an allergic reaction to ACETAMINOPHEN, CODEINE or any other medicine, tell your doctor and pharmacist before you take any of this medicine.

How to Use This Medicine

Time of Administration

If you are taking this medicine to help relieve pain, do not wait until the pain becomes severe. This medicine works best if you take it when the pain first occurs. If your doctor has prescribed this medicine on a regular schedule, take it as recommended and not on an "as needed" basis.

How to Administer

This medicine may be taken with food or a full glass of water.

For liquid medicines:

• If a spoon is used to measure the dose, it is recommended that you use a medicine spoon or an oral liquid syringe, which you can obtain from your pharmacist. *See* Oral Liquid Syringe (page 17) and Medicine Spoon (page 22).

Special Instructions

Length of Therapy

Do not take any more of this medicine than your doctor has prescribed. When used in large doses for a long period of time, these medicines can become habit-forming and less effective.

Call your doctor if you feel you need the medicine more often than was prescribed. Do not take a larger dose without your doctor's approval.

Do not stop taking this medicine suddenly without the approval of your doctor. It may be necessary for your doctor to reduce your dose slowly. This will depend on the dose, length of therapy and the specific medicine you have been taking.

Pregnancy/Breastfeeding

Women who are pregnant, breastfeeding or planning to become pregnant should tell their doctor before taking this medicine.

Drug Interactions

It is important that you obtain the advice of your doctor or pharmacist before taking any other prescription or nonprescription medicines, including pain relievers, sleeping pills, tranquilizers or medicines for depression, cough, cold or allergies. Some of these drugs may cause increased drowsiness if taken with this medicine.

Do not take any other medicine containing ACETAMINOPHEN without consulting your doctor or pharmacist while you are taking this medicine because you could take too much of this drug. Since many nonprescription drugs contain ACETAMINOPHEN, check the labels of any nonprescription drugs you may have and call your pharmacist if you have any questions about the contents.

There are other drug interactions that can occur. If you are taking any other medicines, be sure to check first with your pharmacist or doctor.

Alcohol

Do not drink alcoholic beverages while taking this drug without the approval of your doctor because the combination could cause drowsiness. One drink may have the same effect that 2 or 3 drinks normally would have.

In addition, high doses of ACETAMINOPHEN taken for a long time in combination with large amounts of alcohol may cause liver damage.

Do Not Store Drugs in Bathroom

Medicines should not be stored in the traditional bathroom medicine cabinet. The bathroom often becomes hot and steamy and the heat and humidity can destroy some drugs.

Some medicines must be stored in the refrigerator. If this is the case, there will be a "Keep Refrigerated" label on the prescription container. Do not store any medicines in the refrigerator unless specified by your pharmacist. The cold temperature and high humidity can destroy some drugs.

In general, a cool, dry place is the best storage place for most medications. Always keep your medicines in a place that is away from the reach or sight of children.

Special Precautions

If you feel nauseated when you first start taking the medicine, it may help if you lie down for a few minutes.

In some people, this drug may cause dizziness or drowsiness. Do not drive a car, pilot an airplane, operate dangerous machinery or do jobs that require you to be alert if you are dizzy or drowsy. You should also be careful going up and down stairs. Get up slowly after you have been sitting or lying down. Sit or lie down at the first sign of dizziness. Tell your doctor if dizziness or drowsiness continues.

This medicine may cause some people to become constipated. To help prevent constipation, try increasing the amount of bulk in your diet (for example, bran, fresh fruits and salads), exercising more often or drinking more fluids (unless otherwise directed). Call your doctor if the constipation continues.

When to Call Your Doctor

Call your doctor if the medicine does not relieve your symptoms or if they get worse.

Most people experience few or no side effects from this drug. However, any medicine can sometimes cause unwanted effects. Call your doctor if you develop nausea or vomiting, stomach pain, diarrhea, unexplained sore throat or fever, unusual weakness or tiredness, unusual bruising or bleeding, a yellow color to the skin or eyes, confusion, depression, severe nervousness, severe drowsiness or trembling.

Get emergency help at once if you think that anyone has taken an overdose of this medicine. Overdoses can be very serious and treatment may need to be started even before the symptoms of an overdose appear, because the symptoms of liver damage may not appear until 4 to 6 days after the overdose has been taken. Overdose symptoms include nausea, vomiting, loss of appetite, diarrhea, stomach cramps, swelling of abdomen, increased sweating, fever or a yellow color to the skin or eyes.

Allergic Reactions

Call your doctor immediately if you think you may be allergic to the medicine or if you develop a skin rash, hives, itching, fever, swelling of the face or difficulty in breathing. If you cannot reach your doctor, phone a hospital emergency department.

Storage

Store the medicine in a cool, dark place.

▶ **ACETOHEXAMIDE (ORAL)**
DIMELOR

CHLORPROPAMIDE
APO-CHLORPROPAMIDE, DIABINESE, NOVOPROPAMIDE

GLICLAZIDE
DIAMICRON

GLYBURIDE
ALPHA-GLIBENCLAMIDE, DIABETA, EUGLUCON

METFORMIN
GLUCOPHAGE

TOLBUTAMIDE
APO-TOLBUTAMIDE, MOBENOL, NOVOBUTAMIDE, ORINASE

Purpose

This medicine is used in the treatment of diabetes. When you have diabetes, the body either is not producing enough insulin or is not able to use what is produced. Insulin is needed for the body's proper use of food, especially sugar. In a person with diabetes, the sugar in the blood can build up to dangerous levels and is passed out in the urine. Your doctor has prescribed this medicine to help keep your blood sugar at nearly normal levels.

Allergies/Warnings

If you have ever had an allergic reaction to any medicine or if you have a heart, liver or kidney condition, tell your doctor and pharmacist before you take any of this medicine.

How to Use This Medicine

Time of Administration

Do not take this medicine at bedtime unless your doctor tells you to.

It is very important that you take this medicine exactly as your doctor has prescribed. Do not miss any doses and take the medicine even if you feel well. Try to take this medicine at the same time(s) every day so that you have a constant level of medicine in your body. Do not take extra doses without your doctor's approval.

How to Administer

If you were prescribed ACETOHEXAMIDE, CHLORPROPAMIDE *or* TOLBUTAMIDE:
- This medicine may be taken with food if it upsets your stomach. Call your doctor if you continue to have stomach upset.

If you were prescribed GLYBURIDE, GLICLAZIDE *or* METFORMIN:
- It is best to take this medicine with food or immediately after meals.

If you were prescribed ORINASE:
- You may swallow the tablet whole or mix it with a glass of water. If you mix it with water, allow the tablet to dissolve in a glass of water, stir and drink immediately. Add more water to the glass, stir any remaining particles of medicine and drink immediately.

Special Instructions

Length of Therapy

This medicine will not cure your diabetes but will help to control it. In order to receive the full benefit of the drug, you must take it as long as your doctor feels you need it. It may be necessary for you to take medicine for your diabetes the rest of your life.

Pregnancy/Breastfeeding

Women who are pregnant or planning to become pregnant should not take this medicine.

Women who are breastfeeding should tell their doctor before taking this medicine.

Drug Interactions

Do not start or stop taking any drugs you are currently taking without first consulting your doctor. This includes both prescription and nonprescription medicine.

Before you purchase any nonprescription medicine (for example, cough and cold medicines), ask your pharmacist if the medicine is safe for patients with diabetes to use. Some liquid nonprescription medicines contain a lot of sugar that could interfere with the control of your diabetes.

It is recommended that patients not take products containing ASA, salicylates or large doses of vitamin C because the combination could cause hypoglycemia (low blood sugar). It is recommended that patients avoid the use of sodium bicarbonate (baking soda).

Alcohol

It is recommended that you avoid the use of alcoholic beverages until you have discussed this with your doctor. Some people who drink alcohol while taking this medicine react and develop low blood sugar early after ingestion and then high blood sugar several hours later. A pounding headache, flushing or upset stomach can also occur.

Special Precautions

Follow the special diet your doctor has prescribed for you.

Test your urine or blood regularly for sugar and, if your doctor recommends, test it for acetone. This is especially important during the first few weeks of treatment. Give the results of these tests to your doctor at every office visit unless he or she wants them more often.

See **General Instructions for Patients with Diabetes** (Appendix B) for signs of low blood sugar and high blood sugar, and proper foot care.

When to Call Your Doctor

Call your doctor if you feel sick and have a fever, an infection, nausea or vomiting.

Most people experience few or no side effects from this drug. However, any medicine can sometimes cause unwanted effects. Call your doctor if you develop a skin rash, sore throat, fever, mouth sores, dark-colored urine, increased sensitivity to sunlight or if you get a sunburn, a yellow color to the skin or eyes, unusual bruising or bleeding, unusual tiredness, diarrhea, light-colored stools or stomach pain.

If you are taking CHLORPROPAMIDE:
- Also call your doctor if you develop any of these additional side effects: headache, swelling of the face, hands or legs, muscle cramps or weakness.

If you are taking METFORMIN:
- Also call your doctor if you develop vomiting, a metallic taste in the mouth, stomach upset, diarrhea or loss of appetite.

Allergic Reactions

Call your doctor immediately if you think you may be allergic to this medicine or if you develop a skin rash, hives, itching, swelling of the face or difficulty in breathing. If you cannot reach your doctor, phone a hospital emergency department or emergency medical service.

Refills

Do not stop taking this medicine without your doctor's approval and do not go without medicine between prescription refills. Call your pharmacist for a refill 2 or 3 days before you will run out of the medicine.

Discuss with your pharmacist the implications of dispensing all your refills for this medicine with the same manufacturer's product. (*See* Generic Drugs, page 13.)

Miscellaneous

Carry an identification card (*see* Medicine Card) or wear a medical alert bracelet indicating that you have diabetes and that you are taking this medicine. Always tell your pharmacist, dentist and other doctors who are treating you that you are taking this medicine (especially if you are scheduled for surgery).

When Insulin-Dependent Diabetics Travel through Time Zones

When a diabetic patient who takes insulin travels by airplane through time zones, the dosage of insulin will have to be adjusted to allow for the rapid time changes.

A simple rule is:

When flying east, the insulin dose should be decreased.

- For example, if a man is flying from Ottawa to London, he will lose 6 hours of time, which is equivalent to $\frac{1}{4}$ of a day. When he arrives in London, the first injection of insulin should be decreased by $\frac{1}{4}$. On the second day in London, he should return to his normal insulin dose.

When flying west, the insulin dose should be increased.

- When he flies back to Ottawa from London, he should increase the insulin dosage by $\frac{1}{4}$, since he will be gaining six hours. He should return to his normal dosage on the following day.

These guidelines will have to be tailored by the doctor in order to consider any factors, such as time of departure and meals served on the plane, that require additional adjustments. Therefore, if you have diabetes and take insulin, check with your doctor about your insulin dose before you travel through several time zones.

▶ **ACYCLOVIR (ORAL)**

ZOVIRAX

Purpose

This medicine is used to help shorten the duration and relieve the symptoms of initial episodes of herpes infections due to genital herpes. The drug attacks the herpes virus-infected cells and prevents spread of the virus to other cells. The drug does not act on normal cells that are not infected.

The drug is also used to manage recurrent herpes infections of the genitals. When given continuously to help prevent recurrences, the drug "stands by" in the cells and may stop the virus from spreading.

ACYCLOVIR will not cure genital herpes but it can help to reduce some of the pain and itching and help speed the healing of any sores. It can also help to reduce the number of attacks.

The Glove Compartment Is Not a Medicine Cabinet

Medications should not be stored in automobile glove compartments because the solar-heating effect causes excessively high temperatures which can destroy the drug.

According to the *Journal of the American Medical Association*, temperatures in glove compartments between April and October in the northern hemisphere are up to 28°C (82°F) *higher* than outdoor temperatures. This means that medicines stored inside the glove compartment could be exposed to temperatures reaching 66°C (164°F). The temperature of floor areas shielded from direct sunlight was approximately 11°C (52°F) less. The study was conducted in California.

In general, medications should not be stored in the glove compartments of automobiles during the summer months because of the heat. If you are traveling during the summer, the best way to store medications in a car is in an insulated container on the floor of the car and shielded from direct sunlight. In addition, medications should not be stored in automobiles during the winter months in Canada because the extreme cold could freeze the medications.

Allergies/Warnings

If you have ever had an allergic reaction to ACYCLOVIR, tell your doctor and pharmacist before you take any of this medicine.

How to Use This Medicine

Time of Administration

The medicine must be taken at regularly spaced intervals in order to be effective. Do not miss any doses.

In the treatment of recurrent herpes infections using 5-day treatments, start taking the medicine at the first sign of a recurrence, e.g., tingling, itching or pain. This helps prevent the virus from multiplying and destroying the skin cells.

If you were prescribed this medicine on a daily basis for long-term therapy, try not to miss any doses, so that you have enough drug in the body at all times to prevent the virus from growing and multiplying.

How to Administer

Take the tablets with a full glass of water. The drug may also be taken at the same time as food.

Special Instructions

Length of Therapy

The length of treatment will depend on the severity of the infection and whether it is the first episode (10 days' treatment) or a recurrent episode.

If you have recurrent genital herpes, your doctor will decide whether short-term (5 days) or long-term treatment (up to 12 months) is best for you.

The safety and effectiveness of continuous use of this drug have been established only for up to 12 months.

Pregnancy/Breastfeeding

Women who are pregnant, breastfeeding or planning to become pregnant should tell their doctor before taking this medicine.

Special Precautions

The herpes virus is contained in the blisters. When the blisters break, the infection will spread very easily. If you touch your skin sores, wash your hands immediately and do not touch other parts of your body until your hands are cleaned.

Genital herpes is a sexually transmitted disease and patients should avoid having sex when lesions (blisters) are present because there is a possibility of infecting the other person. The use of a condom will help prevent the spread of genital herpes. *The drug will NOT help prevent you from spreading the disease to others.*

Women with genital herpes should have yearly Pap smears because there appears to be a higher incidence of cancer of the cervix in women with genital herpes.

Do not share the medication with others.

Do not take a higher dose or take the medicine for longer periods of time than prescribed by your doctor.

Some patients may have worsening of symptoms after the first treatment has been completed. If this happens, call your doctor.

If you become dizzy, sit or lie down at the first sign of dizziness. Do not drive a car, pilot an airplane, operate dangerous machinery or do jobs that require you to be alert until you know how you are going to react to the drug. Tell your doctor if the dizziness continues.

It is important to drink adequate amounts of fluids while taking this medicine.

When to Call Your Doctor

Most people experience few or no side effects from this drug. However, any medicine can sometimes cause unwanted effects.

If you are taking the medicine for a *short time* (5 to 10 days), call your doctor if you develop severe nausea or vomiting, unusual headaches, diarrhea, painful urination, skin rash or leg pain.

If you are taking the medicine for a *long time*, call your doctor if you develop any of the previously listed symptoms or joint pain, muscle cramps, rapid heartbeats, insomnia, acne, back pain, swollen glands, hair loss, menstrual abnormalities or depression.

Allergic Reactions

Call your doctor immediately if you think you may be allergic to the medicine or if you develop a skin rash, hives, itching, swelling of the face or difficulty in breathing. If you cannot reach your doctor, phone a hospital emergency department.

Refills

Because of the importance of starting the drug at the first sign of a recurrence, it is a good idea to have at least one or two extra days' supply on hand. If you do not have at least one extra day's supply on hand, ask your doctor to prescribe it for you.

▶ ACYCLOVIR (TOPICAL)
Zovirax

Purpose

This ointment is used to treat initial herpes infections in the genital area. ACYCLOVIR will not cure herpes infections but it can help to reduce some of the pain and help speed the healing of the sores.

This ointment is *not* effective in the treatment of recurrent genital herpes infections.

Allergies/Warnings

If you have ever had an allergic reaction to ACYCLOVIR, or to polyethylene glycol, which is an inactive ingredient in the ointment, tell your doctor and pharmacist before you take any of this medicine.

How to Use This Medicine

Time of Administration

Start applying the ointment at the first sign of an attack (e.g., tingling, itching or pain).

The ointment is usually applied 4 to 6 times daily for up to 10 days. It is important not to miss any doses or the medication may be less effective.

How to Administer

Use a disposable rubber glove or finger cot to apply the ointment. Throw the glove or finger cot away after use. This will help prevent spreading of the infection to other parts of the body or to other people.

Cover all the sores (blisters) with a sufficient quantity of ointment.

Special Instructions

Length of Therapy

The usual length of treatment is 10 days.

Pregnancy/Breastfeeding

Women who are pregnant, breastfeeding or planning to become pregnant should tell their doctor before using this medicine.

Special Precautions

The herpes virus is contained in the blisters. When the blisters break, the infection will spread very easily. If you touch your skin sores, wash your hands immediately and do not touch other parts of your body until your hands are clean.

Genital herpes is a sexually transmitted disease and you should avoid having sex when lesions (blisters) are present because there is a possibility of infecting the other person. The use of a condom will help prevent the spread of genital herpes. *The drug will NOT help prevent you from spreading the disease to others.*

Women with genital herpes should have yearly Pap smears because there appears to be a higher incidence of cancer of the cervix in women with genital herpes.

Do not share the medication with others.

Do not use this ointment in the eyes. It is meant only for application to the skin and mucous membranes.

The ointment normally causes a mild discomfort (e.g., tingling, itching or burning) when it is applied because the herpes lesions are very sensitive and tender.

When to Call Your Doctor

Most people experience few or no side effects from this drug. However, any medicine can sometimes cause unwanted effects. Call your doctor if you develop skin rash, redness or itching of the affected area.

Also call your doctor if your condition does not improve in 10 days.

Allergic Reactions

Call your doctor immediately if you think you may be allergic to the medicine or if you develop a skin rash, hives, itching, swelling of the face or difficulty in breathing. If you cannot reach your doctor, phone a hospital emergency department.

▶ ## ALLOPURINOL (ORAL)
ALLOPRIN, APO-ALLOPURINOL, NOVOPUROL, PURINOL, ZYLOPRIM

Purpose
This medicine is used in the treatment and prevention of gout. It will not be effective in relieving an attack that has already started. It is useful in treating certain types of kidney stones. It is also used in other conditions in which the body has high levels of uric acid.

Allergies/Warnings
If you have ever had an allergic reaction to ALLOPURINOL or if you have kidney or liver problems, tell your doctor and pharmacist before you take any of this medicine.

Drugs That Cause Sexual Problems

More than 100 medications can interfere with sexual function in both men and women. They can cause decreased sex drive, interfere with erection or ejaculation in men and delay or prevent orgasm in women. Some of the drugs that may cause sexual problems are:

Antihypertensives/Heart Drugs	CAPTOPRIL
	GUANETHIDINE
	HYDRALAZINE
	METHYLDOPA
	PHENOXYBENZAMINE
	PROPRANOLOL
	RESERPINE
Tranquilizers	CHLORDIAZEPOXIDE
	DIAZEPAM
	MEPROBAMATE
Antidepressants	AMITRIPTYLINE
	IMIPRAMINE
	DESIPRAMINE
Antipsychotic Drugs	THIORIDAZINE
	CHLORPROMAZINE
Stomach Drugs	CIMETIDINE
	ATROPINE
	BELLADONNA
	PROPANTHELINE
Cancer Drugs	
Diuretics	SPIRONOLACTONE
	CHLORTHALIDONE
	THIAZIDES
Cholesterol-Reducing Drugs	CLOFIBRATE
Alcohol	

It is recommended that patients discuss any sexual problems they are having with their doctor rather than blaming themselves or their partners. These problems can often be solved simply by reducing the dosage or switching to another drug.

In some cases, sexual problems may be due to illnesses such as diabetes, heart disease, alcoholism, depression, fatigue, etc., which will require medical treatment.

How to Use This Medicine

Time of Administration

It is very important that you take this medicine exactly as your doctor has prescribed. Do not miss any doses, and take the medicine even if you feel well. Try to take this medicine at the same time(s) every day so that you will have a constant level of medicine in your body. Do not take extra tablets without your doctor's approval.

How to Administer

Take this medicine with food or a glass of milk or after meals to help prevent stomach upset. Call your doctor if you continue to have stomach upset.

Special Instructions

Length of Therapy

It may be necessary to take this medicine up to 2 to 6 weeks before you feel its full benefits.

Do not stop taking the medicine without your doctor's approval.

Pregnancy/Breastfeeding

Women who are pregnant or planning to become pregnant should tell their doctor before taking this medicine.

Women who are breastfeeding should tell their doctor before taking this medicine. This medicine may pass into the breast milk and cause side effects in the baby.

Look-Alike and Sound-Alike Drugs in Canada

Pharmacists are especially careful when dispensing medications that either look alike on written prescriptions or sound alike when the prescription is received over the telephone.

Examples of such drugs are:

ATARAX	.... IDARAC
BUSCOPAN	.... BUSPAR
CAPOTEN	.... COPTIN
CEFOXITIN	.... CEFOTAXIME
CHLOROQUINE	.... CHLORPROPAMIDE
CLOMIPHENE	.... CHLORPROMAZINE
CORTONE	.... CORDARONE

DANAZOL	....	DIANABOL
DIPHENHYDRAMINE	....	DIMENHYDRINATE
DIPYRIDAMOLE	....	DISOPYRAMIDE
DONNATAL	....	DONNAGEL
DOXEPIN	....	DOXIDAN
ETRAFON	....	ENTROPHEN
FLUZONE	....	FLUTONE
HALCION	....	HALDOL
KAO-CON	....	KAON
KEFLEX	....	KEFLIN
KEMADRIN	....	COUMADIN
K-LOR	....	CECLOR
KOFFEX	....	KEFLEX
LEUCOVORON	....	LEUKERAN
LORATIDINE	....	LERITINE
LOXEPINE	....	DOXEPIN
MODITEN	....	MONITAN
MODULON	....	MODURET
NORPRAMIN	....	NORIPRAMINE
NORTRIPTYLINE	....	NOVOTRIPTYN
PERPHENAZINE	....	PROCYCLIDINE
QUININE	....	QUINIDINE
SELDANE	....	FELDENE
SERENTIL	....	SURMONTIL
STELAZINE	....	STEMETIL
THYROLAR	....	THYTROPAR
TRENTAL	....	TRANDATE
TRIAZOLAM	....	DIAZEPAM
TRIFLUOPERAZINE	....	PROCHLORPERAZINE
VINBLASTINE	....	VINCRISTINE
ZADITEN	....	AZATADINE
ZANTAC	....	XANAX
ZOVIRAX	....	ZOSTRIX
ZYLOPRIM	....	PROLOPRIM

Drug Interactions

Do not take vitamin C supplements without the approval of your doctor while you are taking this medicine. Vitamin C (ascorbic acid) may make the urine more acidic and promote the development of kidney stones in people taking this medicine.

Special Precautions

Be sure to keep your regular doctor's appointments so that he or she can make sure that the medicine is working correctly and that your gout is under control.

To help prevent the formation of new kidney stones, drink at least 10 to 12 full (8-oz or 240 mL) glasses of water or other fluids every day while you are taking this medicine unless directed otherwise by your doctor. If the medicine is for a child, ask your doctor how much water the child should drink each day.

In some people, this drug may cause drowsiness. Do not drive a car, pilot an airplane, operate dangerous machinery or do jobs that require you to be alert until you know how you are going to react to the drug.

When to Call Your Doctor

Stop taking the drug and call your doctor immediately if you develop pain when you urinate (pass your water), blood in the urine, irritation of the eyes, swelling of the lips or mouth, a skin rash or red-purple spots that look like bruises. The skin rash has been reported to appear as late as 3 months after the medicine has been stopped.

Also call your doctor if you develop a sore throat, fever, chills, unusual bruising or bleeding, unusual tiredness or weakness, muscle aching, stomach pain, numbness, tingling or pain in the hands or feet, a yellow color to the skin or eyes, changes in vision or blurred vision or low back pain.

Allergic Reactions

Call your doctor immediately if you think you may be allergic to the medicine or if you develop a skin rash, hives or itching.

▶ ALPRAZOLAM (ORAL)
XANAX

BROMAZEPAM
LECTOPAM

CHLORDIAZEPOXIDE HCl
APO-CHLORDIAZEPOXIDE, LIBRIUM, MEDILIUM, NOVOPOXIDE, SOLIUM

CLONAZEPAM
RIVOTRIL

CLORAZEPATE DIPOTASSIUM
Novoclopate, Tranxene

DIAZEPAM
Apo-Diazepam, Meval, Novodipam, Valium, Vivol

LORAZEPAM (ORAL and SUBLINGUAL)
Apo-Lorazepam, Ativan, Novolorazem, PMS Lorazepam

OXAZEPAM
Apo-Oxazepam, Novoxapam, PMS Oxazepam, Serax, Zapex

Purpose
This medicine (except CLONAZEPAM) is used to help relieve moderate to severe anxiety and tension and to treat some nervous conditions. It should not be used to treat nervousness or tension from the normal pressures of day-to-day living. DIAZEPAM is also used in some conditions to help relieve muscle cramps.

CLONAZEPAM is used in some patients to help prevent seizures. Some of the drugs are used to treat the symptoms of alcohol withdrawal.

Allergies/Warnings
If you have ever had an allergic reaction to any medicine or if you have any medical problem, tell your doctor and pharmacist before you take any of this medicine.

How to Use This Medicine
How to Administer
This medicine may be taken without regard to meals. Take it either with food or on an empty stomach.

For Ativan *sublingual tablets:*
• *See* Sublingual Tablets (page 23).

Special Instructions
Length of Therapy
Do not take this medicine more often or longer than recommended by your doctor. If large doses are taken for long periods of time (months), the drug can become habit-forming.

Do not stop taking this medicine suddenly without the approval of your doctor. It may be necessary for your doctor to reduce your dose slowly since your body may need time to adjust.

Check with your doctor if you develop any of the following symptoms while you are slowly stopping or after you have stopped the medicine: nausea or vomiting, trembling, seizures, muscle cramps, stomach cramps, unusual sweating, trouble sleeping. Also call your doctor if you become confused, irritable or nervous.

Pregnancy/Breastfeeding

Women who are pregnant, breastfeeding or planning to become pregnant should tell their doctor before taking this medicine. Generally, this medicine should not be used during pregnancy and is not recommended during breastfeeding.

Drug Interactions

It is important that you obtain the advice of your doctor or pharmacist before taking any other prescription or nonprescription medicines, including pain relievers, antacids, sleeping pills, tranquilizers or medicines for depression, cough, cold or allergies.

There are other drug interactions that can occur. If you are taking any other medicines, be sure to check first with your pharmacist or doctor.

Alcohol

Do not drink alcoholic beverages while taking this drug or for a few days after you have stopped taking the drug without the approval of your doctor. The combination could cause drowsiness. One drink may have the same effect that 2 or 3 drinks normally would have.

Special Precautions

In some people, this drug may cause dizziness or drowsiness. Do not drive a car, pilot an airplane, operate dangerous machinery or do jobs that require you to be alert if you are dizzy or drowsy. You should also be careful going up and down stairs. Sit or lie down at the first sign of dizziness. Tell your doctor if the dizziness or drowsiness continues.

When to Call Your Doctor

Most people experience few or no side effects from this drug. However, any medicine can sometimes cause unwanted effects. Call your doctor if you develop a sore throat, fever, mouth sores, a staggering walk, a yellow color to the skin or eyes, slow heartbeats or shortness of breath, unusual tiredness or nervousness, stomach pain, unusual bruising or bleeding, confusion or depression, hallucinations, trouble sleeping, slurred speech or severe drowsiness.

If you are taking this medicine to treat epilepsy, call your doctor if you have an increase in the frequency of seizures.

Allergic Reactions

Call your doctor immediately if you think you may be allergic to the medicine or if you develop a skin rash, hives, itching, swelling of the face or difficulty in breathing. If you cannot reach your doctor, phone a hospital emergency department.

Do Not Remove Prescription Labels

You should always keep your medicines in the containers in which they were dispensed by the pharmacist.

Do *not* remove the label until all the medication is taken.

The information on the label is necessary to properly identify the patient, the physician, the drug, the instructions for use and the date the prescription was dispensed.

This information is important when you need a refill of the prescription or in the event of an emergency.

▶ **AMCINONIDE (TOPICAL)**
CYCLOCORT

BECLOMETHASONE
PROPADERM

BETAMETHASONE
BEBEN, BETACORT SCALP LOTION, BETADERM, BETADERM SCALP LOTION, BETAGEL, BETNOVATE, CELESTODERM-V, CELESTODERM-V/2, DIPROLENE, DIPROSONE, ECTOSONE MILD, ECTOSONE REGULAR, ECTOSONE SCALP LOTION, NOVOBETAMET, PREVEX B, TOPILENE, TOPISONE, VALISONE SCALP LOTION

CLOBETASOL PROPIONATE
DERMOVATE

CLOBETASONE
EUMOVATE

DESONIDE
TRIDESILON

DESOXIMETASONE
TOPICORT

DIFLORASONE
FLORONE, FLUTONE

DIFLUCORTOLONE
NERISONE

FLUMETHASONE PIVALATE
LOCACORTEN

FLUOCINOLONE ACETONIDE
FLUODERM, FLUONIDE, SYNALAR, SYNAMOL

FLUOCINONIDE
LIDEMOL, LIDEX, LYDERM, TOPSYN GEL

FLURANDRENOLIDE
DRENISON, DRENISON TAPE

HALCINONIDE
HALOG

HYDROCORTISONE
ALOCORT, BARRIERE-HC, CORTACET, CORTATE, CORTICREME, CORTODERM, EMO-CORT, HYDERM, NOVOHYDROCORT, PREVEX HC, SARNA HC 1.0%, TEXACORT, UNICORT, WESTCORT

HYDROCORTISONE-NEOMYCIN
NEO-CORTEF

METHYLPREDNISOLONE
MEDROL TOPICAL

METHYLPREDNISOLONE-NEOMYCIN
NEO-MEDROL TOPICAL

TRIAMCINOLONE
ARISTOCORT C, ARISTOCORT D, ARISTOCORT R, KENALOG, KENALOG SPRAY, TRIADERM

Purpose

This medicine is used to help relieve pain, itching, redness and swelling of certain types of skin conditions. NEO-CORTEF and NEO-MEDROL Topical contain NEOMYCIN (an antibiotic) and are used to help prevent and treat skin infections.

Do not use this medicine for any other skin problems without checking with your doctor.

Allergies/Warnings

Be sure to tell your doctor and pharmacist if you are allergic to any medicine or have any other medical condition.

Children may absorb larger amounts of this medicine and should have frequent checkups by their doctors while using this medicine. Do not use tight-fitting diapers or plastic pants on infants when using this medication unless instructed by your physician.

How to Use This Medicine

How to Administer

For cream, ointment, gel, solution and lotion:
- *See* Creams, Ointments, Gels, Solutions and Lotions (page 36).

If you were prescribed HALOG, SYNALAR *or* TEXACORT SOLUTION:
- Each time you apply the medicine, wash your hands with water unless otherwise directed by your doctor. Do not allow the skin to dry completely. Pat with a clean towel until slightly damp.
- Apply a small amount of the drug, drop by drop, to the affected area and spread lightly. Do not bandage unless otherwise directed by your doctor.
- In hairy areas, the hair should be parted before applying in order to get the medicine on the affected skin area.

For KENALOG SPRAY:
- *See* Aerosol Sprays (page 36) in How to Administer Medications, except hold the container 7 to 15 cm (3 to 6 inches) away from the skin.
- To cover an area about the size of a hand, spray the area for only about 2 seconds.

For DRENISON TAPE:

- Each time you apply the tape, wash your hands and gently cleanse the skin area well with mild soap and water unless otherwise directed by your doctor. Allow the skin to dry 1 hour. The skin should be *clean* and *completely dry* before the tape is applied. If showers or tub baths are to be taken, they should be completed before applying the tape.
- In hairy areas, shave or clip the hair to allow good contact with the skin and easy removal of the tape.
- Remove the tape from the package and cut a piece slightly larger than the area to be covered. Round off the corners.
- The tape should always be cut—never tear it.
- Remove the paper liner from the back of the transparent tape. Be careful that the tape does not bend and stick to itself.
- Apply the tape and press it into place so that the surface is smooth.
- Unless otherwise directed by your doctor, replace the tape every 12 hours. Cleanse the skin and allow it to dry 1 hour before applying a new tape. If the tape loosens before the end of the 12-hour period, remove and replace it.
- If an irritation or infection develops, remove the tape and call your doctor.

Special Instructions

Length of Therapy

Do not use the drug more frequently or in larger quantities than prescribed by your doctor. Overuse of this medicine may cause you to absorb too much of the drug and increase the risk of side effects.

If the problem does not clear up within 10 to 14 days or if it reappears soon after treatment, see your doctor.

Pregnancy/Breastfeeding

Women who are pregnant, breastfeeding or planning to become pregnant should tell their doctor before using this medicine.

Drug Interactions

Do not apply cosmetics or lotions on top of the drug unless your doctor approves.

Do not use nonprescription creams or ointments (including those containing hydrocortisone) while using this medicine without first consulting with your doctor.

Special Precautions

Do not use this medicine for any other skin conditions that arise or on any other parts of your body without consulting your doctor or pharmacist.

This medicine is for external use only. Do not swallow it.

Some of the medicines may cause a temporary stinging sensation after they are applied. This will usually disappear within a few minutes.

Do not bandage the treated area unless your doctor has told you to do so. Do not apply this medicine to open wounds.

Keep the medicine away from the eyes, nose and mouth because it could cause serious side effects (e.g., cataracts or glaucoma).

When to Call Your Doctor

Call your doctor if the condition for which this drug is being used continues or becomes worse, or if you have a constant irritation such as itching or burning that was not present before you started using this medicine or signs of a skin infection. Also call your doctor if you are using the medicine on the face, under the arms or between the legs and if you develop abnormal red-purple lines, easy bruising or thinning of the skin in these areas, increased facial hair or loss of scalp hair.

Storage

For KENALOG SPRAY:

• *See* Aerosol Sprays in How to Administer Medications (page 36).

Miscellaneous

Tell any other doctors you are seeing that you are using this medicine.

▶ AMILORIDE (ORAL)
MIDAMOR

AMILORIDE-HYDROCHLOROTHIAZIDE
MODURET

Purpose

This medicine is used to help the body get rid of excess fluids and to decrease swelling. The medicine does this by increasing the amount of urine and is commonly called a "water pill" or "fluid pill." It is used to treat high blood pressure and other medical conditions.

It's Up to You

Taking prescription drugs at the correct times is like staying on a diet. You must motivate yourself and decide that you want to take the medications as they were prescribed.

Allergies/Warnings

Be sure to tell your doctor or pharmacist if you are allergic to any medicine.

How to Use This Medicine

Time of Administration

Try to take this medicine at the same time(s) every day so that you have a constant level of the medicine in your body.

When you first start taking this medicine, you will probably urinate (pass your water) more often and in larger amounts than usual. Therefore, if you are to take 1 dose each day, take it in the morning after breakfast. Do not initially take a dose at bedtime or you may have to get up during the night to go to the bathroom.

If you are to take more than 1 dose each day, take the last dose approximately 6 hours before bedtime so that you will not have to get up during the night to go to the bathroom. This effect will usually lessen after you have taken the drug for a while.

How to Administer

Take this medicine with food, meals or milk.

Special Instructions

Length of Therapy

For patients with high blood pressure:

- High blood pressure (hypertension) is a long-term condition and it will probably be necessary for you to take the drug for a long time even if you feel better. If high blood pressure is not treated, it can lead to serious problems such as heart failure, strokes, blood vessel problems or kidney problems.

It is very important that you take this medicine as your doctor has directed and not miss any doses. Otherwise, you cannot expect the drug to keep your blood pressure down or remove excess fluid.

Pregnancy/Breastfeeding

Women who are pregnant, breastfeeding or planning to become pregnant should tell their doctor before taking this medicine.

Drug Interactions

Some nonprescription drugs can aggravate high blood pressure. Do not take any of the following without the approval of your doctor or pharmacist: cough, cold or sinus products; asthma or allergy products, since they may increase your blood pressure.

Read the label of the nonprescription drug product to see if there is a warning. If there is, check with your doctor or pharmacist before using the product.

Alcohol

Be careful drinking alcoholic beverages while taking this medicine because it could make the possible side effect of dizziness worse.

Special Precautions

If this medicine causes dizziness or lightheadedness, you should be careful going up or down stairs and you should not change positions too rapidly. Lightheadedness is more likely to occur if you stand up suddenly—this is due to blood collecting in the legs and lasts for a few seconds. Therefore, get up from a sitting or lying position more slowly and tighten and relax your leg muscles or wiggle your toes to help promote circulation. In the morning, get out of bed slowly and dangle your feet over the edge of the bed for a few minutes before standing up. Sit or lie down at the first sign of dizziness. Do not drive a car, pilot an airplane, operate dangerous machinery or do jobs that require you to be alert if you are dizzy. Tell your doctor if you have been dizzy.

In order to help prevent dizziness or fainting, your doctor may also recommend that you avoid strenuous exercise, standing for long periods of time (especially in hot weather), hot showers, hot baths or saunas.

People more than 65 years of age may be more sensitive to the side effect of dizziness.

This medicine may make some people more sensitive to sunlight and some tanning lamps. When you begin taking this medicine, try to avoid too much sun until you see how you are going to react. If your skin does become more sensitive to sunlight, tell your doctor and try not to stay in direct sunlight for extended periods of time. While in the sun, wear protective clothing and sunglasses. You may wish to ask your pharmacist about suitable sunscreen products. Call your doctor if you become sunburned.

This medicine does not cause your body to lose potassium as some other types of *water pills* do. Therefore, it is not usually necessary for you to eat foods rich in potassium. In fact, too much potassium while you are taking this medicine could be harmful. Call your doctor if you develop any of the warning signs of too much potassium: irregular heartbeats; numbness or tingling in the hands, feet or lips; confusion; difficulty breathing; unusual tiredness or weakness; unexplained nervousness; weakness or a feeling of heaviness in the legs. Since not all patients develop these symptoms, your doctor may want to check your blood occasionally to see if the potassium level is normal.

Do not use salt substitutes, low-salt milk or low-salt soups without the approval of your doctor. They may contain large amounts of potassium, which could affect the way you respond to this medicine.

If you are a diabetic and were prescribed MODURET:
- This medicine may cause your blood sugar to rise. Carefully test your blood or urine for sugar while you are taking this medicine. Call your doctor if you think your blood sugar is higher than normal or harder to control.

When to Call Your Doctor
Most people experience few or no side effects from this drug. However, any medicine can sometimes cause unwanted effects. Call your doctor if you develop nausea, vomiting, a skin rash, headaches, diarrhea, weakness, tiredness, muscle cramps, numbness or tingling of the hands, feet or lips, a yellow color to the skin or eyes or dark yellow-colored urine.

Also call your doctor if you feel sick or develop persistent vomiting or diarrhea.

If you were prescribed MODURET:
- Also call your doctor if you develop sharp joint pain or unusual bruising or bleeding.

Allergic Reactions
Call your doctor immediately if you think you may be allergic to the medicine or if you develop a skin rash, hives, itching, swelling of the face or difficulty in breathing. If you cannot reach your doctor, phone a hospital emergency department.

Refills

Do not stop taking this medicine without your doctor's approval and do not go without medicine between prescription refills. Call your pharmacist for a refill 2 or 3 days before you will run out of the medicine.

Refill Your Prescriptions on Time

You should tell your doctor if you did not have a prescription filled or if you did not take your medicine exactly as prescribed.

Otherwise, your doctor will think that the medicine was not effective and prescribe another medicine that is used to treat the same condition but could have more side effects or be less effective.

▶ **AMINOPHYLLINE (ORAL)**
PALARON, PHYLLOCONTIN, PHYLLOCONTIN-350

OXTRIPHYLLINE
APO-OXTRIPHYLLINE, CHOLEDYL, CHOLEDYL SA, NOVOTRIPHYL, ROUPHYLLINE

THEOPHYLLINE
ELIXOPHYLLIN, PMS THEOPHYLLINE ELIXIR, PULMOPHYLLINE, QUIBRON-T/SR, QUIBRON-T LIQUID, SLO-BID, SOMOPHYLLIN-12, THEOCHRON, THEO-DUR, THEOLAIR, THEOLAIR-SR, THEO-SR, UNIPHYL

AMINOPHYLLINE (RECTAL)
COROPHYLLIN

Purpose

This medicine is used to help open the bronchioles (air passages in the lungs) to make breathing easier and to relieve wheezing and shortness of breath. It is used in the treatment of bronchial asthma, bronchitis, emphysema and other lung conditions.

Allergies/Warnings

If you have ever had an allergic reaction to caffeine or any medicine for lung conditions, tell your doctor and pharmacist before you take any of this medicine.

How to Use This Medicine

Time of Administration

This medicine should be taken with a glass of water.

Many of these medicines can be taken with food but you should check with your pharmacist or doctor for instructions on your particular medicine. Whether you take it with or without food, it is important that you *always take it the same way all the time* so that the same amount of medicine reaches the bloodstream.

Take the medicine in a sitting or upright position. Do not lie down immediately after taking the drug in order to ensure that the medicine reaches the stomach.

For UNIPHYL:
- Most patients only have to take this medicine once a day. Take it with food or within 1 to 2 hours of eating food. It is best to take the medicine later in the day, with or shortly after the evening meal.

   Space your doses of the medicine as equally as possible around the clock (throughout the entire day of 24 hours). For example, if you are to take 3 doses each day, try to space the doses as close as possible to 8 hours apart. This will keep a constant level of the medicine in your body. It is very important to *always* take this medicine at the same time(s) every day. Do not take extra doses without your doctor's approval and try not to miss any doses. If you miss doses, the amount of THEOPHYLLINE in your blood will fall and you will not get the full benefit of this medicine.

   Try not to take doses more than 1/2 hour before their scheduled time.

How to Administer

If you were prescribed CHOLEDYL SA, QUIBRON-T/SR, SLO-BID, THEOCHRON, THEOLAIR-SR, THEO-SR, UNIPHYL:
- This medicine is long-acting and must be swallowed whole. Do not crush or chew.

If you were prescribed SOMOPHYLLIN-12:
- These capsules may be swallowed whole, or the capsule may be opened and the contents sprinkled on a small amount of soft food just before taking. The contents of the capsule should *not* be chewed or crushed.
- Hold the capsule horizontally just above a spoonful of cool, soft food that is easy to swallow such as applesauce, fruit puree, pudding or ice cream.

- Turn both ends of the capsule in opposite directions and gently pull apart.
- Sprinkle the contents of the capsule onto the food.
- Do not chew the drug/food mixture but swallow it immediately. Then drink some water.
- Do not save or reuse any of the medicine that has been sprinkled on any food.
- If you spill any of the beads while sprinkling, start over to make sure that you get the right dose.

If you were prescribed PHYLLOCONTIN TABLETS *or* THEO-DUR TABLETS:
- This medicine is long-acting. Do not crush or chew. The tablets may be swallowed whole or cut in half.

For liquid medicines:
- If a spoon is used to measure the dose, it is recommended that you use a medicine spoon or an oral liquid syringe, which you can obtain from your pharmacist. *See* Oral Liquid Syringe (page 17) and Medicine Spoon (page 22).

For COROPHYLLIN SUPPOSITORIES:
- *See* Rectal Suppositories (page 39).

Special Instructions

Length of Therapy
Do not take this medicine more often or longer than recommended by your doctor. To do so may increase your chance of developing side effects. Do not stop taking this medicine without your doctor's permission. If you suddenly stop taking this medicine, you may have an asthmatic attack. You should discuss the length of therapy with your doctor.

Pregnancy/Breastfeeding
Women who are pregnant, breastfeeding or planning to become pregnant should tell their doctor before taking this medicine.

Drug Interactions
Some nonprescription drugs can aggravate your condition. Do not take any of the following without the approval of your doctor or pharmacist: cough, cold or sinus products; ASA-containing medicines; asthma or allergy products. Read the label of the product to see if there

is a warning. If there is, check with your doctor or pharmacist before using the product.

Do not take this medicine at the same time as a nonprescription drug containing AMINOPHYLLINE or THEOPHYLLINE without the approval of your doctor.

Avoid drinking large amounts of coffee, tea, cocoa (chocolate) or cola drinks, or eating large amounts of foods containing chocolate while you are on this medicine, because you could be more sensitive to the caffeine in these beverages.

Do not smoke while you are on this medicine because smoking can make the drug less effective. If you insist on smoking, be sure to tell your doctor so that he or she can take this into consideration when adjusting your doses.

The effect of this medicine can be decreased by a diet low in carbohydrates, high in protein or with a high frequency of charcoal-broiled foods. On the other hand, a diet high in carbohydrates and low in protein can cause unwanted higher levels of the medicine. Check with your doctor if you have any questions about your diet.

Blood tests for THEOPHYLLINE can be made inaccurate by previous ingestions of coffee, tea, cola beverages, chocolate and medicines containing ACETAMINOPHEN.

Alcohol

Do not drink alcoholic beverages or take nonprescription drugs containing alcohol while taking this drug without the approval of your doctor.

Special Precautions

If your mouth becomes dry, drink water, suck ice chips or a hard, sour candy (sugarless) or chew gum (sugarless). Sugarless products are recommended in order to avoid dental problems. You may wish to ask your pharmacist about special solutions, called artificial saliva, that can also be used to help restore moisture in the mouth. It is especially important to brush and floss your teeth regularly if you develop a dry mouth, to help prevent gum problems.

In some people, this drug may cause dizziness. This side effect is more common in people over 60 years of age and people with lung conditions. Do not drive a car, pilot an airplane, operate dangerous machinery or do jobs that require you to be alert if you are dizzy or drowsy. You should also be careful going up and down stairs. Sit or lie down at the first sign of dizziness. Tell your doctor if the dizziness continues.

Be sure to keep your appointments with your doctor after you first start taking this medicine. People respond to this drug at different rates and your doctor must examine you in order to determine the best dose for you.

If your doctor wants to check the level of this medicine in your blood (a simple blood test), be sure to tell him or her if you have missed a dose of the medicine in the last 2 days. The test will have to be done another time because it will not be accurate if you have missed taking the drug. Also, be sure to have the blood tests done at the times recommended by your doctor. If the blood test is not done at the correct time, the test results may not be accurate.

Do not change the dose of any other asthma or bronchitis medicines except on the advice of your doctor.

When to Call Your Doctor

Call your doctor if you develop flu symptoms, a fever or diarrhea.

Most people experience few or no side effects from this drug. However, any medicine can sometimes cause unwanted effects. Call your doctor if you develop a skin rash, hives, sore throat, fever, mouth sores, vomiting of blood or material resembling coffee grounds, stomach pain or red or black stools, fast or irregular heartbeats, confusion, unusual tiredness, convulsions or agitation, tremor, difficulty sleeping, restlessness or thirst, headaches, muscle twitching or increased urination (passing your water).

If you are using rectal suppositories, contact your doctor also if you develop burning or irritation of the skin in the rectal area.

Refills

Do not stop taking this medicine without your doctor's approval and do not go without medicine between prescription refills. Call your pharmacist for a refill 2 or 3 days before you will run out of the medicine.

Discuss with your pharmacist the implications of dispensing all your refills for this medicine with the same manufacturer's product. (*See* Generic Drugs, page 13.)

▶ **5-AMINOSALICYLIC ACID (ORAL)**
ASACOL, MESASAL, PENTASA, SALOFALK

OLSALAZINE
DIPENTUM

5-AMINOSALICYLIC ACID (RECTAL)
MESASAL, SALOFALK

Purpose
This medicine is used to treat conditions of the intestines causing diarrhea (loose bowel movements), such as ulcerative colitis.

Allergies/Warnings
If you have ever had an allergic reaction to salicylates, ASA or sulfas, or have stomach ulcers, liver disease or kidney disease, tell your doctor or pharmacist before you take any of this medicine.

How to Use This Medicine

How to Administer
This medicine has a special coating and must be swallowed whole. Do not crush, chew or break the tablet into pieces.

If you were prescribed suppositories:
• *See* Rectal Suppositories (page 39).

If you were prescribed an enema:
• *See* Rectal Enemas (page 40).

Time of Administration
If you were prescribed ASACOL, MESASAL:
• Take with a glass of water on an empty stomach.

If you were prescribed PENTASA, DIPENTUM 500 mg Tablets *or* SALOFALK Tablets:
• Take 30 minutes before meals and at bedtime with a glass of water, juice or other fluids.

If you were prescribed DIPENTUM 250 mg Tablets:
• Take with food or a snack.

Special Instructions

Length of Therapy
It is important to take all of this medicine plus any refills that your doctor has prescribed. Do not stop taking this medicine earlier than your doctor has recommended even if you feel better. Otherwise, you cannot expect the drug to work for you.

Pregnancy/Breastfeeding

Women who are pregnant, breastfeeding or planning to become pregnant should tell their doctor before taking this medicine.

Special Precautions

Be sure to keep your appointments with your doctor so that your progress can be checked regularly and to make sure you are getting the most benefit from this medicine.

If you become dizzy, you should be careful going up and down stairs. Do not drive a car, pilot an airplane, operate dangerous machinery or do jobs that require you to be alert until you know how you are going to react to the drug. Sit or lie down at the first sign of dizziness. Tell your doctor if the dizziness continues.

When to Call Your Doctor

Most people experience few or no side effects from this drug. However, any medicine can sometimes cause unwanted side effects. Call your doctor if your symptoms worsen or do not improve within 1 month of starting this medicine.

Allergic Reactions

Call your doctor immediately if you think you may be allergic to the medicine or if you develop a skin rash, hives, itching, fever, dizziness or difficulty in breathing. If you cannot reach a doctor, phone a hospital emergency department.

Storage

The tablets and capsules should be stored at room temperature away from heat and light.

The suppositories and enemas should be stored in a cool place.

▶ AMIORDARONE (ORAL)
CORDARONE

Purpose

This medicine is used to help make the heart beat at a regular and normal rate.

Allergies/Warnings

If you have ever had an allergic reaction to any medication, tell your doctor and pharmacist before you take this medicine. Also tell your doctor if you have ever had liver, thyroid or lung disease.

How to Use This Medicine

Time of Administration

It is best to take this medication with food or a glass of milk to help prevent stomach upset. If stomach upset occurs, call your doctor.

Space doses of this medicine around the clock (throughout the entire day of 24 hours). For example, if you take 3 doses each day, space the doses 8 hours apart.

Special Instructions

Length of Therapy

It is very important that you take this medicine exactly as your doctor has prescribed. Do not miss any doses. Take the medicine even if you feel well. Try to take this medicine at the same time(s) every day so that you will have a constant level of medicine in your body. Do not take extra tablets without your doctor's approval.

Do not stop taking this medicine suddenly without your doctor's approval. It will be necessary for your doctor to reduce your dose slowly since your body will need time to adjust. It could be harmful to you and make your condition worse if you suddenly stopped taking the medicine.

Pregnancy/Breastfeeding

Women who are pregnant, breastfeeding or planning to become pregnant should tell their doctor before taking this medicine.

Drug Interactions

Some prescription drugs can interact with this medicine. Therefore, do not start or stop taking any drugs you are currently taking without first consulting your doctor.

Special Precautions

If this medicine causes dizziness or lightheadedness, you should be careful going up and down stairs and you should not change positions too quickly. This medicine may also cause drowsiness. Do not drive a car, pilot an airplane, operate dangerous machinery or do jobs that require you to be alert if you are dizzy or drowsy.

This medicine may make some people more sensitive to sunlight and various tanning lamps. When you begin taking this medicine, try to avoid too much sun until you see how you are going to react. If your skin does become more sensitive to sunlight, tell your doctor and try not to stay in direct sunlight for extended periods of time. While in the sun, wear protective clothing and sunglasses. You may wish to ask your pharmacist about suitable sunscreen products. Call your doctor if you become sunburned.

When some people first start taking this medicine, they develop nausea, vomiting, headaches, constipation, an unusual taste in the mouth, fatigue, dizziness, nightmares or sleeplessness. These effects may disappear as the body adjusts to the medicine. If you develop any of these effects and if they continue or become bothersome, talk to your doctor about them.

Any imbalance in the level of potassium in your blood may alter the effect of this medicine. Your doctor may prescribe some medicine to adjust your potassium level or may recommend certain changes to your diet. Do not change your diet unless prescribed by your doctor.

When to Call Your Doctor

Some people may experience side effects from this drug. Call your doctor if you develop cough, chest pain, difficulty in breathing, weight loss or weight gain, weakness, visual halos, changes in eyesight (blurred vision), a yellow color in skin or eyes, dark yellow-colored urine, blue-gray skin discoloration, tremor, fatigue, eye discomfort, loss of hair, skin problems or irregular or rapid heartbeats.

Allergic Reactions

Call your doctor immediately if you think you may be allergic to the medicine or if you develop skin rash, hives, itching, swelling of the face or difficulty in breathing. If you cannot reach your doctor, phone a hospital emergency department.

Refills

Do not stop taking this medicine without your doctor's approval and do not go without medicine between refills. Call your pharmacist for a refill 2 or 3 days before you will run out of the medicine.

Miscellaneous

Carry an identification card in your wallet or wear a medical alert bracelet indicating that you are taking this medicine, as well as the names and phone numbers of your doctors. If you do not already carry such a card, complete the Medicine Card in this book. Always tell your dentist, pharmacist and other doctors who are treating you that you are taking this medicine.

▶ **AMITRIPTYLINE HCI (ORAL)**
APO-AMITRIPTYLINE, ELAVIL, LEVATE, NOVOTRIPTYN, PMS
AMITRIPTYLINE

AMOXAPINE
ASENDIN

CLOMIPRAMINE
ANAFRANIL

DESIPRAMINE
NORPRAMIN, PERTOFRANE

DOXEPIN
SINEQUAN, TRIADAPIN

IMIPRAMINE
APO-IMIPRAMINE, IMPRIL, NOVOPRAMINE, PMS IMIPRAMINE,
TOFRANIL

MAPROTILINE
LUDIOMIL

NORTRIPTYLINE
AVENTYL

PROTRIPTYLINE
TRIPTIL

TRAZODONE
DESYREL, DESYREL DIVIDOSE

TRIMIPRAMINE
APO-TRIMIP, SURMONTIL

Purpose
This medicine is used to help relieve the symptoms of depression and may be used to treat other nervous conditions.

IMIPRAMINE and AMITRIPTYLINE are also used to treat bedwetting in children.

Allergies/Warnings
If you have ever had an allergic reaction to any medicine, or if you have high blood pressure, seizures, heart problems, enlarged prostate,

difficulty urinating (passing your water), Parkinson's disease, thyroid problems or glaucoma, tell your doctor and pharmacist before you take any of this medicine.

How to Use This Medicine

How to Administer

If you develop stomach upset while taking this medicine, take it with food or immediately after a snack, unless otherwise directed.

For ELAVIL Syrup:

- Shake the bottle well each time before pouring so that you will measure an accurate dose.
- If a spoon is used to measure the dose, it is recommended that you use a medicine spoon or an oral liquid syringe, which you can obtain from your pharmacist. *See* Oral Liquid Syringe (page 17) and Medicine Dropper (page 21).

For DESYREL DIVIDOSE:

- To break the tablet, hold it between your thumbs and index fingers, close to the correct groove. Hold the tablet with the groove facing upward, and gently apply pressure to break the tablet along the groove.

Special Instructions

Length of Therapy

It is important that you take the medicine regularly and that you do not miss any doses. The full effect of the medicine may not be noticed immediately, but usually takes 10 days or up to several weeks. Early signs of improvement are increased appetite, better sleep, increased energy and improved mood. *Do not stop taking* the medicine when you first feel better or you may feel worse in 3 or 4 days.

Since the medicine does not have an immediate effect on your mood, do not attempt to adjust the dose according to your moods but continue to take the dose prescribed for you. Do NOT take an extra dose if you are having a bad day.

Do not stop taking this medicine suddenly without the approval of your doctor. It will be necessary for your doctor to reduce your dose slowly since your body will need time to adjust. It could make your condition worse if you suddenly stopped taking the medicine. After you have stopped taking this medicine, you must continue to observe the following precautions (*see* "Alcohol" below) for 1 to 2 weeks since some of the medicine will still be in your body.

If you take this medicine only at bedtime and miss a dose, do not take the missed dose the next morning until you check with your doctor. Depending on your dose, the drug may cause some unwanted effects during the day if you take the whole dose the next morning.

Pregnancy/Breastfeeding

Women who are pregnant, breastfeeding or planning to become pregnant should not use this medicine without their doctor's approval.

Drug Interactions

It is important that you obtain the advice of your doctor or pharmacist before taking any prescription or nonprescription medicines, including pain relievers, sleeping pills, tranquilizers or other medicines for depression, cough, cold or allergies.

There are other drug interactions that can occur. If you are taking any other medicines, be sure to check first with your pharmacist or doctor.

Alcohol

Do not drink alcoholic beverages while taking this drug without the approval of your doctor. The combination could irritate your stomach and could cause drowsiness or dizziness. One drink may have the same effect that 2 or 3 drinks normally would have.

If you have been taking this medicine regularly for several days or weeks, it is recommended not to drink alcohol for 2 weeks *after* you have stopped taking the medicine. Depending on your dose, it may take this long for the drug to be eliminated from your body.

Special Precautions

Any medicine has a few unwanted side effects. Many of these side effects are annoying but you should try to keep taking the medicine unless your doctor tells you to stop it. Because this medicine takes a few weeks to work, the side effects show the doctor that the drug is starting to work. Most of these side effects will go away as your body adjusts to the medicine but some may not.

If this medicine causes dizziness or lightheadedness, you should be careful going up and down stairs and you should not change positions too rapidly. Lightheadedness is more likely to occur if you stand up suddenly—this is due to blood collecting in the legs and lasts for a few seconds. Therefore, get up from a sitting or lying position more slowly and tighten and relax your leg muscles or wiggle your toes to help promote circulation. In the morning, get out of bed slowly and dangle your feet over the edge of the bed for a few minutes before standing up. Sit or lie down at the first sign of dizziness. Tell your doctor if you have been dizzy. In order to help prevent dizziness or fainting, your doctor may also recommend that you avoid strenuous exercise, standing for long periods of time (especially in hot weather), hot showers, hot baths, saunas, or Jacuzzis.

Make sure you know how you are going to react to this medicine and whether it will make you dizzy or drowsy. Do not drive a car, pilot an airplane, operate dangerous machinery or do jobs that require you to be alert if you are dizzy or drowsy. The drowsiness may decrease over time.

An urge to urinate (pass your water) with an inability to do so sometimes occurs with this drug. Urinating before taking the drug each time may help relieve this problem. Tell your doctor if you are having this problem.

If your mouth becomes dry, drink water, suck ice chips or a hard, sour candy (sugarless) or chew gum (sugarless). Sugarless products are recommended in order to avoid dental problems. You may wish to ask your pharmacist about special solutions, called artificial saliva, that can also be used to help restore moisture in the mouth. Call your doctor if your mouth becomes extremely dry.

It is especially important to brush and floss your teeth regularly if you develop a dry mouth to help prevent gum problems.

This medicine may cause some people to become constipated. To help prevent constipation, try increasing the amount of bulk in your diet (for example, bran, fresh fruits and salads), exercising more often or drinking more fluids (unless otherwise directed). Call your doctor if the constipation continues.

This medicine (except TRAZODONE) may make some people more sensitive to sunlight and sunlamps. When you begin taking this medicine, try to avoid too much sun until you see how you are going to react. If your skin does become more sensitive to sunlight, tell your doctor and try to stay out of direct sunlight for extended periods of time. While in the sun, wear protective clothing and sunglasses. You may wish to ask your pharmacist about suitable sunscreen products. Call your doctor if you become sunburned.

There have been some reports that smoking may decrease the effect of this drug.

This medicine may cause nasal congestion (stuffy nose). Do not try to treat this yourself with cold or allergy medicines. Check with your doctor.

When to Call Your Doctor

Any medicine can cause unwanted side effects. Call your doctor if you develop a sore throat, fever, mouth sores, eye pain or blurred vision, difficulty in urinating (passing your water), dizziness or drowsiness, difficulty speaking, unexplained nervousness, unusually high energy or irritability, a yellow color in the skin or eyes, fast heartbeats, difficulty breathing, a skin rash, nausea or vomiting, confusion, fainting spells, seizures or shakiness, or convulsions.

For patients prescribed AMOXAPINE:
* Also call your doctor if you develop tremors, drooling, unusual muscle stiffness, shuffling walk, inability to sit still or sleep, unexplained fever, shakiness or unusual movements of the face, tongue or hands, stiffness of the face or body, irregular menstrual periods (in women), pain or discharge from the breasts, numbness or tingling of the hands or feet.

For patients prescribed TRAZODONE:
* Call your doctor if you develop a skin rash, confusion, chest pain, nausea and vomiting, shortness of breath, blood in the urine, dizziness, fainting, trembling or severe drowsiness, changes in sexual ability, fast or slow heartbeats or confusion.

For men:
* Stop taking the drug and call your doctor *immediately* if you develop a painful, long-lasting erection. Immediate treatment is necessary to help avoid serious problems.

Refills

Do not stop taking this medicine without your doctor's approval and do not go without medicine between prescription refills. Call your pharmacist for a refill 2 or 3 days before you will run out of the medicine.

Discuss with your pharmacist the implications of dispensing all your refills for this medicine with the same manufacturer's product. (*See* Generic Drugs, page 13.)

Miscellaneous

Carry an identification card in your wallet or wear a medical alert bracelet indicating that you are taking this medicine, as well as the names and phone numbers of your doctors. If you do not already carry such a card, complete the Medicine Card in this book. Always tell your dentist, pharmacist and other doctors who are treating you that you are taking this medicine.

▶ **AMITRIPTYLINE-PERPHENAZINE (ORAL)**
ELAVIL PLUS, ETRAFON 2-10, ETRAFON-A, ETRAFON-D, ETRAFON-F, PMS LEVAZINE, PROAVIL, TRIAVIL

Purpose

This medicine is used to help relieve the symptoms of anxiety and depression and certain other types of emotional conditions.

Allergies/Warnings

If you have ever had an allergic reaction to any medicine or if you have high blood pressure, seizures, heart problems, enlarged prostate, difficulty urinating (passing your water), Parkinson's disease, thyroid problems, glaucoma or any other medical condition, tell your doctor and pharmacist before you take any of this medicine.

How to Use This Medicine

How to Administer

If you develop stomach upset while taking this medicine, take it with food or immediately after a snack, unless otherwise directed.

Special Instructions

Length of Therapy

It is important that you take the medicine regularly and that you do not miss any doses. The full effect of the medicine may not be noticed immediately, but may take from a few days to several weeks. Early signs of improvement are increased appetite, better sleep, increased energy and improved mood. *Do not stop taking the medicine* when you first feel better or you may feel worse in 3 or 4 days.

Since the medicine does not have an immediate effect on your mood, do not attempt to adjust the dose according to your moods but continue to take the dose prescribed for you. Do NOT take an extra dose if you are having a bad day.

Do not stop taking this medicine suddenly without the approval of your doctor. It will be necessary for your doctor to reduce your dose slowly since your body will need time to adjust. It could make your condition worse if you suddenly stopped taking the medicine. After you have stopped taking this medicine, you must continue to observe the following precautions for 1 to 2 weeks since some of the medicine will still be in your body.

What If My Drug Causes A Dry Mouth?

Research has shown that poor dental hygiene during treatment with a medicine that causes a dry mouth can lead to periodontal disease.

Some helpful hints to help prevent dental problems if you have a dry mouth are:

- Suck bitter or lemon-flavored *sugarless* candies. This will help to stimulate the flow of saliva.
- Avoid gums and candies that contain sugar because they can promote dental cavities.
- Brush your teeth after each meal and floss your teeth daily to remove the plaque on your teeth. Remember the plaque can build up more quickly if you have a dry mouth and plaque is responsible for many gum problems.
- Small sips of water and ice chips will help to moisturize a dry mouth.
- Bland mouth rinses such as salt and sodium bicarbonate may soothe, lubricate and moisturize dry, irritated mouths.
- Spraying the mouth with warm water from a small atomizer can be very soothing.
- Ask your doctor or dentist about the use of lubricating products that can be purchased in a pharmacy. Though they lack the infection-fighting substances and digestive enzymes of natural saliva, they do help to lubricate the mouth.

Pregnancy/Breastfeeding

Women who are pregnant, breastfeeding or planning to become pregnant should not use this medicine without their doctor's approval.

Drug Interactions

It is best not to take this medicine at the same time as an antacid or an anti-diarrhea medicine containing aluminum. Try to space them 2 hours apart if you must take them while you are on this medicine.

It is important that you obtain the advice of your doctor or pharmacist before taking any prescription or nonprescription medicines, including pain relievers, sleeping pills, tranquilizers or medicines for depression, cough, cold or allergies.

There are other drug interactions that can occur. If you are taking any other medicines, be sure to check first with your pharmacist or doctor.

Alcohol

Do not drink alcoholic beverages while taking this drug without the approval of your doctor. The combination could irritate your stomach and could cause drowsiness or dizziness. One drink may have the same effect that 2 or 3 drinks normally would have.

If you have been taking this medicine regularly for several days or weeks, it is recommended not to drink alcohol for 2 weeks *after* you have stopped taking the medicine. Depending on your dose, it may take this long for the drug to be eliminated from your body.

Special Precautions

Any medicine has a few unwanted side effects. Many of these side effects are annoying but you should try to keep taking the medicine unless your doctor tells you to stop it. Because this medicine takes a few weeks to work, the side effects show the doctor that the drug is starting to work. Most of these side effects will go away as your body adjusts to the medicine but some may not.

If this medicine causes dizziness or lightheadedness, you should be careful going up and down stairs and you should not change positions too rapidly. Lightheadedness is more likely to occur if you stand up suddenly—this is due to blood collecting in the legs and lasts for a few seconds. Therefore, get up from a sitting or lying position more slowly and tighten and relax your leg muscles or wiggle your toes to help promote circulation. In the morning, get out of bed slowly and dangle your feet over the edge of the bed for a few minutes before standing up. Sit or lie down at the first sign of dizziness. Tell your doctor if you have been dizzy.

You may become more sensitive to heat because your body may perspire less while you are taking this drug. Be careful not to become overheated during exercise or in hot weather. Try to avoid strenuous exercise, standing for long periods of time (especially in hot weather), hot showers, hot baths, saunas or Jacuzzis while taking this medicine.

Some patients may also become more sensitive to cold and should dress warmly during cold weather and limit exposure to cold temperatures.

This medicine commonly causes drowsiness. Do not drive a car, pilot an airplane, operate dangerous machinery or do jobs that require you to be alert if you are dizzy or drowsy.

If your mouth becomes dry, drink water, suck ice chips or a hard, sour candy (sugarless) or chew gum (sugarless). Sugarless products are recommended in order to avoid dental problems. You may wish to ask your pharmacist about special solutions, called artificial saliva, that can also be used to help restore moisture in the mouth.

It is especially important to brush and floss your teeth regularly if you develop a dry mouth to help prevent gum problems.

This medicine may cause some people to become constipated. To help prevent constipation, try increasing the amount of bulk in your diet (for example, bran, fresh fruits and salads), exercising more often or drinking more fluids (unless otherwise directed). Call your doctor if the constipation continues.

This medicine may make some people more sensitive to sunlight and sunlamps. When you begin taking this medicine, try to avoid too much sun until you see how you are going to react. If your skin does become more sensitive to sunlight, tell your doctor and try to stay out of direct sunlight for extended periods of time. While in the sun, wear protective clothing and sunglasses. You may wish to ask your pharmacist about suitable sunscreen products. Call your doctor if you become sunburned.

There have been some reports that this medicine may cause the urine to turn pink or red in color. This is only temporary and will go away after you have finished taking the medicine.

This medicine may cause nasal congestion (stuffy nose). Do not try to treat this yourself with cold or allergy medicines. Check with your doctor.

An urge to urinate (pass your water) with an inability to do so sometimes occurs with this drug. Urinating before taking the drug each time may help relieve this problem. Tell your doctor you are having this problem.

When to Call Your Doctor

Stop taking the medicine and call your doctor if you become restless or unable to sit still or sleep or if you develop unusually high energy or irritability.

Also call your doctor immediately if you develop a sore throat, fever, mouth sores, eye pain or blurred vision, difficulty in urinating (passing your water), difficulty in breathing, speaking or swallowing, increased sweating, a yellow color in the skin or eyes, dark, yellow-colored urine, irregular heartbeats, a skin rash, unusual bruising or bleeding, nausea or vomiting, unusual tiredness, confusion, nightmares, fainting spells, unusual muscle stiffness, drooling, seizures or shakiness or unusual movements of the face, tongue or hands.

If you develop painful muscle spasms, call your doctor or go to the hospital emergency room since treatment can be given to provide rapid relief of this problem.

Refills

Do not stop taking this medicine without your doctor's approval and do not go without medicine between prescription refills. Call your pharmacist for a refill 2 or 3 days before you will run out of the medicine.

Discuss with your pharmacist the implications of dispensing all your refills for this medicine with the same manufacturer's product. (*See* Generic Drugs, page 13.)

Miscellaneous

Carry an identification card in your wallet or wear a medical alert bracelet indicating that you are taking this medicine, as well as the names and phone numbers of your doctors. If you do not already carry such a card, complete the Medicine Card in this book. Always tell your dentist, pharmacist and other doctors who are treating you that you are taking this medicine.

Smoking Can Affect Medications

Cigarette smoke contains substances that can alter enzymes in the liver and cause some drugs to be less effective. People who smoke more than 20 cigarettes a day tend to experience these drug interactions more often than those who smoke fewer cigarettes per day. Little is known about drug interactions that may occur with pipe or cigar smoking.

Smoking has been shown to interfere with the effects of the following drugs:

- Pain Relievers such as PENTAZOCINE and PROPOXYPHENE
- Oral Contraceptives
- Tricyclic Antidepressants such as AMITRIPTYLINE, DESIPRAMINE, IMIPRAMINE and NORTRIPTYLINE
- Antianxiety Drugs such as CHLORDIAZEPOXIDE and DIAZEPAM
- HEPARIN (a "blood thinner")
- Phenothiazine Drugs such as CHLORPROMAZINE
- PROPRANOLOL, especially if used to treat angina
- THEOPHYLLINE

If you smoke cigarettes, be sure to tell your doctor and pharmacist so that they can watch for any signs that smoking is adversely affecting your response to the medications.

The Canadian Pharmaceutical Association was the first pharmacy association to join Health and Welfare Canada in the fight for a "Generation of Non-Smokers." Over the past two years, almost 3,500 pharmacists have participated in the program and have made information available to help people stop smoking.

Because of the success of this program and the dangers of smoking, the Canadian Pharmaceutical Association has started a new program called "Pharmacists Against Cigarette and Tobacco Sales." Many Canadian pharmacists are refusing to sell cigarette and tobacco products because they feel it is time to take an even harder line against the leading cause of preventable death in the developed world.

▶ **AMOBARBITAL (ORAL)**
AMYTAL

AMOBARBITAL-SECOBARBITAL
TUINAL

BUTABARBITAL
BUTISOL SODIUM

PHENOBARBITAL

SECOBARBITAL
SECONAL SODIUM

PENTOBARBITAL (ORAL and RECTAL)
NEMBUTAL, NOVA-RECTAL

Purpose
This medicine is used in the treatment of some sleep disorders and some nervous problems.

PHENOBARBITAL is also used in the long-term treatment of certain types of seizures.

Allergies/Warnings
If you have ever had an allergic reaction to any medicine or have liver or lung problems, tell your doctor and pharmacist before you take any of this medicine.

How to Use This Medicine

Time of Administration
If you are taking this medicine to help you sleep:
- Take the medicine about 20 minutes before you want to fall asleep. Go to bed after you have taken the medicine.
- If you do not fall asleep after taking the prescribed amount, do *not* take another dose unless advised by your physician.
- Do not smoke in bed after you have taken this medicine because you could fall asleep and cause a fire.

If you are taking this medicine to treat seizures or nervous problems:
- Take the medicine at the times prescribed by your doctor.

How to Administer
For tablets and capsules:
- This medicine may be taken either with food or on an empty stomach.

For liquid medicines:
- If a spoon is used to measure the dose, it is recommended that you use a medicine spoon or an oral liquid syringe, which you can obtain from your pharmacist. *See* Oral Liquid Syringe (page 17) and Medicine Spoon (page 22).

For suppositories:
- *See* Rectal Suppositories (page 39).

Special Instructions

Length of Therapy
Sleeping medicines are only useful for a short time. If too much is used, they could become habit-forming. Do not take any more of this medicine than your doctor has prescribed.

Do not stop taking this medicine suddenly without the approval of your doctor. It may be necessary for your doctor to slowly reduce your dose since your body may need time to adjust.

If you are taking PHENOBARBITAL to control seizures, suddenly stopping the medicine could cause seizures.

Check with your doctor if you develop any of the following while you are slowly stopping the medicine: nausea or vomiting, feeling faint, trembling, seizures, changes in vision or trouble sleeping. You may have a sleep problem on the first night or two after stopping the drug. This is not a reason for restarting the drug.

Pregnancy/Breastfeeding
Women who are pregnant, breastfeeding or planning to become pregnant should not take this medicine without their doctor's permission.

Drug Interactions
It is important that you obtain the advice of your doctor or pharmacist before taking any other prescription or nonprescription medicines, including pain relievers, anticoagulants (blood thinners), drugs used to treat epilepsy, sleeping pills, other tranquilizers or medicines for depression, cough, cold or allergies.

If you have problems sleeping, you should avoid caffeinated beverages, certain cold decongestants and strenuous exercise in the evenings, as they make it more difficult to fall asleep.

There are other drug interactions that can occur. If you are taking any other medicines, be sure to check first with your pharmacist or doctor.

There have been some reports that oral contraceptives (birth control pills) may not work as well while you are taking this medicine. Unplanned pregnancies may occur. Ask your doctor about using another form of birth control or adjusting the dose of your birth control pill while you are taking this medicine. Also call your doctor if you develop spotting or breakthrough bleeding since these can be signs of decreased birth control effect.

Alcohol

Do not drink alcoholic beverages while taking this drug, or for a few days after you have stopped taking the drug, without the approval of your doctor. The combination could cause drowsiness. One drink (even during the day) may have the same effect that 2 or 3 drinks normally would have.

If you are taking PHENOBARBITAL on a long-term basis to control epilepsy, check with your doctor to see what amount of alcohol (if any) you can drink safely. Be careful because the combination can cause severe drowsiness and increase the frequency of seizures.

Special Precautions

If this medicine causes dizziness or drowsiness the day after you take it, do not drive a car, pilot an airplane, use a sewing machine, operate dangerous machinery or do jobs that require you to be alert if you are dizzy or drowsy. You should also be careful going up and down stairs. Sit or lie down at the first sign of dizziness.

If this hangover drowsiness becomes bothersome, call your doctor.

When to Call Your Doctor

Call your doctor if you do not feel that the drug is working. Do not increase your dose without your doctor's approval.

Most people experience few or no side effects from this drug. However, any medicine can sometimes cause unwanted effects. Call your doctor if you develop a sore throat, fever, mouth sores, a staggering walk, a yellow color to the skin or eyes, unusual bruising or bleeding, muscle or joint pain, slow heartbeats or shortness of breath, bothersome sleepiness or tiredness during the day, unusual nervousness, confusion or depression, hallucinations, trouble sleeping, nightmares or slurred speech.

Allergic Reactions

Call your doctor immediately if you think you may be allergic to the medicine or if you develop a skin rash, hives, itching, swelling of the face or difficulty in breathing. If you cannot reach your doctor, phone a hospital emergency department.

Storage

Do not store this medicine by the bedside. Keep it out of the reach of children.

For suppositories:
• *See* Rectal Suppositories (page 39).

Do You Know the Warning Signs of Drug Dependence?

Drug dependence most commonly occurs with pain relievers, sleeping pills, tranquilizers and diet pills.

Call your doctor immediately if you suspect you are becoming dependent on a medication. The warning signs are:

• You need a larger dose to produce the desired effect.
• You start taking the medication automatically without considering whether it is needed.

▶ **AMOXICILLIN TRIHYDRATE (ORAL)**
AMOXIL, APO-AMOXI, NOVAMOXIN

AMOXICILLIN-POTASSIUM CLAVULANATE
CLAVULIN

Purpose

This medicine is an antibiotic used to treat certain types of infections.

Your doctor has prescribed this antibiotic for your present infection only. Do not use it for other infections or give it to other people.

Caffeine and Insomnia

Does the caffeine in coffee, tea and cola beverages cause you to stay awake at night?

If so, you should be aware that caffeine is contained in more than 100 nonprescription drugs and more than 65 commonly prescribed drugs. A cup of drip coffee contains approximately 146 mg caffeine. Some nonprescription drugs contain up to 200 mg per tablet or capsule. Always read the labels of nonprescription products before you purchase them.

If you are sensitive to caffeine, tell your doctor and pharmacist so that they can make sure you are not prescribed a medicine that contains caffeine.

Anyone who suffers from insomnia due to caffeine should not take any beverage or medicine containing caffeine within 6 hours of bedtime.

Allergies/Warnings

If you have ever had an allergic reaction to penicillin, a cephalosporin or any other medicine, or if you have any allergies (for example, asthma or hay fever), tell your doctor and pharmacist before you take any of this medicine.

How to Use This Medicine

Time of Administration

This medicine may be taken with meals or on an empty stomach.

It has been suggested that when CLAVULIN is taken with food, nausea occurs less often.

Space your doses of the medicine around the clock (throughout the entire day of 24 hours). For example, if you are to take 3 doses each day, space the doses 8 hours apart. This will keep a constant level of the medicine in your body.

How to Administer

For tablets or capsules:

• If you were prescribed AMOXIL Chewable Tablets, chew or crush the tablets well before swallowing. Do not swallow them whole. *After* you have chewed and swallowed the small pieces of the tablet, you may wish to drink some water.

- Take the other brands of tablets or capsules with a full glass of water (8 oz or 240 mL) unless otherwise directed. Swallow them whole.

For liquid medicines:
- If you were prescribed a *suspension*, shake the bottle well each time before pouring so that you can measure an accurate dose.
- If a dropper is used to measure the dose and you do not fully understand how to use it, *see* Medicine Dropper (page 21).
- If a spoon is used to measure the dose, it is recommended that you use a medicine spoon or an oral liquid syringe, which you can obtain from your pharmacist. *See* Oral Liquid Syringe (page 17) and Medicine Spoon (page 22).

Special Instructions

Length of Therapy

It is important to take all of this medicine plus any refills that your doctor told you to take. Do not stop taking this medicine earlier than your doctor has recommended even if you begin to feel better. If you stop taking the medicine too soon, the infection may return.

This is especially important if you are taking the medicine to cure a strep infection because if the infection is not completely cleared up, serious heart problems could develop later. After treatment for a strep infection, your doctor may want to do a test to make sure that the infection is gone.

Pregnancy/Breastfeeding

Women who are pregnant or planning to become pregnant should tell their doctor before taking this medicine.

Women who are breastfeeding should tell their doctor before taking this medicine. This medicine can pass into the breast milk and may cause unwanted side effects in the baby.

Drug Interactions

There have been some reports that oral contraceptives (birth control pills) may not work as well while you are taking this medicine. Unplanned pregnancies may occur. Ask your doctor about using another form of birth control while you are taking this medicine. Also call your doctor if you develop spotting or breakthrough bleeding since these can be signs of decreased birth control effect.

Special Precautions
If you develop diarrhea, do not treat it yourself without first checking with your doctor or pharmacist.

When to Call Your Doctor
Call your doctor if your symptoms do not improve within a few days or if they become worse.

Most people experience few or no side effects from this drug. However, any medicine can sometimes cause unwanted effects. Call your doctor if you develop fever, chills, severe watery diarrhea, yellow-green stools, nausea or vomiting, abdominal or stomach cramps, bloating, unusual thirst, unusual weakness or unusual weight loss. These effects are rare and may occur even after the medicine has been stopped. Also call your doctor if you develop rectal itching or, in women, vaginal itching or a vaginal discharge that was not present before you started taking the medicine.

Allergic Reactions
Call your doctor immediately if you think you may be allergic to the medicine or if you develop a skin rash, hives, itching, swelling of the face or difficulty in breathing. If you cannot reach your doctor, phone a hospital emergency department.

Storage
For liquid medicines:
• Store the bottle of medicine in a refrigerator unless otherwise directed. Do not freeze.

If for some reason you cannot take all of the medicine, take the unused portion back to your pharmacist. You should discuss why you cannot finish the medicine with your pharmacist. Do not take any unused medicine after the discard (expiration) date on the bottle.

Refills
Do not go without medicine between prescription refills. Call your pharmacist for a refill 2 or 3 days before you will run out of the medicine.

Is the Family Pet the Source of Your "Strep" Infections?

Bacterial infections can be transmitted to people by their pets.

If a family has repeated episodes of *streptococcal pharyngitis* and if they have a pet, they should have a veterinarian test the pet for *streptococcal* infection. According to the *American Family Physician*, it is possible that the animal has a "strep" infection and is reinfecting the family members.

Animals often develop infections in skin lesions after prolonged scratching. A child with atopic eczema can also develop a *staphylococcal* or *streptococcal* infection from a pet with an infected eczemoid condition.

If the pet does have a *streptococcal* infection, it should be treated with an antibiotic such as penicillin.

▶ **AMPICILLIN (ORAL)**
Apo-Ampi, Novo-Ampicillin, Nu-Ampi, Penbritin

BACAMPICILLIN
Penglobe

CLOXACILLIN
Apo-Cloxi, Novocloxin, Nu-Cloxi, Orbenin

DICLOXACILLIN
Dynapen

FLUCLOXACILLIN
Fluclox

PIVAMPICILLIN
Pondocillin

Purpose

This medicine is an antibiotic used to treat certain types of infections.

Your doctor has prescribed this antibiotic for your present infection only. Do not use it for other infections or give it to other people.

Allergies/Warnings

If you have ever had an allergic reaction to penicillin or a cephalosporin, or any other medicine, or if you have any allergies (for example, asthma or hay fever), tell your doctor and pharmacist before you take any of this medicine.

How to Use This Medicine

Time of Administration

For APO-AMPI, APO-CLOXI, DYNAPEN, FLUCLOX, NOVO-AMPICILLIN, NOVOCLOXIN, NU-AMPI, NU-CLOXI, ORBENIN, PENBRITIN:

- It is best to take this medicine on an empty stomach 1 hour before (or 2 hours after) meals or food unless otherwise directed by your doctor. Take it at the proper time even if you skip a meal.
- Space your doses of the medicine around the clock (throughout the entire day of 24 hours). For example, if you are to take 4 doses each day, space the doses 6 hours apart. This will keep a constant level of the medicine in your body.

For PENGLOBE and PONDOCILLIN only:

- This medicine may be taken without regard to meals. Take it with food or on an empty stomach.

How to Administer

For tablets or capsules:

- Take the tablets or capsules with a full glass of water (8 oz or 240 mL) unless otherwise directed.

For liquid medicines:

- If you were prescribed a *Suspension*, shake the bottle well each time before pouring so that you can measure an accurate dose.
- If a spoon is used to measure the dose, it is recommended that you use a medicine spoon or an oral liquid syringe, which you can obtain from your pharmacist. See Oral Liquid Syringe (page 17) and Medicine Spoon (page 22).

Special Instructions

Length of Therapy

It is important to take all of this medicine plus any refills that your doctor told you to take. Do not stop taking this medicine earlier than your doctor has recommended even if you begin to feel better.

If you stop taking the medicine too soon, the infection may return. This is especially important if you are taking the medicine to cure a strep infection because if the infection is not completely cleared up, serious heart problems could develop later. After treatment for a strep infection, your doctor may want to do a test to make sure that the infection is gone.

Pregnancy/Breastfeeding

Women who are pregnant or planning to become pregnant should tell their doctor before taking this medicine.

Women who are breastfeeding should tell their doctor before taking this medicine. This medicine can pass into the breast milk and may cause unwanted side effects in the baby.

Drug Interactions

There have been some reports that oral contraceptives (birth control pills) may not work as well while you are taking this medicine. Unplanned pregnancies may occur. Ask your doctor about using another form of birth control while you are taking these antibiotics. Also call your doctor if you develop spotting or breakthrough bleeding since these can be signs of decreased birth control effect.

When to Call Your Doctor

Call your doctor if your symptoms do not improve within a few days or if they become worse.

This medicine sometimes causes diarrhea. Call your doctor if the diarrhea becomes severe or lasts for more than two days. Do not try to treat the diarrhea yourself without first checking with your doctor or pharmacist.

Most people experience few or no side effects from this drug. However, any medicine can sometimes cause unwanted effects. Call your doctor if you develop fever, chills, nausea or vomiting, yellow-green stools, abdominal or stomach cramps, bloating, unusual thirst, unusual weakness or unusual weight loss. These effects are rare and may occur even after the medicine has been stopped. Also call your doctor if you develop rectal itching or, in women, vaginal itching or a vaginal discharge that was not present before you started taking the medicine.

Allergic Reactions

Call your doctor immediately if you think you may be allergic to the medicine or if you develop a skin rash, hives, itching, swelling of the face or difficulty in breathing. If you cannot reach your doctor, phone a hospital emergency department.

Storage

For APO-AMPI, FLUCLOX, NOVO-AMPICILLIN, NU-AMPI, *and* PENBRITIN *liquid medicines:*

- Store the bottle of medicine in a refrigerator unless otherwise directed. Do not freeze.

If for some reason you cannot take all of the medicine, take the unused portion back to your pharmacist. You should discuss why you cannot finish the medicine with your pharmacist. Do not take any unused medicine after the discard (expiration) date on the bottle.

Refills

Do not go without medicine between prescription refills. Call your pharmacist for a refill 2 or 3 days before you will run out of the medicine.

Does the Medicine Taste Bad?

Some helpful hints to make bad-tasting medicines taste better:

- If the medicine is a liquid, it may help to chill the medicine in the refrigerator for a few minutes before it is taken.

- If the medicine is a tablet, place the tablet closer to the front of the tongue. The taste buds on the tongue that detect bitter tastes are located near the back of the tongue. By placing the tablet near the front of the tongue, you are placing it on the sweet taste buds and there is less perception of the bitter taste.

- Suck some ice chips before taking a bitter medication. This will help numb the taste buds.

- It may help to hold your nose as you swallow the medicine. The sense of smell is involved in the sensation of taste, and if you decrease your ability to smell the medicine, it may not taste as bad.

- Ask your pharmacist if it is safe to dilute your liquid medicine with juice or some other liquid. Some medicines interact with some liquids and it is important not to dilute your medicine with one that interacts with your drug.

- Drink some water after taking the medicine to help get rid of the aftertaste—unless you are taking a cough syrup which acts by coating the throat to soothe it.

- It may also help to gargle or rinse your mouth or suck a hard candy after taking the medicine.

► **ASA-BUTALBITAL-CAFFEINE (ORAL)**
FIORINAL, TECNAL

ASA-BUTALBITAL-CAFFEINE-CODEINE
FIORINAL-C 1/4, FIORINAL-C 1/2, TECNAL C 1/4, TECNAL C 1/2

ASA-PHENAPHEN-CODEINE
PHENAPHEN NO. 2, PHENAPHEN NO. 3, PHENAPHEN NO. 4

Purpose
This medicine is used to help relieve pain associated with muscle tension (e.g., tension headache).

Allergies/Warnings
If you have a stomach ulcer, hay fever, asthma or nasal polyps or have ever had an allergic reaction to ASA (acetylsalicylic acid), codeine, caffeine, a barbiturate or any other medicine, tell your doctor and pharmacist before you take any of this medicine.

Check with your doctor before giving *any* medicine containing ASA or salicylates to children, teenagers and young adults with chickenpox, flu or other viral infections. Studies have shown a possible link between ASA/salicylate products and Reye's Syndrome, a rare but serious disease. The first symptoms of Reye's Syndrome are usually vomiting, tiredness and loss of concentration, which may lead to delirium and coma.

How to Use This Medicine

Time of Administration
Do not wait until the pain becomes severe. This medicine works best if you take it at the beginning of the pain.

How to Administer
This medicine should be taken with food or a full glass of water to help prevent stomach upset.

Do not take this medicine if it smells strongly like vinegar, since this may mean the ASA is not fresh and may be losing strength.

Special Instructions

Length of Therapy
If your doctor has prescribed this medicine to be taken on a regular schedule, take it as recommended and not on an "as needed" basis.

Do not take any more of this medicine than your doctor has prescribed. When used for a long period of time, the drug can become less effective. These products contain codeine and/or a barbiturate and, when used in large doses for a long period of time, these drugs can become habit-forming. Call your doctor if you feel you need the medicine more often than was prescribed. Do not take a larger dose without your doctor's approval.

If you have been taking this medicine in large doses or for several weeks, do not stop taking this medicine suddenly without the approval of your doctor. It may be necessary for your doctor to reduce your dose slowly. This will depend on the dose and the specific medicine you have been taking.

Pregnancy/Breastfeeding

Women who are pregnant, breastfeeding or planning to become pregnant should tell their doctor before taking this medicine.

Drug Interactions

It is important that you obtain the advice of your doctor or pharmacist before taking any other prescription or nonprescription medicines, including other pain relievers, sleeping pills, tranquilizers or medicines for depression, cough or cold, allergy medicines or blood thinners.

There are other drug interactions which can occur. If you are taking any other medicines, be sure to check first with your pharmacist or doctor.

Alcohol

Do not drink alcoholic beverages while taking this drug because the combination could cause dizziness or drowsiness. One drink may have the same effect that 2 or 3 drinks normally would have. The combination could also cause stomach problems.

Special Precautions

If you feel nauseated when you first start taking the medicine, it may help if you lie down for a few minutes.

In some people, this drug may cause dizziness or drowsiness. Do not drive a car, pilot an airplane, operate dangerous machinery or do jobs that require you to be alert if you are dizzy or drowsy. You should also be careful going up and down stairs. Get up slowly after you have been sitting or lying down. Sit or lie down at the first sign of dizziness. Tell your doctor if the dizziness or drowsiness continues.

This medicine may cause some people to become constipated. To help prevent constipation, try increasing the amount of bulk in your diet (for example, bran, fresh fruits and salads), exercising more often or drinking more fluids (unless otherwise directed). Call your doctor if the constipation continues.

ASA can thin the blood and prolong bleeding time; therefore, you may have to stop taking it before surgery or dental work. Check with your doctor or dentist at least one week before you have any surgery or dental work.

When to Call Your Doctor

Call your doctor if the medicine does not relieve your symptoms or if they get worse.

Most people experience few or no side effects from this drug. However, any medicine can sometimes cause unwanted effects. Call your doctor if you develop stomach pain, vomiting, vomiting of blood or material that looks like coffee grounds, bloody or black stools, blood in the urine, ringing or buzzing in the ears or difficulty hearing, a feeling of fullness in the ears, severe drowsiness or dizziness, bothersome sleepiness or laziness during the day, nightmares, staggering walk, a slow heartbeat, unusual nervousness, confusion, unusual bruising or bleeding, a yellow color to the skin or eyes or severe diarrhea.

Allergic Reactions

Call your doctor immediately if you think you may be allergic to the medicine or if you develop a skin rash, hives, itching, unexplained fever, swelling of the face or difficulty in breathing. If you cannot reach your doctor, phone a hospital emergency department.

Storage

Store the medicine in a cool, dark place.

Miscellaneous

Carry an identification card in your wallet or wear a medical alert bracelet indicating that you are taking this medicine, as well as the names and phone numbers of your doctors. If you do not already carry such a card, complete the Medicine Card in this book. Always tell your dentist, pharmacist and other doctors who are treating you that you are taking this medicine.

► ASA-CAFFEINE-CODEINE (ORAL)
AC&C, Anacin with Codeine, Ancasal 8, Ancasal 15, Ancasal 30, 222, 282, 292, 293, C2 with Codeine, C2 Buffered with Codeine

ASA-CODEINE
Coryphen-Codeine

ASA-OXYCODONE
Endodan, Oxycodan, Percodan, Percodan-Demi

Purpose
This medicine is used to help relieve pain and fever.

Allergies/Warnings
If you have a stomach ulcer, asthma, hay fever or nasal polyps or have ever had an allergic reaction to ASA (acetylsalicylic acid), codeine, caffeine or any other medicine, tell your doctor and pharmacist before you take any of this medicine.

Check with your doctor before giving *any* medicine containing ASA or salicylates to children, teenagers and young adults with chickenpox, flu or other viral infections. Studies have shown a possible link between ASA/salicylate products and Reye's Syndrome, a rare but serious disease. The first symptoms of Reye's Syndrome are usually vomiting and tiredness and loss of concentration, which may lead to delirium and coma.

How to Use This Medicine

Time of Administration
Do not wait until the pain becomes severe. This medicine works best if you take it at the beginning of the pain.

How to Administer
This medicine should be taken with food or a full glass of water to help prevent stomach upset.

Do not take this medicine if it smells strongly like vinegar since this may mean the ASA in it is not fresh and may be losing strength.

If you were prescribed 293 Tablets:
- These tablets are long-acting and must be swallowed whole. Do not crush, chew or break them into pieces.

Do Not Place ASA Tablets Directly on a Sore Tooth or Gum

ASA tablets should not be sucked or placed directly on a canker sore, sore gum or sensitive tooth and allowed to dissolve.

ASA is an acidic drug, and if it is left in one spot and allowed to dissolve, there is a good chance that it will irritate the sore area even more. With continued use, the ASA could even cause a severe chemical burn and destroy that area of the skin. When this happens, the skin will turn white and slough off leaving a painful ulceration known as *aspirin burn*.

Special Instructions

Length of Therapy

Do not take any more of this medicine than your doctor has prescribed. When used for a long period of time, the drug can become less effective. These products contain codeine and/or a barbiturate and when used in large doses for a long period of time, the drug can become habit-forming. Call your doctor if you feel you need the medicine more often than was prescribed. Do not take a larger dose without your doctor's approval.

If you have been taking this medicine in large doses or for several weeks, do not stop taking this medicine suddenly without the approval of your doctor. It may be necessary for your doctor to reduce your dose slowly. This will depend on the dose and the specific medicine you have been taking.

Pregnancy/Breastfeeding

Women who are pregnant, breastfeeding or planning to become pregnant should tell their doctor before taking this medicine.

Drug Interactions

It is important that you obtain the advice of your doctor or pharmacist before taking any other prescription and nonprescription medicines, including other pain relievers, sleeping pills, tranquilizers or medicines for depression, cough, cold or allergies.

There are other drug interactions which can occur. If you are taking any other medicines, be sure to check first with your pharmacist or doctor.

Alcohol

Do not drink alcoholic beverages while taking this drug without the approval of your doctor because the combination could cause dizziness or drowsiness. One drink may have the same effect that 2 or 3 drinks normally would have. The combination could also cause stomach problems.

Special Precautions

If you feel nauseated when you first start taking the medicine, it may help if you lie down for a few minutes.

In some people, this drug may cause dizziness or drowsiness. Do not drive a car, pilot an airplane, operate dangerous machinery or do jobs that require you to be alert if you are dizzy or drowsy. You should also be careful going up and down stairs. Get up slowly after you have been sitting or lying down. Sit or lie down at the first sign of dizziness. Tell your doctor if the dizziness and drowsiness continue.

This medicine may cause some people to become constipated. To help prevent constipation, try increasing the amount of bulk in your diet (for example, bran, fresh fruits and salads), exercising more often or drinking more fluids (unless otherwise directed). Call your doctor if the constipation continues.

ASA can thin the blood and prolong bleeding time; therefore, you may have to stop taking it before surgery or dental work. Check with your doctor or dentist at least one week before you have any surgery or dental work.

When to Call Your Doctor

Call your doctor if the medicine does not relieve your symptoms or if they get worse.

Most people experience few or no side effects from this drug. However, any medicine can sometimes cause unwanted effects. Call your doctor if you develop stomach pain, vomiting, vomiting of blood or material that looks like coffee grounds, bloody or black stools, blood in the urine, ringing or buzzing in the ears or difficulty hearing, a feeling of fullness in the ears, severe drowsiness or dizziness, bothersome sleepiness or laziness during the day, sweating, unusual nervousness, severe constipation, diarrhea, confusion or depression.

Allergic Reactions

Call your doctor immediately if you think you may be allergic to the medicine or if you develop a skin rash, hives, itching, unexplained fever, swelling of the face or difficulty in breathing. If you cannot reach your doctor, phone a hospital emergency department.

Storage
Store the medicine in a cool, dark place.

Miscellaneous
Carry an identification card in your wallet or wear a medical alert bracelet indicating that you are taking this medicine, as well as the names and phone numbers of your doctors. If you do not already carry such a card, complete the Medicine Card in this book. Always tell your dentist, pharmacist and other doctors who are treating you that you are taking this medicine.

A Bad Combination: Aspirin and Alcohol

ASA and alcohol should not be taken together.

Both ASA and alcohol are capable of irritating the lining of the stomach, and when they are taken together, there is a chance that the double irritation could cause bleeding. ASA can also thin the blood and prolong bleeding time. This unwanted effect will not happen in everyone, but it is especially important in people who have or have had peptic ulcers.

Whenever possible, avoid ASA use within 8 to 10 hours of heavy alcohol use. Taking ASA the morning after alcoholic overindulgence would seem less likely to cause difficulty than taking ASA before retiring, since the gastric irritation caused by the alcohol would have been at least partially relieved by the next morning.

▶ **ASTEMIZOLE (ORAL)**
HISMANAL

LORATIDINE
CLARITIN

TERFENADINE
SELDANE

Purpose

This medicine is used to help relieve the symptoms of certain types of allergic conditions (such as hay fever) as well as to treat certain types of allergic skin conditions.

Allergies/Warnings

If you have ever had an allergic reaction to any medicine, tell your doctor and pharmacist before you take any of this medicine.

How to Use This Medicine

Time of Administration

For HISMANAL:

- This medicine should be taken on an empty stomach.

For CLARITIN and SELDANE:

- This medicine may be taken without regard to meals. Take it either with food or on an empty stomach.

How to Administer

For tablets or caplets:

- Take the medicine with a full glass of water unless otherwise directed.

For liquid medicines:

- Shake the bottle well each time before pouring so that you can measure an accurate dose of medicine.
- It is recommended that a medicine spoon be used to measure the dose. An average household spoon is not accurate. *See* Medicine Spoon (page 22).

Special Instructions

Length of Therapy

For HISMANAL:

- After you start taking this medicine, it may take up to 3 days before you notice relief from your symptoms. It is important to take this medicine daily even though you may not feel any immediate benefit. Hismanal will also continue to work for a few days after you have stopped taking it.

The Canadian Pharmaceutical Association
"Drugs and Driving Program"

Any medicine that causes blurred vision, drowsiness, dizziness, hearing problems, decreased reflexes, inability to concentrate, or muscle incoordination has the potential to impair your ability to drive a car safely.

In the past few years, increased attention has been focused on the dangers of drinking and driving. Governments have set strict limits on blood alcohol concentrations at which a driver's performance could be considered to be "impaired." Until recently, little attention has been given to the effect of medications on driving. There are some medications that are capable of decreasing a person's mental alertness and physical coordination and thereby lessening that person's ability to drive a car safely.

The Canadian Pharmaceutical Association, with the support of interested consumer groups, has undertaken "A Drugs and Driving Program: Take Care." This is a project designed to help make consumers more aware of medicines that can adversely affect driving skills. A booklet, "Drugs and Driving," may be obtained by writing: The Canadian Pharmaceutical Association, 1785 Alta Vista Drive, Ottawa, Ontario K1G 3Y6.

Other sources of information are also available. The Drug Caution Code, a program developed by pharmacists in Manitoba and available in Saskatchewan, Newfoundland and Alberta, informs consumers about the hazards of over-the-counter medicines and driving. The individual prescription drug monographs in *Understanding Canadian Prescription Drugs* contain information on prescription drugs that may impair a person's ability to drive a car or do tasks that require mental alertness.

The best advice is to ask your doctor or pharmacist about possible side effects that could affect your driving performance whenever you are prescribed a medication. Not everyone will respond the same way to a medication. Some people will experience these side effects and others will not. Until you know how you are going to respond to the medication, your doctor or pharmacist may advise you to refrain from, or minimize, driving for a few days after starting the medication. In this way, you can assess whether it will be safe for you to drive, or do any task requiring mental alertness, while undergoing the treatment.

Pregnancy/Breastfeeding

Women who are pregnant, breastfeeding or planning to become pregnant should tell their doctor before taking this medicine.

When to Call Your Doctor

Call your doctor if your symptoms do not improve after a few days or if they become worse.

▶ **ATROPINE-SCOPOLAMINE-HYOSCYAMINE-PHENOBARBITAL (ORAL)**
DONNATAL

Purpose

This medicine is used to help relieve cramps and spasms of the bowels and as an aid to treating some cases of duodenal ulcers by lowering the stomach acid secretions.

Allergies/Warnings

If you have ever had an allergic reaction to atropine, bromides, barbiturates or any other drug, or if you have glaucoma, enlarged prostate, difficulty urinating (passing your water) or any other medical condition, tell your doctor and pharmacist before you take any of this medicine.

How to Use This Medicine

Time of Administration

Take this medicine approximately 30 minutes to 1 hour before a meal unless otherwise directed.

The DONNATAL EXTENTABS are usually taken in the morning and at night since they are long-acting.

How to Administer

If you were prescribed DONNATAL EXTENTABS:

- These tablets are long-acting and must be swallowed whole. Do not crush, chew or break them into pieces.

For liquid medicines:

- If a spoon is used to measure the dose, it is recommended that you use a medicine spoon or an oral liquid syringe, which you can obtain from your pharmacist. These are more accurate than the average household teaspoon. *See* Oral Liquid Syringe (page 17) and Medicine Spoon (page 22).

Special Instructions

Length of Therapy

Do not take this medicine more often or longer than recommended by your doctor. To do so may increase your chance of developing side effects.

Do not stop taking this medicine suddenly without the approval of your doctor.

Pregnancy/Breastfeeding

Women who are pregnant, breastfeeding or planning to become pregnant should tell their doctor before taking this medicine.

Drug Interactions

It is important that you obtain the advice of your doctor or pharmacist before taking any other prescription or nonprescription medicines, including pain relievers, sleeping pills, tranquilizers or medicines for depression, cough, cold or allergies.

Do not take antacids or medicines for diarrhea within 1 hour of taking this medicine because they could make this medicine less effective.

There are other drug interactions that can occur. If you are taking any other medicines, be sure to check first with your pharmacist or doctor.

Alcohol

Do not drink alcoholic beverages while taking this drug without the approval of your doctor because the combination could cause severe drowsiness. One drink may have the same effect that 2 or 3 drinks normally would have.

Special Precautions

If your mouth becomes dry, drink water, suck ice chips or a hard, sour candy (sugarless) or chew gum (sugarless). Sugarless products are recommended in order to avoid dental problems. You may wish to ask your pharmacist about special solutions, called artificial saliva, that can also be used to help restore moisture in the mouth.

It is especially important to brush and floss your teeth regularly if you develop a dry mouth, to help prevent gum problems.

In some people, this drug may cause dizziness, drowsiness or blurred vision. Do not drive a car, pilot an airplane, operate dangerous machinery or do jobs that require you to be alert until you know how you are going to react to this drug. You should also be careful going up and down stairs. Sit or lie down at the first sign of dizziness. Tell your doctor if these problems continue.

If your eyes become more sensitive to sunlight, it may help to wear sunglasses.

An urge to urinate (pass your water) with an inability to do so sometimes occurs with this drug. Urinating before taking the drug each time may help relieve this problem. Tell your doctor if you are having this problem.

This medicine will often cause you to sweat less and you may become more sensitive to heat. Be careful not to become overheated during exercise or to stand for long periods of time, especially if the weather is hot. Avoid hot showers, hot baths, Jacuzzis or saunas while taking this medicine.

This medicine may cause some people to become constipated. This side effect occurs more often in people over 65 years of age. To help prevent constipation, try increasing the amount of bulk in your diet (for example, bran, fresh fruits and salads), exercising more often or drinking more fluids (unless otherwise directed). Call your doctor if the constipation continues.

When to Call Your Doctor

Most people experience few or no side effects from this drug. However, any medicine can sometimes cause unwanted effects. Call your doctor if you develop a skin rash, difficulty in breathing, diarrhea, unusual restlessness, flushing, eye pain or changes in vision, a sore throat, fever, headache, nausea or vomiting, bothersome constipation, a yellow color to the skin or eyes, easy bruising or bleeding, unusual tiredness, a change in the heart rate, difficulty in urinating (passing your water), confusion or slurred speech.

Allergic Reactions

Call your doctor immediately if you think you may be allergic to the medicine or if you develop a skin rash, hives, itching, swelling of the face or difficulty in breathing. If you cannot reach your doctor, phone a hospital emergency department.

The Herbal Tea You Drink May Be Toxic

All herbal teas are not necessarily "healthy" teas. Some herbal teas contain toxins that may cause serious medical problems ranging from dermatitis to sudden liver failure and death.

The following herbal teas are commercially available yet have varying levels of toxicity.

- Teas made from tonka beans, woodruff, or melilot interfere with blood clotting. Patients taking anticoagulant drugs ("blood thinners") should not drink these teas.
- Tea made from hops has caused internal bleeding.
- Teas brewed from buckthorn and senna contain anthraquinones that can cause severe diarrhea. One person developed gastroenteritis, bloody diarrhea and severe hypertension after drinking one cup of poke root tea.
- Comfrey, groundsel and gordolobo teas are responsible for the epidemic tea poisonings in Jamaica, South Africa and India.
- Comfrey and sassafras are unsafe and can cause cancer of the liver.

Do not self-treat with herbal teas without first checking with your doctor or pharmacist. Some herbal teas are not safe and some could be contraindicated because of your medical problems or drugs you are taking.

Miscellaneous

Carry an identification card in your wallet or wear a medical alert bracelet indicating that you are taking this medicine as well as the names and phone numbers of your doctors. If you do not already carry such a card, complete the Medicine Card in this book. Always tell your dentist, pharmacist and other doctors who are treating you that you are taking this medicine.

▶ **BACITRACIN (OPHTHALMIC)**
BACIGUENT

POLYMYXIN
AEROSPORIN OPHTHALMIC

POLYMYXIN B-BACITRACIN
POLYSPORIN EYE OINTMENT

POLYMYXIN B-GRAMICIDIN
POLYSPORIN EYE/EAR DROPS

POLYMYXIN B-NEOMYCIN COMBINATIONS
NEOSPORIN EYE AND EAR SOLUTION, NEOSPORIN EYE OINTMENT

POLYMYXIN B-NEOMYCIN-STEROID COMBINATIONS
CORTISPORIN EYE/EAR DROPS, CORTISPORIN EYE OINTMENT,
MAXITROL EYE DROPS, MAXITROL EYE OINTMENT

Purpose
This medicine is an antibiotic used to treat certain types of eye infections and used after eye surgery. It is to be used *only* for the eye infection you have now and should not be used for *any* eye infections that may develop later.

CORTISPORIN and MAXITROL eye medicines contain a steroid that helps relieve redness and irritation of certain eye conditions.

Allergies/Warnings
Be sure to tell your doctor and pharmacist if you are allergic to neomycin or any medicine.

How to Use This Medicine

How to Administer
For eye drops:
- *See* Eye Drops (page 24).

For eye ointment:
- *See* Eye Ointments (page 26).

For ear drops:
- *See* Ear Drops (page 27).

Special Instructions

Length of Therapy
It is important to use all of this medicine, plus any refills that your doctor told you to use. Do not stop using it earlier than your doctor has recommended in spite of the fact that your symptoms seem to have improved. Otherwise, the infection may return.

Pregnancy/Breastfeeding

Women who are pregnant, breastfeeding or planning to become pregnant should tell their doctor before taking this medicine.

Drug Interactions

Do not use this medicine at the same time as any other eye medicine without the approval of your doctor. Some medicines cannot be mixed.

Special Precautions

If you are being treated for only 1 infected eye, do not touch the healthy eye, to avoid spreading the infection.

Vision may be blurred for a few minutes after you use the eye medicine, especially after the eye ointments. Do not drive a car or operate dangerous machinery or do jobs that require you to be alert until your vision has cleared.

If you are prescribed CORTISPORIN or MAXITROL eye medicines for a long time, your doctor will want to do eye tests at regular intervals.

When to Call Your Doctor

Contact your doctor if the eye infection for which you are using this medicine does not begin to improve in 3 to 4 days, if increased eye redness or eye pain develops, if you develop any changes in vision or if the eye becomes irritated by the eye medicine for more than a few minutes. Many eye medicines sting for a short time immediately after use.

Miscellaneous

This medicine is for external use only. Do not swallow it.

Do not share this eye medication with family members or friends. The infection could be transferred.

▶ BECLOMETHASONE (INHALATION)

BECLODISK DISKHALER, BECLOFORTE INHALER, BECLOVENT INHALER, BECLOVENT ROTACAPS, VANCERIL ORAL INHALER

FLUNISOLIDE

BRONALIDE AEROSOL

Purpose

This medicine is a steroid (cortisone) and is used to help prevent asthmatic attacks. It is not effective in treating an asthma attack that has already begun and should not be used during an attack.

Allergies/Warnings

If you have ever had an allergic reaction to any steroid (cortisone) medicines or inhalation spray medicines, tell your doctor and pharmacist before you use any of this medicine.

How to Use This Medicine

How to Administer

BECLOVENT ROTOCAPS must *not* be swallowed. The capsules are to be used with the BECLOVENT ROTAHALER. Follow the instructions that come with the ROTAHALER.

The BECLODISKS must be used with the BECLODISK DISKHALER. Follow the instructions that come with the DISKHALER. Do not pierce a blister until you are ready to use it.

For aerosol inhaler:

- Follow the specific instructions for your brand of inhaler on the sheet that comes with the medicine. Also *see* Metered-Dose Inhalers (page 31) for general instructions.
- If your doctor has prescribed a second dose, wait about 1 minute before shaking the container again and repeating this procedure.
- Rinse your mouth and gargle with lukewarm water after you have used the inhaler. This will help prevent your throat from becoming dry or sore, your voice from becoming hoarse, and will help prevent an infection.
- The VANCERIL INHALER has a "dosage reminder" at the top of the canister to help you remember to take each dose. Each time you take a dose, set the number of your dose opposite the arrow on the plastic shell.

Special Instructions

Length of Therapy

Patients vary in the dose they require, and your doctor will determine the dosage that is best for you. Take the medicine regularly. It may take 1 to 4 weeks before you feel the full benefit of this medicine. If you develop difficulty in breathing, contact your doctor immediately.

Do not take any more of this medicine than your doctor has prescribed and do not stop taking this medicine suddenly without the approval of your doctor. If you should suddenly stop taking it or reduce the dose, you may experience a worsening of your asthma.

Since this drug is used to help prevent asthma attacks, you may need to take it for a prolonged period of time. Discuss the length of therapy with your doctor.

Pregnancy/Breastfeeding

Women who are pregnant, breastfeeding or planning to become pregnant should tell their doctor before taking this medicine.

Drug Interactions

Some nonprescription drugs can aggravate your condition. Do not take any of the following without the approval of your doctor or pharmacist: cough, cold or sinus products; asthma or allergy products; or ASA-containing products. Read the label of the product to see if there is a warning. If there is, check first with your doctor or pharmacist before using the product.

Do not take other inhaled medicines that have not been prescribed by your doctor while you are using this medicine.

Special Precautions

Do not change the dose of your regular asthma or bronchitis medicines except on the advice of your doctor.

If you are also using another inhaler medicine (bronchodilator) that opens up the air passages in the lungs, use it several minutes before using this medicine as directed by your doctor. The bronchodilator will help open up the air passages in the lungs and increase the amount of this steroid medicine that can get into the lungs.

When to Call Your Doctor

Call your doctor if you develop difficulty breathing or coughing when you use the medicine, if your sputum turns yellow or green in color or if you develop an infection of the mouth, throat or lungs, fever, congestion, skin rash, hives, fast heartbeats, or white curdlike patches inside the mouth.

Also call your doctor if you develop a soreness in the mouth or throat, a bad taste in the mouth that will not go away, insomnia or hoarseness, or if your asthma gets worse.

Storage

For inhalers:
• See Metered-Dose Inhalers (page 31).

Miscellaneous

Carry an identification card in your wallet or wear a medical alert bracelet indicating that you are taking this medicine, as well as the

names and phone numbers of your doctors. If you do not already carry such a card, complete the Medicine Card in this book. Always tell your dentist, pharmacist and other doctors who are treating you that you are taking this medicine.

▶ BECLOMETHASONE (NASAL)
BECONASE, BECONASE AQUEOUS NASAL SPRAY, VANCENASE NASAL INHALER

FLUNISOLIDE
RHINALAR

Purpose
This medicine is used in the treatment of hay fever and to help prevent or relieve the symptoms of nasal stuffiness and runny nose associated with allergic conditions.

Allergies/Warnings
If you have ever had an allergic reaction to any cortisone medicines or inhalation spray medicines, tell your doctor and pharmacist before you take any of this medicine.

What Does "Hypoallergenic" Mean?

You see it on cosmetic packaging everywhere: "Hypoallergenic." But what does it mean?

Hypoallergenic products have a reduced potential to cause allergic reactions because they are "fragrance-free." Researchers have found that scent in cosmetics is the main culprit in causing skin irritations and allergic reactions. To determine how fragrance-free the product actually is, just smell it. Also consider the manufacturer's reputation. Many manufacturers make it a point to omit fragrances, avoid known irritants and test their products for allergic reactions.

In the end, no makeup company can say its products are totally allergen-free. There is not a chemical available to which someone is not allergic.

How to Use This Medicine

How to Administer

Follow the special instructions for your specific brand on the sheet that comes with the medicine.

It is very important that you use this medicine regularly as your doctor has prescribed. It will not relieve your symptoms immediately. It is not like ordinary nasal decongestants that you take only when you feel it is necessary.

Children should use the nasal medicine under the supervision of an adult who is aware of its proper use.

For BECONASE AEROSOL:
- As with most inhaled medications in aerosol canisters, the effect of the medication may decrease when the canister is cold.

Special Instructions

Length of Therapy

Do not take any more of this medicine than your doctor has prescribed and do not stop taking this medicine suddenly without the approval of your doctor. If you suddenly stop taking it or reduce the dose, you may experience a worsening of your symptoms.

If this medicine is going to work for your condition, you should notice an improvement in your symptoms, usually in a few days to 2 weeks, when you use it regularly.

Pregnancy/Breastfeeding

Women who are pregnant, breastfeeding or planning to become pregnant should tell their doctor before taking this medicine.

When to Call Your Doctor

Call your doctor if you develop an infection of the nose, sinuses, mouth, throat or lungs. It may be necessary to stop this medicine until you have recovered.

Most people experience few or no side effects from this drug. However, any medicine can sometimes cause unwanted effects. Call your doctor if you develop unexplained nosebleeds, blood in the mucus, sore throat, sneezing attacks, headaches, burning or soreness in the nose or if your condition does not improve within 2 or 3 weeks.

Storage

For BECONASE *and* VANCENASE:
- Store the nasal inhaler at room temperature. Do not place it in hot water or near radiators, stoves or other sources of heat. Do not puncture, burn or incinerate the container (even when it is empty).

For BECONASE AQUEOUS NASAL SPRAY:
- Discard 3 months after first using the spray.

Miscellaneous

Carry an identification card in your wallet or wear a medical alert bracelet indicating that you are taking this medicine, as well as the names and phone numbers of your doctors. If you do not already carry such a card, complete the Medicine Card in this book. Always tell your dentist, pharmacist and other doctors who are treating you that you are taking this medicine.

▶ **BENDROFLUMETHIAZIDE (ORAL)**
NATURETIN

CHLORTHALIDONE
APO-CHLORTHALIDONE, HYGROTON, NOVOTHALIDONE, URIDON

HYDROCHLOROTHIAZIDE
APO-HYDRO, DIUCHLOR H, HYDRODIURIL, NEO-CODEMA, NOVOHYDRAZIDE

INDAPAMIDE
LOZIDE

METHYCLOTHIAZIDE
DURETIC

METOLAZONE
ZAROXOLYN

Purpose

This medicine is used to treat high blood pressure and heart and kidney problems. It helps rid the body of excess fluids and decreases swelling. The medicine works by increasing the amount of urine and is commonly called a water pill or fluid pill.

Allergies/Warnings

Be sure to tell your doctor and pharmacist if you are allergic to sulfa drugs, thiazide diuretics or any other medicine or if you have a history of gout.

How to Use This Medicine

Time of Administration

Try to take this medicine at the same time(s) every day so that you have a constant level of the medicine in your body.

When you first start taking this medicine, you will probably urinate (pass your water) more often and in larger amounts than usual. Therefore, if you are to take 1 dose each day, take it in the morning after breakfast. Do not initially take a dose at bedtime or you may have to get up during the night to go to the bathroom. If you are to take more than 1 dose each day, take the last dose approximately 6 hours before bedtime so that you will not have to get up during the night to go to the bathroom. This effect will usually lessen after you have taken the drug for awhile.

How to Administer

Take this medicine with food, meals or milk if it upsets your stomach.

Special Instructions

Length of Therapy

For patients with high blood pressure:

• High blood pressure (hypertension) is a long-term condition and it will probably be necessary for you to take the drug for a long time even if you feel better. If high blood pressure is not treated, it can lead to serious problems such as heart failure, strokes, blood vessel problems or kidney problems.

It is very important that you take this medicine as your doctor has directed and that you do not miss any doses. Otherwise, you cannot expect the drug to keep your blood pressure down or remove excess fluid.

Pregnancy/Breastfeeding

Women who are pregnant, breastfeeding or planning to become pregnant should tell their doctor before taking this medicine.

Drug Interactions

Some nonprescription drugs can aggravate high blood pressure. Do not take any of the following without the approval of your doctor or pharmacist: cough, cold or sinus products; asthma or allergy products, since they may increase your blood pressure. Read the label of the nonprescription drug product to see if there is a warning. If there is, check with your doctor or pharmacist before using the product.

Alcohol

Be careful drinking alcoholic beverages while taking this medicine because it could make the possible side effect of dizziness worse.

Special Precautions

This medicine normally causes your body to lose potassium. The body has warning signs to let you know if too much potassium is being lost. Call your doctor if you become unusually thirsty or if you develop leg cramps, unusual weakness, fatigue, vomiting, confusion or an irregular pulse. Since these symptoms may not be present in all patients, your doctor may wish to check your blood occasionally to see if it is low in potassium. Depending upon your dose, your doctor may prescribe some medicine to replace the potassium or he or she may recommend that you regularly eat foods that contain a lot of potassium (see Appendix A). *Do not change your diet unless your doctor tells you to.*

If this medicine causes dizziness or lightheadedness, you should be careful going up and down stairs and you should not change positions too rapidly. Lightheadedness is more likely to occur if you stand up suddenly—this is due to blood collecting in the legs and lasts for a few seconds. Therefore, get up from a sitting or lying position more slowly and tighten and relax your leg muscles or wiggle your toes to help promote circulation. In the morning, get out of bed slowly and dangle your feet over the edge of the bed for a few minutes before standing up. Sit or lie down at the first sign of dizziness. Do not drive a car, pilot an airplane, operate dangerous machinery or do jobs that require you to be alert if you are dizzy. Tell your doctor if you have been dizzy.

In order to help prevent dizziness or fainting, your doctor may also recommend that you avoid strenuous exercise, standing for long periods of time (especially in hot weather), hot showers, hot baths, Jacuzzis or saunas.

People more than 65 years of age may be more sensitive to the side effects of dizziness and potassium loss.

This medicine may make some people more sensitive to sunlight and some tanning lamps. When you begin taking this medicine, try to avoid too much sun until you see how you are going to react. If your skin does become more sensitive to sunlight, tell your doctor and try not to stay in direct sunlight for extended periods of time. While in the sun, wear protective clothing and sunglasses. You may wish to ask your pharmacist about suitable sunscreen products. Call your doctor if you become sunburned.

For patients with diabetes:
- This medicine may cause your blood sugar to rise. Carefully test your blood or urine for sugar while you are taking this medicine. Call your doctor if you think your blood sugar is higher than normal or harder to control.

When to Call Your Doctor

Most people experience few or no side effects from this drug. However, any medicine can sometimes cause unwanted effects. Call your doctor if you develop an unexplained sore throat or fever, sharp stomach pain, sharp joint pain, unusual bruising or bleeding, a yellow color to the skin or eyes, unusual weakness or tiredness or a sudden weight gain of 5 pounds (2.5 kg) or more. Also call your doctor if you feel sick or develop persistent vomiting or diarrhea.

Allergic Reactions

Call your doctor immediately if you think you may be allergic to the medicine or if you develop a skin rash, hives, itching, swelling of the face or difficulty in breathing. If you cannot reach your doctor, phone a hospital emergency department.

Refills

Do not stop taking this medicine without your doctor's approval and do not go without medicine between prescription refills. Call your pharmacist for a refill 2 or 3 days before you will run out of the medicine.

Discuss with your pharmacist the implications of dispensing all your refills for this medicine with the same manufacturer's product. (*See* Generic Drugs, page 13.)

▶ BENZTROPINE MESYLATE (ORAL)
APO-BENZTROPINE, COGENTIN, PMS BENZTROPINE

Purpose
This medicine is used to improve various symptoms of Parkinson's disease such as tremors, uncontrolled shaking movements, muscle rigidity or problems in walking.

Allergies/Warnings
If you have ever had an allergic reaction to any medicine or if you have glaucoma, enlarged prostate, difficulty urinating (passing your water), high blood pressure or any other medical condition, tell your doctor and pharmacist before you take any of this medicine.

This medicine should not be given to children less than 3 years of age and should be used with caution in older children.

How to Use This Medicine

Time of Administration
Take this medicine with food or immediately after meals to help prevent stomach upset unless otherwise directed.

Your doctor may prescribe the medicine at bedtime to help prevent drowsiness during the day.

Special Instructions

Length of Therapy
Do not take this medicine more often or longer than recommended by your doctor. To do so may increase your chance of developing side effects.

Do not stop taking this medicine suddenly without the approval of your doctor. It may be necessary for your doctor to reduce your dose slowly since your body may need time to adjust. It could be harmful and make your condition worse if you suddenly did not receive the medicine.

Pregnancy/Breastfeeding
Women who are pregnant, breastfeeding or planning to become pregnant should tell their doctor before taking this medicine.

Drug Interactions

It is important that you obtain the advice of your doctor or pharmacist before taking any other prescription or nonprescription medicines including pain relievers, sleeping pills, tranquilizers, medicine for seizures, muscle relaxants, anesthetics, medicines for depression or medicines for allergies, colds or sinus conditions. Combining this medication with some of these drugs could cause drowsiness or dizziness.

Do not take antacids or diarrhea medicines within 1 hour of taking this medicine as it could make this medicine less effective.

There are other drug interactions that can occur. If you are taking any other medicines, be sure to check first with your pharmacist or doctor.

Alcohol

Do not drink alcoholic beverages while taking this drug without the approval of your doctor because the combination could cause severe drowsiness or dizziness. One drink may have the same effect that 2 or 3 drinks normally would have.

Special Precautions

People over 60 years of age may be more sensitive to some of these side effects.

If your mouth becomes dry, drink water, suck ice chips or a hard, sour candy (sugarless) or chew gum (sugarless). Sugarless products are recommended in order to avoid dental problems. You may wish to ask your pharmacist about special solutions, called artificial saliva, that can also be used to help restore moisture in the mouth.

It is especially important to brush and floss your teeth regularly if you develop a dry mouth to help prevent gum problems.

If your mouth becomes extremely dry and you have difficulty swallowing or speaking or if you lose your appetite, call your doctor. It may be necessary to lower your dose.

In some people, this drug may cause dizziness, drowsiness or blurred vision, particularly during the first 2 weeks of use. This will usually go away as your body adjusts to the medicine. Do not drive a car, pilot an airplane, operate dangerous machinery or do jobs that require you to be alert until you know how you are going to react to the drug.

If this medicine causes dizziness or lightheadedness, you should be careful going up and down stairs and you should not change positions too rapidly. Lightheadedness is more likely to occur if you stand up suddenly—this is due to blood collecting in the legs and lasts for a few seconds. Therefore, get up from a sitting or lying position more slowly and tighten and relax your leg muscles or wiggle your toes to help promote circulation. In the morning, get out of bed slowly and dangle your feet over the edge of the bed for a few minutes before standing up. Sit or lie down at the first sign of dizziness. Tell your doctor if you have been dizzy.

You may become more sensitive to heat because your body may perspire less while you are taking this drug. Be careful not to become overheated during exercise or in hot weather. Try to avoid strenuous exercise, standing for long periods of time (especially in hot weather), hot showers, hot baths, saunas or Jacuzzis while taking this medicine.

This medicine may cause some people to become constipated. To help prevent constipation, try increasing the amount of bulk in your diet (for example, bran, fresh fruits and salads), exercising more often or drinking more fluids (unless otherwise directed). Call your doctor if the constipation continues.

If your eyes become more sensitive to sunlight, it may help to wear sunglasses.

An urge to urinate (pass your water) with an inability to do so sometimes occurs with this drug. Urinating before taking the drug each time may help relieve this problem. Tell your doctor if you are having this problem.

When to Call Your Doctor

Most people experience few or no side effects from this drug. However, any medicine can sometimes cause unwanted effects. Call your doctor if you develop a skin rash, eye pain, difficulty reading, fainting spells, fast heartbeats, shortness of breath or difficulty breathing, confusion, unusual restlessness, seizures, abdominal pain, muscle weakness, severe constipation or continued difficulty urinating.

Allergic Reactions

Call your doctor immediately if you think you may be allergic to the medicine or if you develop a skin rash, hives, itching, swelling of the face or difficulty in breathing. If you cannot reach your doctor, phone a hospital emergency department.

Refills

Do not stop taking this medicine without your doctor's approval and do not go without medicine between prescription refills. Call your pharmacist for a refill 2 or 3 days before you will run out of the medicine.

▶ **BETAMETHASONE (ORAL)**
BETNESOL, CELESTONE

CORTISONE
CORTONE

DEXAMETHASONE
DECADRON, DERONIL, DEXASONE, HEXADROL, ORADEXON

HYDROCORTISONE
CORTEF

METHYLPREDNISOLONE
MEDROL

PREDNISONE
APO-PREDNISONE, DELTASONE, NOVOPREDNISONE, WINPRED

TRIAMCINOLONE
ARISTOCORT

Purpose

This medicine is a hormone (corticosteroid) used to help decrease inflammation. This then relieves pain, redness and swelling. It is used to treat certain kinds of arthritis, severe allergies or skin conditions as well as a variety of other medical conditions. If you do not know why you were prescribed this medicine, ask your doctor.

Allergies/Warnings

If you have ever had an allergic reaction to any medicine or if you have or have had tuberculosis (TB), a positive skin test for TB, an infection, ulcers, high blood pressure or any other medical condition, tell your doctor and pharmacist before you take any of this medicine.

How to Use This Medicine

Time of Administration

If your doctor has prescribed only *one* dose of this medicine every day or every other day, it is best to take it before 9 A.M. or with breakfast.

Try to take this medicine at the same time(s) every day so that you will have a constant level of medicine in your body. The time of day affects the way your body responds to this medicine. It is important to follow your doctor's directions as closely as possible.

How to Administer

Take this medicine after meals or with a snack in order to help prevent stomach upset. Call your doctor if you develop stomach upset, stomach pain, heartburn (especially if it awakens you during the night) or if your stools become black and tarry. Do *not* try to treat these problems yourself.

If you were prescribed CELESTONE REPETABS:
- These tablets are long-acting and must be swallowed whole. Do not crush, chew or break them into pieces.

If you were prescribed BETNESOL TABLETS:
- These are effervescent tablets and must be dissolved in a full glass of water before taking. Let the bubbles disappear before drinking the solution.

If you were prescribed BETNESOL PELLETS:
- These tablets should be placed close to the ulcer in the mouth and allowed to dissolve.

For liquid medicines:
- If a spoon is used to measure the dose, it is recommended that you use a medicine spoon or an oral liquid syringe, which you can obtain from your pharmacist. *See* Oral Liquid Syringe (page 17) and Medicine Spoon (page 22).

Special Instructions

Length of Therapy

Do not take this medicine more often or longer than recommended by your doctor. To do so may increase your chance of developing side effects. Your doctor will want you to take the lowest dose possible.

Do not stop taking this medicine suddenly without the approval of your doctor. It may be necessary for your doctor to reduce your dose slowly since your body will need time to adjust. It could be harmful and make your condition worse if you suddenly stopped taking the medicine. You might then experience symptoms of too rapid withdrawal including nausea, tiredness, loss of appetite, difficulty breathing, fainting, joint and muscle pains.

Pregnancy/Breastfeeding

Women who are pregnant, breastfeeding or planning to become pregnant should tell their doctor before taking this medicine.

Drug Interactions

It is best not to take ASA or medicines containing salicylates while you are taking this medicine without the approval of your doctor or pharmacist. The combination could cause stomach problems.

Alcohol

It is best not to drink alcoholic beverages while you are taking this medicine because the combination could cause stomach problems.

Special Precautions

While you are taking this medicine you may gain some weight. This could be due to an increase in your appetite or to increased water in your body. Your doctor may prescribe a special diet to decrease the number of calories you eat, and/or to lower the amount of sodium or to increase the amount of potassium in your diet. Follow any diet that your doctor may order.

Bruising may occur more easily. Try to protect yourself from all injuries to prevent bruising.

Diabetic patients should regularly check the sugar in their urine or blood and report any unusual levels to their doctor.

It is generally not recommended that patients taking this medicine (especially high doses) receive vaccinations against infectious diseases. The body is not usually able to respond in the normal manner.

When to Call Your Doctor

Call your doctor if you are taking this medicine or have recently stopped taking it and you experience severe stress.

Most people experience few or no side effects from this drug. However, any medicine can sometimes cause unwanted effects. Call your doctor if you develop stomach pain, sore throat, fever, swelling of the legs or ankles, eye pain or changes in vision, frequent urination (passing your water), nightmares or a change in your mood, depression, unusual bruising, changes in the skin, increased facial hair (in women), muscle cramps, stomach or back pain, bloody or black stools, puffy face, irregular heartbeats, dizziness, weakness, unusual thirst, menstrual problems (in women) or an infection that does not clear up as quickly as usual.

Allergic Reactions

Call your doctor immediately if you think you may be allergic to this medicine or if you develop a skin rash, hives, itching, swelling of the face or difficulty in breathing. If you cannot reach your doctor, phone a hospital emergency department.

Refills

Do not stop taking this medicine without your doctor's approval and do not go without medicine between prescription refills. Call your pharmacist for a refill 2 or 3 days before you will run out of the medicine.

Miscellaneous

Carry an identification card in your wallet or wear a medical alert bracelet indicating that you are taking this medicine, as well as the names and phone numbers of your doctors. If you do not already carry such a card, complete the Medicine Card in this book. Always tell your dentist, pharmacist and other doctors who are treating you that you are taking this medicine. This is especially important if you have an infection or injury or if you plan to have an operation, vaccination, skin tests or dental surgery. This medicine can affect the way your body responds to stress, such as surgery. Your doctor may need to adjust your dose.

If you were taking the medicine for a long time, your body's response to stress may take several months to return to normal. It is important to tell your future doctors and dentists this even after you have stopped the medicine for 1 year.

▶ **BETAXOL HCI (OPHTHALMIC)**
BETOPTIC

LEVOBUNOLOL HCI
BETAGAN

TIMOLOL
APO-TIMOP, TIMOPTIC

Purpose

This medicine is used in the treatment of certain types of glaucoma, to lower the pressure in the eye. Increased pressure may lead to a gradual loss of vision.

Allergies/Warnings

If you have ever had an allergic reaction to any medicine or if you have bronchial asthma, bronchitis, thyroid problems, diabetes, emphysema or heart problems, tell your doctor and pharmacist before you take any of this medicine.

BETAGAN contains sulfites. Do not use it if you are allergic to sulfites.

How to Use This Medicine

How to Administer
For eye drops:
- *See* Eye Drops (page 24).
- If more than 1 drop is prescribed, wait 3 to 5 minutes before administering another drop.
- Wait at least 5 minutes before using any other eye drops.

Special Instructions

Length of Therapy
Do not use the eye drops more frequently or in larger quantities than prescribed by your doctor.

Do not stop using the eye drops on your own without talking with your doctor or pharmacist.

Pregnancy/Breastfeeding
Women who are pregnant, breastfeeding or planning to become pregnant should tell their doctor before taking this medicine.

Helpful Hint for Relief of Dry Mouth

The husband of a semiconscious woman discovered an ingenious way to relieve her dry mouth. He filled a small perfume atomizer with fresh water and misted his wife's mouth frequently. According to the *American Journal of Nursing*, the condition of the woman's throat and mouth improved. After the wife recovered, she commented that the misting had been very comforting.

If you decide to use this technique, use fresh water and change the water at least once daily to help prevent bacterial contamination of the water.

Drug Interactions

Do not use this medicine at the same time as any other eye medicine without the approval of your doctor. Some medicines cannot be mixed.

Special Precautions

If you are wearing contact lenses, you must remove them before using the eye drops. Ask your doctor how long you must wait before reinserting the lenses.

Keep your doctor's appointments regularly so that your doctor can make sure that the medicine is working correctly and that your glaucoma is under control.

If you are using BETOPTIC and your eyes become more sensitive to light, wearing sunglasses may help.

When to Call Your Doctor

Contact your doctor if your vision gets worse or if the eye becomes painful or irritated by the medicine for more than a few minutes. Many eye medicines sting and cause tears for a short time immediately after use.

If you were prescribed TIMOPTIC:

- Also call your doctor if you develop unusual tiredness or weakness, slow or irregular heartbeats, wheezing or difficulty breathing, fainting, persistent headaches, confusion, depression, swelling of legs or ankles or sudden weight gain of 5 pounds (2.5 kg) or more.

If you were prescribed BETAGAN:

- Also call your doctor if you develop slow or irregular heartbeats, wheezing, redness of eyes, difficulty breathing or shortness of breath, fainting, swelling of feet, ankles or legs, or sudden weight gain of 5 pounds (2.5 kg) or more. Also call your doctor if you develop unusual tiredness or weakness, confusion, depression or persistent headaches.

If you were prescribed BETOPTIC:

- Also call your doctor if you develop increased sensitivity to light, difficulty sleeping, depression, wheezing or difficulty breathing, fainting, slow or irregular heartbeats, swelling of the legs or ankles, or sudden weight gain of 5 pounds (2.5 kg) or more.

Allergic Reactions

Call your doctor immediately if you think you may be allergic to the medicine or if you develop a skin rash or itching. If you cannot reach your doctor, phone a hospital emergency department.

Miscellaneous

This medicine is for external use only. Do not swallow it.

Carry an identification card in your wallet or wear a medical alert bracelet indicating that you are taking this medicine, as well as the names and phone numbers of your doctors. If you do not already carry such a card, complete the Medicine Card in this book. Always tell your dentist, pharmacist and other doctors who are treating you that you are taking this medicine.

▶ **BROMPHENIRAMINE (ORAL)**
DIMETANE

BROMPHENIRAMINE-PHENYLEPHRINE-PHENYLPROPANOLAMINE
DECONGESTANT ANTIHISTAMINE SYRUP, DIMETAPP, DIMETAPP ELIXIR, DIMETAPP ORAL INFANT DROPS

BROMPHENIRAMINE-PHENYLEPHRINE-PHENYLPROPANOLAMINE-ACETAMINOPHEN
DIMETAPP-A, DIMETAPP-A PEDIATRIC

BROMPHENIRAMINE-PHENYLEPHRINE-PHENYLPROPANOLAMINE-CODEINE
DIMETAPP-C, DIMETAPP WITH CODEINE

BROMPHENIRAMINE-PHENYLEPHRINE-PHENYLPROPANOLAMINE-DEXTROMETHORPHAN
DIMETAPP-DM

BROMPHENIRAMINE-PHENYLEPHRINE-PHENYLPROPANOLAMINE-GUAIFENESIN
DIMETANE EXPECTORANT

BROMPHENIRAMINE-PHENYLEPHRINE-PHENYLPROPANOLAMINE-GUAIFENESIN-CODEINE
DIMETANE EXPECTORANT-C

BROMPHENIRAMINE-PHENYLEPHRINE-PHENYLPROPANOLAMINE-GUAIFENESIN-HYDROCODONE
DIMETANE EXPECTORANT-DC

Purpose

This medicine is used to help relieve or prevent the symptoms of certain types of allergic conditions (such as hay fever), coughs and colds and certain allergic skin conditions.

Allergies/Warnings

If you have ever had an allergic reaction to any medicine or if you have asthma, glaucoma, an enlarged prostate, urinary retention (a type of bladder problem), high blood pressure or diabetes, tell your doctor and pharmacist before you take any of this medicine.

How to Use This Medicine

Time of Administration

This medicine may be taken without regard to meals. Take it either with food or on an empty stomach. If stomach upset occurs, take it with some food or a glass of milk.

How to Administer

If you were prescribed DIMETANE EXTENTABS, DIMETAPP EXTENTABS:
- These tablets must be swallowed whole. Do not crush, chew or break them into pieces. Do not take chipped tablets.

If your child was prescribed DIMETAPP ORAL INFANT DROPS:
- Use the special dropper that comes with the medicine.
- If you do not understand how to use the dropper to measure an accurate dose, *see* Medicine Dropper (page 21).

If you were prescribed DIMETANE ELIXIR, DIMETANE EXPECTORANT, DIMETANE EXPECTORANT-C, DIMETANE EXPECTORANT-DC, DIMETAPP ELIXIR, DIMETAPP-A PEDIATRIC, DIMETAPP-C, DIMETAPP-DM ELIXIR:
- Use a medicine spoon to measure each dose. Household teaspoons are not accurate.

Special Instructions

Length of Therapy

Do not take this medicine more often or longer than recommended by your doctor. To do so may increase your chance of developing side effects.

Prolonged use of DIMETANE EXPECTORANT-C, DIMETANE EXPECTORANT-DC, DIMETAPP-C or DIMETAPP WITH CODEINE should be avoided. Do not use more often than recommended by your physician.

Pregnancy/Breastfeeding

Women who are pregnant, breastfeeding or planning to become pregnant should tell their doctor before taking this medicine. Some of the products should not be taken during pregnancy or while breast-feeding.

Drug Interactions

It is important that you obtain the advice of your doctor or phar-macist before taking any other prescription or nonprescription med-icines including pain relievers, sleeping pills, tranquilizers, medicine for seizures, muscle relaxants, anesthetics, medicines for depression or other medicines for allergies. Combining this medicine with some of these drugs could cause drowsiness or dizziness.

There are other drug interactions that can occur. If you are taking any other medicines, be sure to check first with your pharmacist or doctor.

Alcohol

Do not drink alcoholic beverages while taking this drug without the approval of your doctor because the combination could cause drow-siness. One drink may have the same effect that 2 or 3 drinks normally would have.

Special Precautions

In some people, this drug may initially cause dizziness or drowsi-ness. Do not drive a car, pilot an airplane, operate dangerous ma-chinery or do jobs that require you to be alert until you know how you are going to react to the drug. If you become dizzy or drowsy, you should be careful going up and down stairs. Sit or lie down at the first sign of dizziness. Tell your doctor if the dizziness continues.

People over 65 years of age may be more sensitive to these side effects.

If your mouth becomes dry, drink water, suck ice chips or a hard, sour candy (sugarless) or chew gum (sugarless). Sugarless products are recommended in order to avoid dental problems. You may wish to ask your pharmacist about special solutions, called artificial saliva, that can also be used to help restore moisture in the mouth. It is especially important to brush and floss your teeth regularly if you develop a dry mouth to help prevent gum problems.

When to Call Your Doctor

Most people experience few or no side effects from these drugs. However, any medicine can sometimes cause unwanted effects. Call your doctor if you develop a skin rash, fast or irregular heartbeats, blurred vision, stomach pain, unexplained weakness or tiredness, unexplained sore throat or fever, unusual bruising or bleeding, unexplained nervousness, restlessness or irritability (especially in children), trouble sleeping or difficulty in urinating (passing your water), severe constipation or if mucous (lung secretions) becomes thicker than normal.

▶ **BUSPIRONE (ORAL)**
BUSPAR

Purpose

This medicine is used to help relieve moderate to severe anxiety. It should not be used to treat nervousness and tension from the normal pressures of day-to-day living.

Allergies/Warnings

If you have ever had an allergic reaction to any medicine or you have liver or kidney problems, tell your doctor or pharmacist before you take this medicine.

How to Break Tablets in Half

Most tablets that are intended to be broken in half have an indented line (score line) down the middle. In addition, the tablet surfaces are frequently convexly curved. These two properties make it possible to split the tablet quite easily by using the following procedure:

1. Hold the tablet so the indented line is facing you.
2. Place a thumb on each side of the indented line.
3. Press down firmly until the tablet breaks.

The tablet will usually break along the indented line with very little loss of the drug.

How to Use this Medicine

How to Administer

This medicine may be taken without regard for meals. Take it either with food or on an empty stomach.

Special Instructions

Pregnancy/Breastfeeding

Women who are pregnant, planning to become pregnant or are breastfeeding should tell their doctor before taking this medicine. Generally, this medicine should not be used during pregnancy, and it is not generally recommended during breastfeeding.

Drug Interactions

It is important you obtain the advice of your doctor or pharmacist before taking other prescription medicines. Do not start or stop this medicine without first consulting with your doctor or pharmacist.

Alcohol

It is recommended that you do not drink alcoholic beverages while taking this medicine, as it may cause drowsiness or an unsettled feeling.

Special Precautions

In some people, this drug may cause dizziness or drowsiness. Do not drive a car, pilot an airplane, operate dangerous machinery or do jobs that require you to be alert if you are dizzy or drowsy. You should also be careful going up and down stairs. Sit or lie down at the first sign of dizziness. Tell your doctor if the dizziness continues.

If your mouth becomes dry, drink water, suck ice chips or a hard, sour candy (sugarless) or chew gum (sugarless). Sugarless products are recommended in order to avoid dental problems. You may wish to ask your pharmacist about special solutions, called artificial saliva, that can also be used to help restore moisture in the mouth. Call your doctor if your mouth becomes extremely dry.

This medicine may cause some people to become constipated. To help prevent constipation, try increasing the amount of bulk in your diet (for example, bran, fresh fruits and salads), exercising more often or drinking more fluids (unless otherwise directed). Call your doctor if the constipation continues.

This medicine may cause nasal congestion (stuffy nose). Do not try to treat this yourself with cold or allergy medicines. Check with your doctor.

When to Call Your Doctor

Most people experience few or no side effects from this drug. However, any medicine can sometimes cause unwanted effects. Call your doctor if you develop a skin rash, sore throat, persistent headache, nausea, changes in mood, nightmares, numbness, tingling in the feet or hands, stiff muscles or jerky muscle movements, changes in vision, hearing or speech, unusual bruising, rapid heartbeat or nasal stuffiness.

▶ CAPSAICIN (TOPICAL)
AXSAIN, ZOSTRIX

Purpose

AXSAIN (0.075%) is used for temporary relief of pain due to arthritis or diabetes and after surgery.

ZOSTRIX (0.025%) is used to help relieve the pain during and after herpes zoster ("shingles") infections.

How to Use This Medicine

How to Administer

Apply the cream lightly to the affected area not less than 3 to 4 times daily unless otherwise directed.

Most patients will experience a burning or stinging sensation after applying this medicine. This is a normal effect of the medicine and will usually go away in a few days.

Immediately after applying the cream, wash your hands thoroughly with warm water and soap. Be careful not to touch the eyes or mouth with your hands until after you have washed any medicine off your hands.

Do not apply a bandage over the affected area.

Special Instructions

Length of Therapy

It is important that you use the medicine regularly as prescribed by your doctor. It takes about 2 to 4 weeks for the maximum benefit to occur once you have started using the medicine.

The medicine must be used regularly every day in order to work.

Special Precautions

This medicine is for external use only. It should be applied to affected areas only but not if the skin lesions are moist or crusted. The medicine must NOT be applied to open or blistered skin areas. Do NOT apply the cream near or in the eyes.

When to Call Your Doctor

This medicine may cause a burning sensation immediately after it is applied. This usually disappears as the drug is used more often. If it continues or worsens, contact your doctor. Also call your doctor if the symptoms do not improve after 14 days or if the condition worsens.

▶ **CAPTOPRIL (ORAL)**
Capoten

ENALAPRIL
Vasotec

LISINOPRIL
Prinivil, Zestril

Purpose

This medicine is used to treat high blood pressure and may also be used to treat heart failure.

Allergies/Warnings

Be sure to tell your doctor and pharmacist if you are allergic to any medicine.

How to Use This Medicine

Time of Administration

Try to take this medicine at the same time every day so that you have a constant level of the medicine in your body.

How to Administer

For Capoten:
- Take this medicine with a glass of water on an empty stomach at least 1 hour before or 2 hours after eating food.

For Vasotec, Prinivil and Zestril:
- This medicine is not affected by food and may be taken with food or on an empty stomach.

Special Instructions

Length of Therapy
For patients with high blood pressure:
- High blood pressure (hypertension) is a long-term condition, and it will probably be necessary for you to take the drug for a long time in spite of the fact that you feel better. If high blood pressure is not treated, it can lead to serious problems such as heart failure, strokes, blood vessel problems or kidney problems. It is very important that you take this medicine as your doctor has directed and that you do not miss any doses. Otherwise, you cannot expect the drug to keep your blood pressure down.

Pregnancy/Breastfeeding
Women who are pregnant, breastfeeding or planning to become pregnant must tell their doctor before taking this medicine.

Drug Interactions
Some nonprescription drugs can aggravate your condition. Do not take any of the following without the approval of your doctor or pharmacist: cough, cold, or sinus products; products containing ASA; asthma or allergy products, since they may increase your blood pressure. Read the label of the product to see if there is a warning. If there is, check with your doctor or pharmacist before using the product.

Special Precautions
In order to prevent dizziness or fainting, you should avoid strenuous exercise, standing for long periods of time (especially in hot weather), hot showers, hot baths, Jacuzzis or saunas. If this medicine causes dizziness or lightheadedness, you should be careful going up and down stairs and you should not change positions too rapidly. Sit or lie down at the first sign of dizziness. Do not drive a car, pilot an airplane, operate dangerous machinery or do jobs that require you to be alert if you are dizzy. Tell your doctor if you have been dizzy.

Do not use salt substitutes, low-salt milk or low-salt soups without the approval of your doctor. They may contain large amounts of potassium, which could affect the way you respond to this medicine. Do not start any special diets without first consulting your physician. NEVER take potassium supplements while you are being treated with this medicine.

Is Your Blood Pressure Normal?

Most people with high blood pressure do not have any symptoms.

The only way to determine if your blood pressure is higher than normal is to have it measured.

For CAPOTEN *or* VASOTEC:
- This medicine may cause a temporary loss of taste or metallic taste. This is not harmful and usually disappears after 2 or 3 months of treatment. If it does not disappear, call your doctor.

When to Call Your Doctor

Most people experience few or no side effects from this drug except for a cough. A dry, irritating cough may occur in up to 10% of patients taking any of these medicines. This cough is not associated with any lung abnormality and disappears when the medicine is stopped. There is no way your doctor can tell in advance whether or not you will develop a cough.

Your doctor may want to check your blood occasionally to see if the potassium level is normal, especially if your kidneys are not working at full capacity.

Call your doctor if you feel sick or develop persistent nausea, vomiting or diarrhea or excessive perspiration. These conditions could cause the blood pressure to fall more than desired.

Allergic Reactions

Call your doctor immediately if you think you may be allergic to the medicine or if you develop a skin rash, hives, itching, swelling of the face or difficulty in breathing. If you cannot reach your doctor, phone a hospital emergency department.

Refills

Do not stop taking this medicine without your doctor's approval and do not go without medicine between prescription refills. Call your pharmacist for a refill 2 or 3 days before you will run out of the medicine.

Miscellaneous

Carry an identification card in your wallet or wear a medical alert bracelet indicating that you are taking this medicine, as well as the

names and phone numbers of your doctors. If you do not already carry such a card, complete the Medicine Card in this book. Always tell your dentist, pharmacist and other doctors who are treating you that you are taking this medicine.

Chewable Tablets — How Much Chewing Is Necessary?

Chewable tablets should be completely chewed and broken into very small pieces before being swallowed.

Since the pieces of the tablet must still dissolve in the stomach fluids in order to be absorbed into the bloodstream, the smaller the pieces, the quicker the tablet will dissolve and then be absorbed. Always drink some water after you have chewed and swallowed the small tablet pieces, unless otherwise directed.

▶ CARBAMAZEPINE (ORAL)
APO-CARBAMAZEPINE, MAZEPINE, NOVOCARBAMAZ, PMS CARBAMAZEPINE, TEGRETOL, TEGRETOL-CR

Purpose
This medicine is used to help control convulsions and seizures. It is commonly used in the treatment of epilepsy. It is also used to help relieve a certain type of face pain called trigeminal neuralgia, glossopharyngeal neuralgia and other types of "nerve pain."

Do not take this medicine for ordinary aches and pains. It is *not* an ordinary pain reliever.

Allergies/Warnings
If you have ever had an allergic reaction to an anticonvulsant (seizure medicine) or a medicine for depression or if you have glaucoma, heart disease, anemia or other blood problems, tell your doctor and pharmacist before you take any of this medicine.

How to Use This Medicine

Time of Administration
It is very important that you take this medicine exactly as your doctor has prescribed. Do not miss any doses and take the medicine

even if you feel well. Try to take this medicine at the same time(s) every day so that you will have a constant level of medicine in your body. This is the only way that you can receive the full benefit of the medicine.

How to Administer

Take this medicine after food to help prevent stomach upset and to improve absorption of the drug into the body. Call your doctor if you continue to have stomach upset.

If you were prescribed TEGRETOL-CR:
- This medicine is long-acting and must not be crushed or chewed. Swallow the medicine whole.

If you were prescribed TEGRETOL CHEWTABS:
- These tablets should be swallowed whole or chewed well before swallowing. Always take them the same way so that you receive the same amount of medicine each time.

Special Instructions

Length of Therapy

If you are taking this medicine to treat epilepsy, do not stop taking it suddenly without the approval of your doctor. It will usually be necessary for your doctor to reduce your dose slowly, since your body will need time to adjust. You could develop seizures if you suddenly stopped taking the medicine. The only time this medicine should be stopped quickly is if certain serious side effects develop.

Pregnancy/Breastfeeding

Women who are pregnant, planning to become pregnant or breast-feeding should tell their doctor before taking this medicine.

Drug Interactions

It is important that you obtain the advice of your doctor or pharmacist before taking any other prescription or nonprescription medicines including pain relievers, sleeping pills, birth control pills, erythromycin antibiotics, tranquilizers, medicine for seizures, muscle relaxants, anesthetics, medicines for depression or medicines for allergies. Combining this medicine with some of these drugs could cause drowsiness or dizziness.

There are other drug interactions that can occur. If you are taking any other medicines, be sure to check first with your pharmacist or doctor.

There have been some reports that oral contraceptives (birth control pills) may not work as well while you are taking this medicine. Unplanned pregnancies may occur. Ask your doctor about using another form of birth control or adjusting your dose of birth control pills while you are taking this medicine. Also call your doctor if you develop spotting or breakthrough bleeding since these can be signs of decreased birth control effect.

Alcohol

Do not drink alcoholic beverages while taking this drug without the approval of your doctor because the combination could cause drowsiness.

Special Precautions

Be sure to keep your doctor's appointments so that your doctor can check your progress. This is especially important during the first few months of therapy, when the doctor will decide the best dose of this medicine for your condition. To make sure that your dose is correct, your doctor may wish to take a blood sample periodically to measure the amount of medicine in it.

This medicine may cause dizziness, drowsiness or blurred vision in some people. Do not drive a car, operate dangerous machinery or do jobs that require you to be alert until you know how you are going to react to the drug. If you become dizzy, you should be careful going up and down stairs. Sit or lie down at the first sign of dizziness. Tell your doctor if you are dizzy, drowsy or have blurred vision.

If this medicine is for a child, do not let him or her ride a bike, climb trees, etc. until you can determine how he or she is going to react to this medicine. Children could hurt themselves if they participated in these activities when they were dizzy.

This medicine may make some people more sensitive to sunlight and some tanning lamps. When you begin taking this medicine, try to avoid too much sun until you see how you are going to react. If your skin does become more sensitive to sunlight, tell your doctor and try not to stay in direct sunlight for extended periods of time. While in the sun, wear protective clothing and sunglasses. You may wish to ask your pharmacist about suitable sunscreen products. Call your doctor if you become sunburned.

When to Call Your Doctor

Most people experience few or no side effects from this drug. However, any medicine can sometimes cause unwanted effects. Call your

doctor immediately if you develop a sore throat, fever or mouth sores, chills, swollen glands, fainting, muscle weakness, unexplained coughing, difficulty breathing, unusual bruising or bleeding, dark-colored urine, a yellow color to the skin or eyes, unusual tiredness or weakness, continuous back-and-forth or rolling eye movements, numbness or tingling in the hands or feet, fast or slow heartbeats, chest pain, trembling, abdominal pain, light-colored stools, ringing or buzzing in the ears, confusion, hallucinations, nightmares or depression, swelling of the legs or ankles or if you urinate (pass your water) in smaller amounts than usual.

Call your doctor if you are taking this medicine for seizures and you have an increase in the frequency of seizures.

Allergic Reactions

Call your doctor immediately if you think you may be allergic to the medicine or if you develop a skin rash, hives, itching, swelling of the face or difficulty in breathing. If you cannot reach your doctor, phone a hospital emergency department.

Storage

Protect the medicine from heat and humidity.

Refills

Do not stop taking this medicine without your doctor's approval and do not go without medicine between prescription refills. Call your pharmacist for a refill 2 or 3 days before you will run out of the medicine.

Miscellaneous

Carry an identification card in your wallet or wear a medical alert bracelet indicating that you are taking this medicine, as well as the names and phone numbers of your doctors. If you do not already carry such a card, complete the Medicine Card in this book. Always tell your dentist, pharmacist and other doctors who are treating you that you are taking this medicine.

Ask about Possible Side Effects

When a medicine is prescribed, you should ask the doctor what you should expect to feel and what you can do if a common side effect occurs. Then, if the effect occurs, you will know whether it is a sign that the drug is working or whether you should contact your doctor.

▶ **CEFACLOR (ORAL)**
CECLOR

CEFADROXIL
DURICEF

CEFIXIME
SUPRAX

CEFUROXIME AXETIL
CEFTIN

CEPHALEXIN MONOHYDRATE
APO-CEPHALEX, CEPOREX, KEFLEX, NOVOLEXIN, NU-CEPHALEX

CEPHRADINE
VELOSEF

Purpose

This medicine is an antibiotic used to treat certain types of infections. Your doctor has prescribed this antibiotic for your present infection only. Do not use it for other infections or give it to other people.

Allergies/Warnings

If you have ever had an allergic reaction to penicillin, a cephalosporin or any other medicine or if you have any allergies (for example, asthma or hay fever), tell your doctor and pharmacist before you take any of this medicine.

How to Use This Medicine

Time of Administration

This medicine may be taken with meals or on an empty stomach. However, if you develop an upset stomach after taking the drug, take it with some food. Call your doctor if you continue to have stomach upset.

Space your doses of the medicine around the clock (throughout the entire day of 24 hours). For example, if you are to take 2 doses each day, space the doses 12 hours apart. This will keep a constant level of the medicine in your body.

How to Administer
If you were prescribed CEFTIN:
- It is best to take this medicine after food.
- Swallow these tablets whole. If you have to crush or chew the tablets, they have a very bitter taste and you may wish to mix the crushed tablet in orange juice, grape juice, apple juice or chocolate milk.

For tablets and capsules:
- Take the medicine with a full glass of water unless otherwise directed.

For liquid medicines:
- If you were prescribed a *suspension*, shake the bottle well each time before pouring so that you can measure an accurate dose.
- If a spoon is used to measure the dose, it is recommended that you use a medicine spoon or an oral liquid syringe, which you can obtain from your pharmacist. *See* Oral Liquid Syringe (page 17) and Medicine Spoon (page 22).

Special Instructions

Length of Therapy
It is important to take all of this medicine plus any refills that your doctor told you to take. Do not stop taking this medicine earlier than your doctor has recommended even if you begin to feel better. If you stop taking the medicine too soon, the infection may return.

This is especially important if you are taking the medicine to cure a strep infection, such as a strep throat, because if the infection is not completely cleared up, serious heart problems could develop later. After treatment for a strep infection, your doctor may want to do a test to make sure that the infection is gone.

Pregnancy/Breastfeeding
Women who are pregnant or who are planning to become pregnant should tell their doctor before taking this medicine.

Even though this medicine passes into breast milk, it is considered to be relatively safe for mothers to use when breastfeeding (nursing). However, mothers should tell their doctor that they are nursing before they take this medicine. In addition, if the nursing baby is seen by a doctor while the mother is taking this medicine, the mother should inform the baby's doctor that she is nursing AND taking this medicine.

Special Precautions
For patients with diabetes:
- If you have diabetes, this medicine may interfere with some of the tests for sugar in the urine. Check with your doctor or pharmacist for advice on which test you should use for detecting sugar in the urine while you are taking this antibiotic.

When to Call Your Doctor
Call your doctor if your symptoms do not improve within a few days or if they become worse.

Most people experience few or no side effects from this drug. However, any medicine can sometimes cause unwanted effects. Call your doctor if you develop nausea, vomiting, fever, chills, sore mouth or sore tongue, watery or bloody diarrhea, severe stomach cramps and bloating, unusual weight loss, rectal or genital itching or, in women, a vaginal discharge that was not present before you started taking the medicine.

Allergic Reactions
Call your doctor immediately if you think you may be allergic to the medicine or if you develop a skin rash, hives, itching, swelling of the face or difficulty in breathing. If you cannot reach your doctor, phone a hospital emergency department.

Storage
For liquid medicines except SUPRAX Liquid:
- Store the bottle of medicine in a refrigerator unless otherwise directed. Do not freeze.

For SUPRAX Liquid:
- This medicine may be stored at room temperature. It does not require refrigeration.

If for some reason you cannot take all of the medicine, take the unused portion back to your pharmacist. You should discuss why you cannot finish the medicine with your pharmacist. Do not take any unused medicine after the discard (expiration) date on the bottle.

Do Not Mix an Infant's Medicine with Foods

You should not mix pediatric medicines with infant formulas or foods because:

- If the child detects a strange taste in the food due to the medicine, he or she may refuse that particular food in the future.

- If the infant does not drink all the formula, he or she will not receive the full dose of the medicine.

▶ CHLORDIAZEPOXIDE-CLIDINIUM (ORAL)
APO-CHLORAX, CORIUM, LIBRAX

Purpose
This medicine is used to decrease the amount of acid in the stomach and help relax the muscles of the stomach and bowels.

Allergies/Warnings
If you have ever had an allergic reaction to any medicine or if you have glaucoma, depression, an enlarged prostate, difficulty in urinating (passing your water) or any medical problem, tell your doctor and pharmacist before you take any of this medicine.

How to Use This Medicine

Time of Administration
Take this medicine ½ hour to 1 hour before meals unless otherwise directed by your doctor.

Special Instructions

Length of Therapy
Do not take this medicine more often or longer than recommended by your doctor. If large doses are taken for long periods of time (months), the drug can become habit-forming.

If you are taking the medicine regularly, do not stop taking it suddenly without the approval of your doctor. It may be necessary for your doctor to reduce your dose slowly since your body may need time to adjust.

Check with your doctor if you develop any of the following while you are slowly stopping the medicine: nausea or vomiting, trembling, seizures, muscle cramps, stomach cramps, unusual sweating or trouble sleeping, or if you become confused, irritable or nervous.

Pregnancy/Breastfeeding

Women who are pregnant, breastfeeding or planning to become pregnant should tell their doctor before taking this medicine. This medicine should generally not be used during pregnancy and is not generally recommended during breastfeeding.

Drug Interactions

It is important that you obtain the advice of your doctor or pharmacist before taking any other prescription or nonprescription medicines, including pain relievers, sleeping pills, tranquilizers or medicines for depression, cough, cold or allergies, because the combination could cause drowsiness or confusion.

There are other drug interactions that can occur. If you are taking any other medicines, be sure to check first with your pharmacist or doctor.

Alcohol

Do not drink alcoholic beverages while taking this drug or for a few days after you have stopped taking the drug without the approval of your doctor. The combination could cause drowsiness. One drink may have the same effect that 2 or 3 drinks normally would have.

Special Precautions

In some people, this drug may cause dizziness or drowsiness. Do not drive a car, pilot an airplane, operate dangerous machinery or do jobs that require you to be alert if you are dizzy or drowsy. You should also be careful going up and down stairs. Sit or lie down at the first sign of dizziness. Tell your doctor if the dizziness or drowsiness continues.

If your mouth becomes dry, drink water, suck ice chips or a hard, sour candy (sugarless) or chew gum (sugarless). Sugarless products are recommended in order to avoid dental problems. You may wish to ask your pharmacist about special solutions, called artificial saliva, that can also be used to help restore moisture in the mouth. It is especially important to brush and floss your teeth regularly if you develop a dry mouth, to help prevent gum problems.

You may become more sensitive to heat because your body may

perspire less while you are taking this drug. Be careful not to become overheated during exercise or in hot weather. Try to avoid strenuous exercise, standing for long periods of time (especially in hot weather), hot showers, hot baths, saunas or Jacuzzis while taking this medicine.

When to Call Your Doctor

If you develop constipation, do not try to treat it yourself with nonprescription drugs. Call your doctor.

Most people experience few or no side effects from this drug. However, any medicine can sometimes cause unwanted effects. Call your doctor if you develop a sore throat, fever, mouth sores, a staggering walk, a yellow color to the skin or eyes, slow heartbeats or shortness of breath, unusual tiredness or nervousness, stomach pain, confusion or depression, hallucinations, trouble sleeping, seizures, slurred speech or severe drowsiness. Also call your doctor if you develop constipation, difficulty urinating (passing your water), eye pain or fast heartbeats.

Allergic Reactions

Call your doctor immediately if you think you may be allergic to the medicine or if you develop a skin rash, hives, itching, swelling of the face or difficulty in breathing. If you cannot reach your doctor, phone a hospital emergency department.

▶ **CHLOROTRIANISENE (ORAL)**
TACE

CONJUGATED ESTROGENS
C.E.S., CONGEST, PREMARIN

ESTRADIOL
ESTRACE

ESTROPIPATE
OGEN

ETHINYL ESTRADIOL
ESTINYL

ESTRADIOL (TRANSDERMAL)
ESTRADERM PATCH

ESTROGENS (VAGINAL)
OESTRILIN VAGINAL, ORTHO DIENESTROL CREAM, PREMARIN VAGINAL CREAM

Purpose

This medicine is a hormone commonly used to relieve hot flashes, sleep problems and sweating that may occur during menopause. The medicine has many other uses and the reason it was prescribed depends on your condition. If you do not understand why you are taking it, check with your doctor.

Allergies/Warnings

If you have ever had an allergic reaction to any medicine, tell your doctor and pharmacist before you take any of this medicine.

Also tell your doctor if you have had cancer or problems of the breast or uterus, changes in vaginal bleeding, endometriosis, blood clotting problems, migraine headaches, strokes or liver disease. The medicines should not be used in these conditions.

Also tell your doctor if you have had high blood pressure, heart or kidney disease, asthma, epilepsy, diabetes or depression. This will help your doctor decide whether estrogen therapy should be prescribed.

How to Use This Medicine

How to Administer
For tablets:
- Take the tablets after meals or with a snack if they upset your stomach. Call your doctor if the stomach upset continues.

For vaginal suppositories:
- *See* Vaginal Suppositories (page 44).

For vaginal creams:
- *See* Vaginal Creams, Ointments and Gels (page 42).

For ESTRADERM PATCHES:
- Apply the patch on the same 2 day(s) of the week. If you forget to change the patch on the correct day, change it as soon as you remember and continue to follow your ORIGINAL schedule. The patch is worn continuously for 3 to 4 days and is changed twice weekly.
- Apply the patch to a non-hairy area of the body that is not oily, damaged, irritated or exposed to the sun. Do not apply the patch over skin folds (for example, waistline or under tight clothing) since the patch may fall off. Suggested areas to apply the patch include the side of the torso, lower back or buttocks. Do not apply

ESTRADERM to the breasts or to skin that is exposed to the sun. The skin should be clean and dry so that the patch will stick to the skin.

- Tear open the foil pouch and remove the ESTRADERM PATCH. Do not use scissors to open the pouch since you may accidentally cut the patch.
- Loosen the protective liner on the back of the pouch by sliding the patch sideways between your thumb and index finger. Then remove the protective liner by holding at the edge with one hand and peeling back the liner with the other hand. Do not touch the sticky surface of the pouch.
- Apply the patch immediately by pressing the sticky side onto the chosen area of the skin. Press the patch firmly in place with the palm of your hand for about 10 seconds.
- Water (bath, pool, shower) will not damage the patch; however, very hot water or steam may loosen it.
- When it is time to apply a new patch, select a different area of the skin. You can use the same spot more than once — but not twice in a row.
- When you remove the used patch, fold it in half (with the sticky side inside) and throw it away, safely out of the reach of children.
- If the patch falls off, reapply the SAME patch to a DIFFERENT area of skin that is clean and dry. Continue to follow your ORIGINAL schedule for changing patches. If this patch will not stick to the new area, apply a new patch but continue with your original dosing schedule.
- Be sure to read the booklet "Estraderm and How To Use It" that comes with the medicine.

Special Instructions

Length of Therapy

Do not take this medicine more often or longer than recommended by your doctor. To do so may increase your chance of developing side effects.

Do not stop taking this medicine suddenly without the approval of your doctor.

Pregnancy/Breastfeeding

Women who are pregnant or planning to become pregnant should not take this medicine because it can cause birth defects.

Women who are breastfeeding should tell their doctor before taking this medicine.

Special Precautions

If you are taking the oral medicine for a long time, do not smoke while you are on this medicine, because smoking can increase the incidence of heart attacks and slow down the circulation of the blood.

Diabetic patients should regularly check the sugar in their urine or blood while they are taking this medicine.

If you are taking this medicine for a long time, it is recommended that you visit your doctor every 6 or every 12 months for follow-up to make sure that you are not developing side effects.

Call your doctor if you develop brown, blotchy spots. These spots may disappear or fade after you have stopped taking the drug.

If you were prescribed a vaginal cream or suppository:

• You may wish to wear a sanitary napkin to protect your clothing from the medicine. Do not use tampons while you are using the vaginal cream or suppository.

For additional information, read the leaflet "Information for the Patient" which was given to you by your pharmacist.

When to Call Your Doctor

Most people experience few or no side effects from this drug. However, any medicine can sometimes cause unwanted effects. Call your doctor immediately or go to the nearest hospital emergency department if you develop:

• Sudden, severe headaches.
• Sudden loss of coordination.
• Blurred vision or slurred speech.
• Pain in the calves of the legs or numbness in an arm or leg.
• Chest pain, shortness of breath or coughing of blood.

These side effects are rare but could be a sign that blood clots have formed.

Also call your doctor if you develop a skin rash, white vaginal discharge, abnormal vaginal bleeding, irregular or missed menstrual period, breast tenderness, lumps in the breast, dizziness, skin irritation with ESTRADERM PATCH, severe depression, a yellow color to the skin or eyes or dark-colored urine, severe abdominal pain, weight gain or swelling of the hands or ankles.

If you are using a vaginal cream or suppository:

• Call your doctor if the condition for which the drug is being used persists or becomes worse or if it causes a constant irritation such as itching or burning that was not present before you started using this medicine.

If you are using ESTRADERM PATCHES:
- If you develop bothersome redness or irritation in the area where the patch has been applied, tell your doctor.

Allergic Reactions

Call your doctor immediately if you think you may be allergic to the medicine or if you develop a skin rash, hives, itching, swelling of the face or difficulty in breathing. If you cannot reach your doctor, phone a hospital emergency department.

How Transdermal Patches Work

Some medicines for estrogen replacement, motion sickness and some heart conditions now come in the form of small adhesive bandages. They are called transdermal patches. *See* "How to Administer Transdermal Patches"(page 37).

The medicine is contained in a thin membrane and is slowly released through the skin directly into the bloodstream. Because the medicine bypasses the stomach and liver, lower dosages can be used and fewer side effects occur. This new form of treatment makes it much easier to use medicines since the person does not have to take the medicine as often.

Not every medicine is suitable for this dosage form:
- The molecules of the medicine must be small enough to pass through the skin and must not cause skin irritation.
- The medicine must be released at a rate that will result in correct blood levels. Some medicines are absorbed too slowly and are unsuitable.
- Another important factor is the quality of the person's skin. A young person's skin absorbs medicines differently from an older person's skin.
- Oiliness of the skin can affect the absorption of the drug and this is why the skin area should be cleansed and dried before a patch is applied.
- Hair can also interfere with the ability of the patch to stick and with the absorption of the medicine. For this reason, patches should be applied to non-hairy areas of skin.

Storage

For suppositories:
* *See* Vaginal Suppositories (page 44).

For Estraderm Patches:
* Store the patch in its original pouch at room temperature.

Refills

Do not stop taking this medicine without your doctor's approval and do not go without medicine between prescription refills. Call your pharmacist for a refill 2 or 3 days before you will run out of the medicine.

▶ **CHLORPHENIRAMINE MALEATE (ORAL)**
Chlor-Tripolon, Contac Allergy Formula, Novopheniram

CHLORPHENIRAMINE-PHENYLPROPANOLAMINE
Chlor-Tripolon Decongestant Syrup, Dristan Long Lasting Capsules, Ornade, Ornade-A.F., Triaminic Syrup

CHLORPHENIRAMINE-PHENYLPROPANOLAMINE-DEXTROMETHORPHAN
Ornade-DM 10 Pediatric, Ornade-DM 15, Ornade-DM 30

CHLORPHENIRAMINE-PHENYLPROPANOLAMINE-GUAIFENESIN
Ornade Expectorant

PHENIRAMINE-PHENYLPROPANOLAMINE-PYRILAMINE
Triaminic, Triaminic Oral Infant Drops

PHENIRAMINE-PHENYLPROPANOLAMINE-PYRILAMINE-GUAIFENESIN
Triaminic Expectorant

PHENIRAMINE-PHENYLPROPANOLAMINE-PYRILAMINE-GUAIFENESIN-DEXTROMETHORPHAN
Triaminic-DM

Purpose

This medicine is used to help relieve the symptoms of certain types of allergic conditions (such as hay fever), coughs and colds. Some of the products are also used to treat certain types of allergic skin conditions.

Allergies/Warnings

If you have ever had an allergic reaction to any medicine or if you have asthma, glaucoma, an enlarged prostate, urinary retention (a type of bladder problem), high blood pressure or diabetes, tell your doctor and pharmacist before you take any of this medicine.

How to Use This Medicine

Time of Administration

This medicine may be taken without regard to meals. Take it either with food or on an empty stomach. If stomach upset occurs, take it with some food or a glass of milk.

How to Administer

If you were prescribed a long-acting form of this medicine (CHLOR-TRIPOLON REPETABS, CONTAC ALLERGY FORMULA, DRISTAN LONG LASTING CAPSULES, ORNADE CAPSULES, ORNADE A.F. CAPSULES):

- This medicine lasts approximately 12 hours or longer and must be swallowed whole. Do not crush, chew or break it into pieces.

For liquid medicines:

- It is recommended that a medicine spoon be used to measure the dose. An average household teaspoon is not accurate.

For drops:

- If a dropper is used to measure the dose and you do not fully understand how to use it, *see* Medicine Dropper (page 21). Caution: Some drops are very concentrated. Be sure you know how much to use.

Special Instructions

Length of Therapy

Do not take this medicine more often or longer than recommended by your doctor. To do so may increase your chance of developing side effects.

Pregnancy/Breastfeeding

Women who are pregnant, breastfeeding or planning to become pregnant should tell their doctor before taking this medicine. Some of the products should not be taken during pregnancy or while breastfeeding.

Trouble Swallowing Tablets?

People who have dry mouths will often have trouble swallowing tablets.

This is a common problem in people who sleep with their mouths open, in elderly patients who are dehydrated and in patients taking medicines that can cause a dry mouth. It is very difficult to swallow a tablet if the mouth and throat are dry.

It may be easier to swallow tablets if a drink of water is taken before the medication is put into the mouth. This will moisten and lubricate the mucous membranes of the mouth and make it more slippery. Then put the tablet on the tongue and swallow the medicine with some more water.

Drug Interactions

It is important that you obtain the advice of your doctor or pharmacist before taking any other prescription or nonprescription medicines including pain relievers, sleeping pills, tranquilizers, medicine for seizures, muscle relaxants, anesthetics, medicines for depression or other medicines for allergies. Combining this medicine with some of these drugs could cause drowsiness or dizziness.

Drug interactions can occur. If you are taking any other medicines, be sure to check first with your pharmacist or doctor.

Alcohol

Do not drink alcoholic beverages while taking this drug without the approval of your doctor because the combination could cause drowsiness. One drink may have the same effect that 2 or 3 drinks normally would have.

Special Precautions

In some people, this drug may initially cause dizziness or drowsiness. Do not drive a car, pilot an airplane, operate dangerous machinery or do jobs that require you to be alert until you know how you are going to react to the drug. If you become dizzy or drowsy, you should be careful going up and down stairs. Sit or lie down at the first sign of dizziness. Tell your doctor if the dizziness or drowsiness continues.

People over 65 years of age may be more sensitive to these side effects.

If your mouth becomes dry, drink water, suck ice chips or a hard, sour candy (sugarless) or chew gum (sugarless). Sugarless products are recommended in order to avoid dental problems. You may wish to ask your pharmacist about special solutions, called artificial saliva, that can also be used to help restore moisture in the mouth. It is especially important to brush and floss your teeth regularly if you develop a dry mouth, to help prevent gum problems.

When to Call Your Doctor

Most people experience few or no side effects from this drug. However, any medicine can sometimes cause unwanted effects. Call your doctor if you develop a skin rash, fast or irregular heartbeats, blurred vision, stomach pain, unexplained weakness or tiredness, unexplained sore throat or fever, unusual bruising or bleeding, unexplained nervousness, restlessness or irritability (especially in children), trouble sleeping, difficulty in urinating (passing your water) or if mucous (lung secretions) becomes thicker than usual.

▶ **CHLORPROMAZINE HCl (ORAL and RECTAL)**
CHLORPROMANYL, LARGACTIL, NOVOCHLORPROMAZINE

FLUPHENAZINE HCl
APO-FLUPHENAZINE, MODITEN, PERMITIL

MESORIDAZINE
SERENTIL

METHOTRIMEPRAZINE
NOZINAN

PERPHENAZINE
APO-PERPHENAZINE, PMS PERPHENAZINE, TRILAFON

PROCHLORPERAZINE
PMS PROCHLORPERAZINE, PRORAZIN, STEMETIL

THIORIDAZINE HCl
APO-THIORIDAZINE, MELLARIL, NOVORIDAZINE, PMS THIORIDAZINE

TRIFLUOPERAZINE HCl
APO-TRIFLUOPERAZINE, NOVOFLURAZINE, PMS TRIFLUOPERAZINE, SOLAZINE, STELAZINE

Purpose

This medicine is used in the treatment of anxiety and tension and certain types of emotional problems such as severe anxiety, mood problems, confusion, troubling thoughts and feelings. Some products are also used to treat severe nausea and vomiting and some are used to treat severe hiccups. Check with your doctor if you do not fully understand why you are taking it.

Allergies/Warnings

If you have ever had an allergic reaction to any medicine or if you have high blood pressure, seizures, heart problems, enlarged prostate, difficulty urinating (passing your water), Parkinson's disease, liver disease, glaucoma or any other medical condition, tell your doctor and pharmacist before you take any of this medicine.

How to Use This Medicine

How to Administer
For tablets and capsules:
- If you develop stomach upset while taking this medicine, take it with food or immediately after a snack, unless otherwise directed.

For liquid medicine:
- If a dropper is used to measure the dose and you do not fully understand how to use it, *see* Medicine Dropper (page 21).
- If a spoon is used to measure the dose, it is recommended that you use a medicine spoon or an oral liquid syringe, which you can obtain from your pharmacist. These are more accurate than the average household teaspoon. *See* Oral Liquid Syringe (page 17) and Medicine Spoon (page 22).

For other liquid medicines:
- Check with your pharmacist to see if you can dilute it.

If you were prescribed MELLARIL SUSPENSION:
- Shake the bottle well each time before measuring a dose.

For suppositories:
- *See* Rectal Suppositories (page 39).

Special Instructions

Length of Therapy

The full effect of this medicine may not be noticed immediately and may take several weeks. Be patient. Take the medicine regularly and try not to miss any doses.

Do not stop taking this medicine suddenly without the approval of your doctor. It may be necessary for your doctor to reduce your dose slowly since your body will need time to adjust. It could make your condition worse if you suddenly stopped taking the medicine. After you have stopped taking this medicine, you may have to continue to observe the following precautions for 1 to 2 weeks since some of the medicine may still be in your body.

Pregnancy/Breastfeeding

Women who are pregnant, breastfeeding or planning to become pregnant should not take this medicine without their doctor's approval.

Drug Interactions

It is best not to take this medicine at the same time as an antacid or an anti-diarrhea medicine containing aluminum. Try to space them 2 hours apart if you must take them while you are on this medicine.

It is important that you obtain the advice of your doctor or pharmacist before taking any other prescription or nonprescription medicines, including pain relievers, sleeping pills, other tranquilizers or medicines for depression, cough, cold or allergies.

There have been some reports that caffeine (in coffee, tea, colas and some nonprescription drugs) may decrease the effect of this medicine.

There are other drug interactions that can occur. If you are taking any other medicines, be sure to check first with your pharmacist or doctor.

Alcohol

Do not drink alcoholic beverages while taking this drug without the approval of your doctor. The combination could irritate your stomach and could cause drowsiness or dizziness. One drink may have the same effect that 2 or 3 drinks normally would have.

If you have been taking this medicine regularly for several days or weeks, it is recommended not to drink alcohol for 2 weeks *after* you have stopped taking the medicine. Depending on your dose, it may take this long for the drug to be eliminated from your body.

Special Precautions

If this medicine causes dizziness or lightheadedness, you should be careful going up and down stairs and you should not change positions too rapidly. Lightheadedness is more likely to occur if you stand up suddenly—this is due to blood collecting in the legs and lasts for a few seconds. Therefore, get up from a sitting or lying position more slowly and tighten and relax your leg muscles or wiggle your toes to help promote circulation. In the morning, get out of bed slowly and dangle your feet over the edge of the bed for a few minutes before standing up. Sit or lie down at the first sign of dizziness. Tell your doctor if you have been dizzy.

You may become more sensitive to heat because your body may perspire less while you are taking this drug. Be careful not to become overheated during exercise or in hot weather. Try to avoid strenuous exercise, standing for long periods of time (especially in hot weather), hot showers, hot baths, saunas or Jacuzzis while taking this medicine.

Some patients may also become more sensitive to cold and should dress warmly during cold weather and limit exposure to cold temperatures.

This medicine commonly causes drowsiness, especially during the first week of treatment. Make sure you know how you are going to react to this medicine and whether it will make you dizzy or drowsy. Do not drive a car, pilot an airplane, operate dangerous machinery or do jobs that require you to be alert if you are dizzy or drowsy. The drowsiness may decrease over time.

If your mouth becomes dry, drink water, suck ice chips or a hard, sour candy (sugarless) or chew gum (sugarless). Sugarless products are recommended in order to avoid dental problems. You may wish to ask your pharmacist about special solutions, called artificial saliva, that can also be used to help restore moisture in the mouth. It is especially important to brush and floss your teeth regularly if you develop a dry mouth, to help prevent gum problems.

This medicine often makes some people more sensitive to sunlight and some tanning lamps. When you begin taking this medicine, try to avoid too much sun until you see how you are going to react. If your skin does become more sensitive to sunlight, tell your doctor and try not to stay in direct sunlight for extended periods of time. While in the sun, wear protective clothing and sunglasses. You may wish to ask your pharmacist about suitable sunscreen products. Call your doctor if you become sunburned.

An urge to urinate (pass your water) with an inability to do so sometimes occurs with this drug. Urinating before taking the drug each time may help relieve this problem. Tell your doctor you are having this problem.

There have been some reports that this medicine may cause the urine to turn pink, red or red-brown in color. This is only temporary and will go away after you have finished the medicine.

When to Call Your Doctor

Call your doctor if you become restless, unable to sit still or sleep, or if you develop unusual muscle stiffness, drooling, disturbed gait, shuffling walk, tremors, shakiness or unusual movements of the face, tongue or hands, or stiffness of the face or body. If you develop painful muscle spasms, call your doctor or the hospital emergency room, since treatment can be given to provide rapid relief of this problem.

Check with your doctor if you develop constipation.

Any medicine can sometimes cause unwanted effects. Call your doctor if you develop a sore throat, fever, mouth sores, eye pain or changes in vision, difficulty in urinating (passing your water), difficulty breathing, speaking or swallowing, a yellow color in the skin or eyes, dark yellow-colored urine, fast heartbeats, fever, seizures, a skin rash, fainting spells or decreased sexual ability.

Medicines That Make Some People More Sensitive to Heat

Certain drugs may make a person more vulnerable to heat exhaustion and heatstroke.

Recent summer heat waves have caused thousands of cases of heat-related illness. The most important method of regulating the temperature of the body is sweating. As sweat evaporates on the skin, it has a cooling effect. Sweat must evaporate, however, and when the relative humidity increases, less sweat evaporates. The hotter the temperature, the higher the humidity and the brighter the sun's rays, the greater the risk.

Patients taking any of the following drugs are at greater risk because the medications may:
- impair their ability to sweat or regulate the body temperature
- increase fluid loss

- increase the rate of metabolism of the body, which in turn increases the body temperature

Anticholinergic drugs such as ATROPINE, BENZTROPINE and SCOPOLAMINE

Diuretics ("Water Pills") such as HYDROCHLOROTHIAZIDE and FUROSEMIDE

Phenothiazines such as CHLORPROMAZINE

Tricyclic Antidepressants such as AMITRIPTYLINE, IMIPRAMINE, NORTRIPTYLINE and PROTRIPTYLINE

Monoamine Oxidase Inhibitors such as ISOCARBOXAZID, PHENELZINE and TRANYLCYPROMINE

Beta-Blockers such as PROPRANOLOL

Alcohol

Excessive Laxatives

Sunscreens used while exercising in hot weather

Other Drugs such as AMPHETAMINE, anesthetics, barbiturates and some cancer drugs

Patients taking any medicine that can increase their sensitivity to heat should take the following precautions to stay as cool as possible during heat waves:
- Increase fluid and salt intakes, unless they are restricted because of a medical condition.
- Avoid strenuous exercise.
- Avoid Jacuzzis, hot baths, saunas and hot showers (year-round).
- Contact a physician at the slightest sign of heat illness.

Storage
For liquid medicine:
- Store the liquid medicine in a cool, dark place.

For LARGACTIL LIQUID *or* LARGACTIL ORAL DROPS:
- Throw away the medicine if it turns dark in color.

For MODITEN ELIXIR:
- Do not freeze the medicine.

For suppositories:
- *See* Rectal Suppositories (page 39).

Refills
Do not stop taking this medicine without your doctor's approval and do not go without medicine between prescription refills. Call your pharmacist for a refill 2 or 3 days before you will run out of the medicine.

Discuss with your pharmacist the implications of dispensing all your refills for this medicine with the same manufacturer's product. (*See* Generic Drugs, page 13.)

Miscellaneous
Carry an identification card in your wallet or wear a medical alert bracelet indicating that you are taking this medicine, as well as the names and phone numbers of your doctors. If you do not already carry such a card, complete the Medicine Card in this book. Always tell your dentist, pharmacist and other doctors who are treating you that you are taking this medicine.

▶ CHOLESTYRAMINE RESIN (ORAL)
QUESTRAN, QUESTRAN LIGHT

COLESTIPOL
COLESTID

Purpose
This medicine is used to reduce lipids and cholesterol in the blood.

CHOLESTYRAMINE is also used to control certain types of diarrhea and to relieve itching in some conditions.

Allergies/Warnings
If you have ever had an allergic reaction to any medicine or are taking other medicines to lower cholesterol, tell your doctor and pharmacist before you take any of this medicine.

How to Use This Medicine

How to Administer

If you have been prescribed QUESTRAN *or* QUESTRAN LIGHT:

- This medicine must *not* be taken as a dry powder. Each packet or scoopful of powder must be mixed with 4 to 6 ounces (120 to 180 mL) of liquid such as water, fruit juice, milk or non-carbonated beverages, and mixed well. It may also be mixed with very liquid soups or pulpy foods such as applesauce or crushed pineapple.

If you have been prescribed COLESTID:

- This medicine must *not* be taken as a dry powder. The contents of each packet must be mixed well with at least 3 ounces (90 mL) of liquid such as water, fruit juice, milk or carbonated beverages, and mixed well. It may also be mixed with very liquid soups or pulpy foods such as applesauce or crushed pineapple.

Special Instructions

Length of Therapy

It is very important to take this medicine exactly as your doctor has prescribed. Do not increase or decrease the amount you are taking without first consulting your doctor. Otherwise, you cannot expect the medicine to control your condition.

Pregnancy/Breastfeeding

Women who are pregnant, breastfeeding or planning to become pregnant should tell their doctor before taking this medicine.

Drug Interactions

This medicine may interact with certain other medicines if taken at the same time. Therefore, take any other medicine at least 1 hour before or 4 to 6 hours after taking this medicine. You should talk with your physician or pharmacist to get advice on exactly how to adjust the times to take your medicines. Also, do not stop taking any drugs you are currently taking without first consulting your physician.

Special Precautions

Your doctor may prescribe a special diet while you are taking this medicine. Be sure to follow the diet closely as this will also help to control your condition.

If you are taking this medicine for a long time, your doctor may recommend that you take vitamin supplements.

This medicine may cause some people to become constipated. To prevent constipation, try increasing the amount of bulk in your diet (for example, bran, fresh fruits and salads), exercising more often or drinking more fluids (unless otherwise directed). Call your doctor if the constipation continues.

This medicine may cause a feeling of indigestion, stomach discomfort, gas or mild nausea. These can usually be avoided if the dosage is gradually increased when you start treatment or change dosage.

When to Call Your Doctor

Most people experience few or no side effects from this drug. However, any medicine can sometimes cause unwanted effects. Call your doctor if you develop a skin rash, difficulty in breathing, wheezing, unusual bruising, joint pain, changes in vision, black stools or blood in the stools, or if you continue to have problems with stomach upset or constipation.

Allergic Reactions

Call your doctor immediately if you think you may be allergic to the medicine or if you develop a skin rash, hives, itching, swelling of the face or difficulty in breathing. If you cannot reach your doctor, phone a hospital emergency department.

Refills

Do not stop taking this medicine without your doctor's approval and do not go without medicine between prescription refills. Call your pharmacist for a refill 2 or 3 days before you run out of the medicine.

▶ **CIMETIDINE (ORAL)**
APO-CIMETIDINE, NOVOCIMETINE, PEPTOL, TAGAMET

FAMOTIDINE
PEPCID

NIZATIDINE
AXID

RANITIDINE
APO-RANITIDINE, NOVORANIDINE, ZANTAC, ZANTAC-C

Purpose

This medicine is used in the treatment and prevention of certain types of stomach and duodenal ulcers and in conditions in which the stomach is producing too much acid. The medicine is also used to help relieve both day- and night-time symptoms (e.g., heartburn, sour taste, coughing, choking, etc.) of gastroesophageal reflux disease.

Allergies/Warnings

If you have ever had an allergic reaction to any medicine, tell your doctor and pharmacist before you take any of this medicine.

How to Use This Medicine

How to Administer

This medicine may be taken with or without food depending upon your condition.

If you develop stomach pain between doses of this medicine, ask your doctor if you may take an antacid between doses. The two medicines should not be taken at the same time. Ask your doctor or pharmacist how many hours you must wait before you take the other medicine.

For liquid medicines:

- It is recommended that you use a medicine spoon to measure each dose. A medicine spoon is more accurate than the average household teaspoon. See Medicine Spoon (page 22).

Special Instructions

Length of Therapy

It is very important that you take this medicine for the full length of treatment your doctor has prescribed, even if your symptoms have stopped. Try not to miss any doses because the medicine will not be as effective. It may take several days or a few weeks before you feel the full benefit of this medicine.

Do not stop taking the medicine suddenly without the approval of your doctor.

Pregnancy/Breastfeeding

Women who are pregnant, breastfeeding or planning to become pregnant should tell their doctor before taking this medicine.

Drug Interactions

There have been some reports that antacids may decrease the effect of this medicine. The interaction can probably be avoided by taking them at different times. Ask your doctor or pharmacist how many hours you must wait before you take the other medicine.

Smoking cigarettes appears to decrease the effect of this medicine and lengthen the time it takes an ulcer to heal. Do not smoke while taking this drug.

There are other interactions that can occur. If you are taking any other medicines, be sure to check with your doctor or pharmacist.

Alcohol

Do not drink alcoholic beverages while taking this drug because it may make the ulcer pain worse and interfere with healing of the ulcer.

Special Precautions

People with ulcers should generally avoid medicines that can upset the stomach, such as ASA or salicylates, since they may interfere with healing of the ulcer. Always read the label and check with your pharmacist if you have any questions. Also avoid those foods and beverages that cause your ulcer symptoms to reappear.

Rarely, this drug may cause dizziness. Do not drive a car, pilot an airplane, operate dangerous machinery or do jobs that require you to be alert until you know how you are going to react to the drug. If you become dizzy, you should be careful going up and down stairs. Sit or lie down at the first sign of dizziness. Tell your doctor if the dizziness continues.

For AXID, TAGAMET and ZANTAC:
- Rarely, some people taking this medicine may notice a slight increase in the size of their breasts or some breast soreness. This is temporary and will go away after the treatment has ended. Tell your doctor if you develop this problem.

When to Call Your Doctor

Call your doctor immediately if you are being treated for an ulcer and you develop fainting spells, unusual thirst, dizziness, sweating, vomiting of blood or bloody or black stools. This may mean your condition is getting worse.

Most people experience few or no side effects from this drug. However, any medicine can sometimes cause unwanted effects. Call your doctor if you develop a skin rash, unexplained sore throat, fever, muscle cramps or joint pain, unusual bruising or bleeding, severe diarrhea, changes in sexual ability, bothersome headaches, bothersome constipation or hallucinations, or if you become confused or restless.

Allergic Reactions

Call your doctor immediately if you think you may be allergic to the medicine or if you develop a skin rash, hives, itching, swelling of the face or difficulty in breathing. If you cannot reach your doctor, phone a hospital emergency department.

▶ CIPROFLOXACIN (ORAL)
Cipro

NORFLOXACIN
Noroxin

Purpose

This medicine is an antibiotic used to treat certain types of infections. Your doctor has prescribed this antibiotic for your present infection only. Do not use it for other infections or give it to other people.

Allergies/Warnings

If you have ever had an allergic reaction to medicine used to treat infections or any other medicine, or if you have any allergies (for example, asthma or hay fever), tell your doctor and pharmacist before you take any of this medicine.

How to Use This Medicine

Time of Administration

This medicine is best taken on an empty stomach. However, it may be taken before or after meals. Space the doses of medicine around the clock (throughout the entire day of 24 hours). For example, if you take two doses each day, space the doses 12 hours apart. This will keep a constant level of medicine in your body.

How to Administer

Take the medicine with a full glass of water and try to drink at least 6 to 8 additional glasses of water or other liquids every day, unless otherwise directed by your doctor. This will help prevent unwanted side effects on the kidneys. If the medicine was prescribed to treat a bladder infection, the extra water intake will help wash the bacteria causing the infection out in the urine.

Special Instructions

Length of Therapy

It is important to take all of this medicine plus any refills that your doctor has prescribed. Do not stop taking this medicine earlier than your doctor has recommended, even if you begin to feel better. If you stop taking the medicine too soon, the infection may return.

Pregnancy/Breastfeeding

Women who are pregnant or planning to become pregnant should tell their doctor before taking this medicine.

This medicine should not be given to infants. Mothers who are breastfeeding (nursing) should discuss this with their doctors before taking this medicine and breastfeeding.

Drug Interactions

This medicine may interact with other medicines. If you are taking any other medicine, be sure to check with your doctor or pharmacist.
- Some antacids and laxatives can make this medicine less effective if they are taken at the same time. This includes products which contain aluminum, magnesium or sucralfate. Check with your pharmacist before you purchase any antacids or laxatives. If you must take certain laxatives or antacids, they should not be taken within 2 hours of each other.
- Avoid drinking large amounts of coffee or caffeine-containing beverages while taking this medicine. The effects of caffeine may be increased and last longer when you are taking this medicine.

If you were prescribed CIPRO:
- Iron and zinc medicine or vitamins containing minerals can also make this medicine less effective. If you must take iron, zinc or vitamins containing minerals, take them at least 3 hours before or 2 hours after the medicine.

Special Precautions

If this medicine causes dizziness or lightheadedness, you should be careful going up or down stairs and you should not change positions too rapidly. Sit or lie down at the first sign of dizziness. Do not drive a car, pilot an airplane, operate dangerous machinery or do jobs that require you to be alert if you are dizzy.

This medicine should not be given to children prior to the onset of puberty unless otherwise directed.

This medicine may make some people more sensitive to sunlight and some tanning lamps. When you begin taking this medicine, try to avoid too much sun until you see how you are going to react. If your skin does become more sensitive to sunlight, tell your doctor and try not to stay in direct sunlight for extended periods of time. While in the sun, wear protective clothing and sunglasses. You may wish to ask your pharmacist about suitable sunscreen products. Call your doctor if you become sunburned.

When to Call Your Doctor

Call your doctor if your symptoms do not improve within a few days or if they become worse.

Most people experience few or no side effects from this drug. However, any medicine can sometimes cause unwanted effects. Call your doctor if you develop tremor (shakiness), severe lightheadedness, skin rash, dark-colored tongue, sore throat or tongue, headache, sore or aching joints. Also call your doctor if you develop rectal itching or, in women, a vaginal discharge that was not present before you started taking this medicine.

Allergic Reactions

Call your doctor immediately if you think you may be allergic to the medicine or if you develop a skin rash, hives, itching, swelling of the face or difficulty in breathing. If you cannot reach a doctor, phone a hospital emergency department.

▶ CISAPRIDE
PREPULSID

Purpose
This medicine is used to treat certain types of stomach and intestinal conditions in which there is nausea, vomiting and a persistent feeling of fullness after eating. It is used to treat conditions in which food regurgitates (flows back) from the stomach into the esophagus.

Allergies/Warnings

If you have ever had an allergic reaction to any medicine, tell your doctor and pharmacist before you take any of this medicine.

How to Use This Medicine

Time of Administration

Take this medicine 15 minutes *before* eating food unless otherwise directed.

If your physician prescribes a dose at bedtime, be sure to drink a large glass of water or eat a snack 15 to 30 minutes *after* taking this medicine.

Special Instructions

Pregnancy/Breastfeeding

Women who are pregnant, breastfeeding or planning to become pregnant should tell their doctor before taking this medicine.

Drug Interactions

Do not start or stop taking any medicines that you are currently taking without first consulting your doctor. It is important that you obtain the advice of your doctor or pharmacist before taking any other prescription or nonprescription medicines including sleeping pills, tranquilizers, medicines for seizures, anticoagulants ("blood thinners"), muscle relaxants, pain relievers, medicines for allergies, diarrhea or glaucoma. Combining these drugs with this medicine could cause drowsiness or alter the effect of the medicine.

There are other drug interactions that can occur. If you are taking other medicines, be sure to check first with your doctor or pharmacist.

Alcohol

Do not drink alcoholic beverages while taking this medication because the combination could cause drowsiness. One drink may have the same effect as 2 or 3 drinks.

When to Call Your Doctor

Most people experience few or no side effects from this drug. However, any medicine can sometimes cause unwanted effects. Call your doctor if you develop severe diarrhea, stomach or abdominal cramps or constipation.

Allergic Reactions

Call your doctor immediately if you think you may be allergic to the medicine or if you develop a skin rash, hives, itching, swelling of the face or difficulty in breathing.

Storage

Store the medicine at room temperature, away from heat, moisture and light.

▶ CLOBAZAM (ORAL)
FRISIUM

Purpose

This medicine is used to help control seizures. It is commonly used in the treatment of epilepsy.

Allergies/Warnings

If you have ever had an allergic reaction to any medicine, tell your doctor or pharmacist before taking this medicine.

How to Use This Medicine

Time of Administration

If you take this medicine once a day, take it at bedtime. If you take 2 doses of medicine, take the larger dose at bedtime.

How to Administer

Take this medicine on an empty stomach with a full glass of water.

Special Instructions

Length of Therapy

Do not stop taking this medicine suddenly without the approval of your doctor. It may be necessary for your doctor to reduce your dose slowly since your body may need time to adjust. Check with your doctor if you develop any of the following symptoms while you are slowly reducing the medicine or after you have stopped the medicine: nausea or vomiting, trembling, seizures, muscle cramps, stomach cramps, unusual sweating, difficulty sleeping. Also call your doctor if you become confused, irritable or nervous.

Pregnancy/Breastfeeding

Women who are pregnant, breastfeeding or planning to become pregnant should tell their doctor before taking this medicine. Generally, this medication should not be used during pregnancy and is not recommended during breastfeeding.

Drug Interactions

This medicine may interact with other medicines used to treat seizures. Therefore, do not stop taking this medicine or other anti-seizure medicines without checking first with your doctor or pharmacist.

It is important that you obtain the advice of your doctor or pharmacist before you take any prescription or non-prescription medicine including pain relievers, cough, cold or allergy medicine, sleeping pills, tranquilizers or medicines for depression.

Alcohol

Do not drink alcoholic beverages while taking this medicine or for several days after you have stopped taking this drug, without the approval of your doctor. Use of this medicine with alcohol may cause increased drowsiness, dizziness and irritability (rare).

Special Precautions

In some people, this drug may cause dizziness or drowsiness. Do not drive a car, pilot an airplane, operate dangerous machinery or do jobs that require you to be alert if you are drowsy or dizzy. You should also be careful going up and down stairs. Sit or lie down at the first sign of dizziness. Tell your doctor if the dizziness or drowsiness continues.

Be sure to keep your doctor's appointments so that your doctor can check your progress. This is especially important during the first few months of therapy, when the doctor will decide the best dose of this medicine for your condition. While you are taking this medicine, it is important that you go to have any blood tests which your doctor may recommend.

When to Call Your Doctor

Any medicine can sometimes cause unwanted side effects. Call your doctor if you develop weight gain, blurred vision, severe drowsiness or dizziness, unusual tiredness or nervousness, staggering walk, restlessness or irritability, hostile feelings, confusion or depression. Call your doctor if you have an increase in the frequency of seizures.

Refills

Do not stop taking this medicine without your doctor's approval and do not go without medicine between prescription refills. Call your pharmacist 2 or 3 days before you will run out of the medicine.

Miscellaneous

Carry an identification card in your wallet or wear a medical alert bracelet indicating that you are taking this medicine, as well as the names and phone numbers of your doctor. If you do not already carry such a card, complete the Medicine Card in this book.

▶ **CLOFIBRATE**
ATROMID-S

FENOFIBRATE
LIPIDIL

Purpose

This medicine is used to lower cholesterol and lipids in the blood.

Allergies/Warnings

If you have ever had an allergic reaction to any medicine or are taking any other medicines to lower cholesterol, tell your doctor and pharmacist before you take any of this medicine. Before taking this medicine, tell your doctor if you have ever had liver or kidney problems.

How to Use This Medicine

Time of Administration

This medicine should be taken with meals.

Special Instructions

Pregnancy/Breastfeeding

Women who are pregnant, planning to become pregnant or breastfeeding should tell their doctor before taking this medicine. This medicine is not recommended for patients who are pregnant or breastfeeding.

It is recommended that women taking this medicine use an effective form of birth control in order to avoid becoming pregnant.

Drug Interactions

Some prescription drugs can interact with this medicine. Therefore, do not start or stop taking any medicines you are currently taking without first asking your doctor.

Special Precautions

It is very important to take this medicine exactly as your doctor has prescribed. Otherwise, you cannot expect the medicine to control your condition.

Follow any special diet, exercise and/or weight loss programs prescribed by your doctor.

It is important that you go to have any blood tests which your doctor may recommend while you are taking this medicine.

If this medicine causes dizziness or lightheadedness, you should be careful going up and down stairs and you should not change positions too quickly. This medicine may also cause drowsiness. Do not drive a car, pilot an airplane, operate dangerous machinery or do jobs that require you to be alert if you are dizzy or drowsy.

Medicines Are Not "Candy"

There are many candies that look like medicines and some medicines that look like candies. Parents should not confuse children further by sending mixed signals that their medicines *taste* like candy.

Children are naturally curious and will put virtually everything they can hold into their mouths. Unfortunately, this includes medicines, poisons and objects that can obstruct their airways. If you have young children, watch out for the following items:

- Miniature plastic replicas that look or smell like fruit or candy
- Tiny, compressed sponge toys, often packaged in capsules, that expand in water to form zoo animals
- Medicines that look like candy

As long as candies and toys that look like medicines are available to the public, parents should take steps to protect young children from accidentally swallowing these items.

When to Call Your Doctor

Most people experience few or no side effects from this medicine. However, any medicine can sometimes cause unwanted effects. Call your doctor if you develop severe stomach upset (nausea, vomiting, gas), sore throat, fever, mouth sores, heart palpitations, flu-like symptoms (muscle aches and pains, weakness), sudden decrease in the amount of urine, bloody or cloudy urine, or pain on urinating (passing your water).

Storage

Store this medicine in a cool, dark place away from children.

▶ **CLONIDINE (ORAL)**
CATAPRES, DIXARIT

CLONIDINE-CHLORTHALIDONE (ORAL)
COMBIPRES

Purpose

This medicine is commonly used to treat high blood pressure. DIXARIT is also used to control hot flashes during menopause.

Allergies/Warnings

Be sure to tell your doctor and pharmacist if you are allergic to any medicine.

If you were prescribed COMBIPRES:
• Be sure to tell your doctor and pharmacist if you are allergic to sulfa drugs, thiazide diuretics or any medicine.

How to Use This Medicine

Time of Administration

Try to take the medicine at the same time(s) each day so that you have a constant level of the medicine in your body.

If you were prescribed CATAPRES:
• The last dose of CATAPRES is usually taken immediately before going to bed. This helps to control your blood pressure during the night and also helps to reduce daytime drowsiness.

If you were prescribed COMBIPRES:
- When you first start taking this medicine, you will probably urinate (pass your water) more often and in larger amounts than usual. Therefore, if you are to take 1 dose each day, your doctor may want you to take it in the morning after breakfast. If you take it in the morning, be alert for possible drowsiness and dizziness (*see* Special Precautions).
- If you are to take more than 1 dose each day, ask your doctor if you can take the last dose approximately 6 hours before bedtime so that you will not have to get up during the night to go to the bathroom. This effect will usually lessen after you have taken the drug for awhile.

How to Administer
Take the medicine with food or a glass of water.

Special Instructions

Length of Therapy
If you were prescribed this medicine for high blood pressure:
- High blood pressure (hypertension) is a long-term condition and it will probably be necessary for you to take the drug for a long time in spite of the fact that you feel better. If high blood pressure is not treated, it can lead to serious problems such as heart failure, strokes, blood vessel problems or kidney problems.
- It is very important that you take this medicine as your doctor has directed and that you do not miss any doses. Otherwise, you cannot expect the drug to keep your blood pressure down.

Do not take any more of this medicine than your doctor has prescribed and *do not stop taking this medicine suddenly without the approval of your doctor*. It will be necessary for your doctor to reduce your dose slowly over 2 to 4 days since your body will need time to adjust. It could be harmful and make your condition worse if you suddenly stopped taking the medicine. Call your doctor if you develop any of the following symptoms as you are stopping the medicine: fast heartbeats, chest pain, nausea, vomiting, unexplained nervousness, shaking, headache, flushing or stomach pain.

Pregnancy/Breastfeeding
Women who are pregnant, breastfeeding or planning to become pregnant should tell their doctor before taking this medicine.

Drug Interactions

Do not take any nonprescription drugs without the approval of your doctor or pharmacist. Some of these products can aggravate your condition and some can combine with this medicine and make the drowsiness or dizziness worse. Read the label of the product to see if there is a warning. If there is, check with your doctor or pharmacist before using the product.

Alcohol

You may become more sensitive to alcohol while you are taking this medicine. Do not drink alcoholic beverages while you are on this drug because the combination could make the possible side effects of dizziness and drowsiness worse.

Special Precautions

If this medicine causes dizziness or lightheadedness, you should be careful going up and down stairs and you should not change positions too rapidly. Lightheadedness is more likely to occur if you stand up suddenly—this is due to blood collecting in the legs and lasts for a few seconds. Therefore, get up from a sitting or lying position more slowly and tighten and relax your leg muscles or wiggle your toes to help promote circulation. In the morning, get out of bed slowly and dangle your feet over the edge of the bed for a few minutes before standing up. Sit or lie down at the first sign of dizziness. Tell your doctor if you have been dizzy.

In order to help prevent dizziness or fainting, your doctor may also recommend that you avoid strenuous exercise, standing for long periods of time (especially in hot weather), hot showers, hot baths or saunas.

Do not drive a car, operate dangerous machinery, pilot an airplane or do jobs that require you to be alert if you are dizzy or drowsy.

If your mouth becomes dry, drink water, suck ice chips or a hard, sour candy (sugarless) or chew gum (sugarless). Sugarless products are recommended in order to avoid dental problems. You may wish to ask your pharmacist about special solutions, called artificial saliva, that can also be used to help restore moisture in the mouth. It is especially important to brush and floss your teeth regularly if you develop a dry mouth, to help prevent gum problems.

This medicine may cause some people to become constipated. To help prevent constipation, try increasing the amount of bulk in your diet (for example, bran, fresh fruits and salads), exercising more often or drinking more fluids (unless otherwise directed). Call your doctor if the constipation continues.

The side effects of dizziness, constipation and tiredness usually decrease after you have taken the medicine for 4 to 6 weeks.

Follow any special diet your doctor may have prescribed. It may be necessary to limit the amount of salt in your diet.

Your doctor may want you to have regular eye checkups if you will be taking this medicine for a long period of time.

If your eyes become dry, ask your doctor or pharmacist to recommend artificial tears to wet the eyes. Call your doctor if you experience itching or burning of your eyes.

If you were prescribed COMBIPRES, *the following special instructions also apply:*

- This medicine normally causes your body to lose potassium. The body has warning signs to let you know if too much potassium is being lost. Call your doctor if you become unusually thirsty or if you develop leg cramps, unusual weakness, fatigue, vomiting, confusion or an irregular pulse. Since these symptoms may not be present in all patients, your doctor may wish to check your blood occasionally to see if it is low in potassium. Depending upon your dose, your doctor may prescribe some medicine to replace the potassium or he or she may recommend that you regularly eat foods that contain a lot of potassium (see Appendix A). *Do not change your diet unless your doctor tells you to.*
- This medicine may make some people more sensitive to sunlight and some tanning lamps. When you begin taking this medicine, try to avoid too much sun until you see how you are going to react. If your skin does become more sensitive to sunlight, tell your doctor and try not to stay in direct sunlight for extended periods of time. While in the sun, wear protective clothing and sunglasses. You may wish to ask your pharmacist about suitable sunscreen products. Call your doctor if you become sunburned.
- If you have diabetes, this medicine may cause your blood sugar to rise. Carefully test your blood or urine for sugar while you are taking this medicine. Call your doctor if you think your blood sugar is higher than normal or harder to control.

When to Call Your Doctor

Any medicine can sometimes cause unwanted effects. Call your doctor if you develop paleness or coldness in the fingertips or toes, nightmares, impotence, decreased sexual function, difficulty breathing, unusual tiredness or weakness, swelling of the feet or ankles or depression.

If you were prescribed COMBIPRES:

- In addition to the previous symptoms, also call your doctor if you develop an unexplained sore throat or fever, sharp stomach pain, sharp joint pain, unusual bruising or bleeding, a yellow color to the skin or eyes, or a sudden weight gain of 5 pounds (2.5 kg) or more.

Allergic Reactions

Call your doctor immediately if you think you may be allergic to the medicine or if you develop a skin rash, hives, itching, swelling of the face or difficulty in breathing. If you cannot reach your doctor, phone a hospital emergency department.

Refills

Do not stop taking this medicine without your doctor's approval and do not go without medicine between prescription refills. Call your pharmacist for a refill 2 or 3 days before you will run out of the medicine.

Miscellaneous

Carry an identification card in your wallet or wear a medical alert bracelet indicating that you are taking this medicine, as well as the names and phone numbers of your doctors. If you do not already carry such a card, complete the Medicine Card in this book. Always tell your dentist, pharmacist and other doctors who are treating you that you are taking this medicine.

Always Go to the SAME Pharmacy

You should have all your prescriptions filled at the same pharmacy so that the pharmacist can keep a complete record of your medicines.

This is especially important if you are being treated by more than one doctor. Some drugs can interact with each other and cause serious problems.

Just as your doctor keeps your medical record, pharmacists keep "drug records" or "drug profiles" for their patients. These drug profiles make it possible for the pharmacist to review your drug therapy each time you have a prescription filled and to help prevent you from receiving any drugs which can interact with each other.

▶ **CICLOPIROX OLAMINE (TOPICAL)**
LOPROX

CLOTRIMAZOLE
CANESTEN, CLOTRIMADERM, MYCLO

CLOTRIMAZOLE (VAGINAL)
CANESTEN, CANESTEN 1, CANESTEN 1 COMBI-PAK, CANESTEN 3,
CLOTRIMADERM, MYCLO

Purpose
This medicine is used to treat fungal and yeast infections.

Allergies/Warnings
Be sure to tell your doctor and pharmacist if you are allergic to any medicine.

How to Use This Medicine

Time of Administration
The vaginal medicine is usually used at bedtime when you are lying down so that the drug is less likely to drain out.

How to Administer
For skin cream and solution:
- *See* Creams, Ointments, Gels, Solutions and Lotions (page 36).

For vaginal creams:
- *See* Vaginal Creams, Ointments and Gels (page 42).

For vaginal tablets:
- *See* Vaginal Tablets, Ovules and Inserts (page 43).

For CANESTEN SOLUTION WITH SPRAY:
- Cleanse the affected area well unless otherwise directed by your doctor. Dry the area.

Spray the prescribed amount of solution and massage into the affected and surrounding areas. Do NOT spray the solution on the face.

Special Instructions

Length of Therapy
It is important to use all of this medicine, plus any refills that your doctor told you to use. Do not stop using it earlier than your doctor

has recommended in spite of the fact that your symptoms seem to have improved. Otherwise, the infection may return.

Recurrences are common, and at the first sign of any recurrence, call your doctor. Sometimes it may be necessary to use this medicine long-term, if you have frequent recurrent infections.

Pregnancy/Breastfeeding

Women who are pregnant, breastfeeding or planning to become pregnant should tell their doctor before taking this medicine. The vaginal medicines should not be used during the first 3 months of pregnancy unless otherwise directed by your doctor.

If you are pregnant, check with your doctor before using the applicator to insert the vaginal cream or tablets.

Special Precautions

If you are using this medicine to treat a fungal infection of the feet, it is important to dry the feet (especially between the toes) well after washing.

If you are using this medicine to treat a vaginal infection, you may wish to wear a sanitary napkin to protect your clothing from any drainage of the drug. Do *not* use menstrual tampons without your doctor's approval while using this drug.

In the treatment of vaginal infections, the drug is usually used throughout the menstrual period. Check with your doctor if you can have sexual intercourse or if you can douche during treatment.

It is important to wash all towels, linens, bedding and clothing in hot water after they have been in contact with the affected skin area. If it is not possible to wash them in hot water, they should be dry-cleaned. This will help prevent reinfection.

Keep the affected skin areas as dry as possible. Do not bandage the affected skin area unless directed by your doctor.

When to Call Your Doctor

Call your doctor if the condition for which you are using this medicine has not improved after 1 or 2 weeks or becomes worse or if the medicine causes itching or burning of the skin or vagina for more than a few minutes after instillation.

Also call your doctor if you are using this medicine to treat a vaginal infection and if you develop increased frequency of urination (passing your water) or stomach cramps or pains.

Also call your doctor if you are applying the medicine to the skin and you develop stinging, blistering, swelling, peeling, hives or itching of the skin.

Miscellaneous
For creams, solutions and lotions:
- This medicine is for external use only. Do not swallow it, and keep it away from the eyes.

▶ **CROMOGLYCATE SODIUM (ORAL)**
NALCROM

Purpose
This medicine is used to help prevent food-related allergies and some types of bowel disease.

Allergies/Warnings
If you have ever had an allergic reaction to CROMOGLYCATE, tell your doctor and pharmacist before you take any of this medicine.

How to Use This Medicine

Time of Administration
It is very important that you take this medicine exactly as your doctor has prescribed. Do not miss any doses, and take the medicine even if you feel well. Try to take this medicine at the same time(s) every day so that you will have a constant level of medicine in your body.

Take this medicine 15 to 20 minutes before a meal.

How to Administer
There are 2 ways to take the NALCROM CAPSULES:
- The preferred method is to dissolve the contents of the capsule(s) in a small amount of very hot water and then dilute with about ¼ cup of cold water.

OR
- Take the capsules by swallowing whole with a glass of water.

Special Instructions

Length of Therapy
After you have taken this medicine for awhile, the number of times you will have to use this medicine may be slowly decreased by your doctor.

Do not take any more of this medicine than your doctor has prescribed and do not stop taking this medicine suddenly without the approval of your doctor. It may be necessary for your doctor to slowly reduce your dose since your body may need time to adjust. If you should suddenly stop taking it or reduce your dose, you may experience a worsening of your condition.

Pregnancy/Breastfeeding

Women who are pregnant, breastfeeding, or planning to become pregnant should tell their doctor before taking this medicine.

When to Call Your Doctor

Most people experience few or no side effects from this drug. However, any medicine can sometimes cause unwanted effects. Call your doctor if you develop fever, nausea, unusual headaches, difficulty sleeping, skin rashes or joint pains.

Allergic Reactions

Call your doctor immediately if you think you may be allergic to the medicine or if you develop a skin rash, hives, itching, swelling of the face or difficulty in breathing. If you cannot reach your doctor, phone a hospital emergency department.

Storage

Store the capsules in a cool, dry, dark place.

"Senility" Due to Medicines

If an older person becomes confused or forgetful, thinks more slowly or cannot care for himself or herself, don't jump to the conclusion that it is due to old age.

Emergency Medicine reports that in a research study of 308 elderly patients, adverse reactions to medications were causing symptoms of forgetfulness, confusion, falling down and slow thought processes in 35. The types of medicines causing the problems included sleeping pills, tranquilizers, high blood pressure medicines, ASA, CIMETIDINE and insulin.

If you think an older person is having these symptoms from medicines being taken, discuss the problem with the doctor. However, do not stop taking any medications without medical advice because the problem may not be due to the medicines. Stopping the medicines without a doctor's approval could lead to more serious problems.

▶ **CROMOGLYCATE SODIUM (INHALATION)**
INTAL INHALER, INTAL SPINCAPS, INTAL SYNCRONER, INTAL
NEBULIZER SOLUTION

NEDOCROMIL SODIUM
TILADE

Purpose

This medicine is used to help prevent asthma attacks. It is to be taken
on a continuous basis to prevent symptoms from appearing. The medicine will not help an asthma attack that has already begun—and may
even make the attack worse. If an asthma attack occurs, check with
your doctor regarding treatment. In some cases, the medicine will have
to be changed.

This medicine is also used to help prevent bronchospasm and wheezing caused by exercise or cold air. It is taken shortly before physical
exercise or exposure to cold air.

Allergies/Warnings

If you have ever had an allergic reaction to CROMOGLYCATE or
NEDOCROMIL, tell your doctor and pharmacist before you take any
of this medicine.

How to Use This Medicine

Time of Administration

It is very important that you take this medicine exactly as your
doctor has prescribed. Do not miss any doses, and take the medicine
even if you feel well. Try to take this medicine at the same time(s)
every day so that you will have a constant level of medicine in your
body.

How to Administer

For INTAL SPINCAPS (INHALATION):
- These capsules must be used in the special Spinhaler or Halermatic
  device designed for them. DO NOT SWALLOW THE CAPSULES.
  The medicine must be inhaled in order to work.
- It is important to get the powder as deep as possible into the lungs.
- Follow the special administration instructions that come with these
  capsules. Insert one end of the capsule down into the device. *See*

Metered-Dose Inhalers (page 31) for general instructions on how to hold the head and when to inhale the powder.

- Repeat the inhalation procedure until the capsule is empty.
- Do not breathe out into the Spinhaler or Halermatic device because moisture from the mouth can cause powder to plug up the inhaler.
- A little powder may stick to the Spinhaler or Halermatic device during use. This is normal but the inhalers should be cleaned and dried before reuse. If there are large amounts of powder sticking to the inhaler, you may not be using it correctly.
- Wash the inhalers at least once a week and dry thoroughly. It is recommended that the inhalers be replaced after six months of use. You may obtain a new one from your pharmacist.
- *Special note for parents*: Your doctor or pharmacist can show you how to attach a whistle on the end of the Spinhaler. This could make taking the INTAL more fun for your child and may help him or her learn to use the Spinhaler properly.

For INTAL NEBULIZER SOLUTION:
- A power-operated (not hand-operated) nebulizer machine must be used to administer this solution.
- Be sure you understand how to use the equipment, including the face mask or mouthpiece.

For INTAL INHALER:
- *See* Metered-Dose Inhalers (page 31).
- To test the inhaler, press down on the canister once. The dose can be seen as a fine white mist. This mist should never be seen to escape from the mouth or nose during a treatment. If it is seen, you are not using the inhaler correctly.
- Keep the cap on the inhaler when it is not in use. This will keep dirt out of the inhaler.
- The inhaler should be cleaned approximately once a week. Remove the canister from the plastic mouthpiece. Wash the mouthpiece in warm water and dry thoroughly before replacing the canister.

For TILADE INHALER:
- Pull the dust cap off the inhaler.
- *See* Metered-Dose Inhalers (Method I. Closed-Mouth Instructions, page 32).
- DO NOT BREATHE OUT THROUGH THE INHALER. Moisture from the mouth could plug the inhaler.

- Cleaning Instructions: It is very important to keep the plastic mouth-piece clean. Wash the mouthpiece every day or at least twice a week in hand-hot water. Shake off any excess water. Allow the mouthpiece to dry *overnight*. Then replace the canister and dust cap.

Special Instructions

Length of Therapy

It may take 1 to 4 weeks before you feel the full benefit of this medicine. If you are also using another inhaler containing a bron-chodilator to open up the air passages in your lungs, use the bron-chodilator several minutes before you use this inhaler.

After you have taken this medicine for awhile and your asthma symptoms have decreased, the number of times you will have to use this medicine may be slowly reduced by your doctor.

Do not take any more of this medicine than your doctor has pre-scribed and do not stop taking this medicine suddenly without the approval of your doctor. It may be necessary for your doctor to slowly reduce your dose since your body may need time to adjust. If you suddenly stop taking it or reduce your dose, you may experience a worsening of your asthma.

Pregnancy/Breastfeeding

Women who are pregnant, breastfeeding or planning to become pregnant should tell their doctor before taking this medicine.

Special Precautions

Drinking a few sips of water or gargling after each inhalation may help decrease mild throat irritation, cough or hoarseness which may be caused by the powder.

This medicine may cause a bitter taste after use. This is a normal side effect. Some patients may develop headache, nausea or vomiting that usually disappears after using the medicine for awhile. If these side effects persist, contact your physician.

If you develop coughing or wheezing after using this drug, check with your doctor. Use of a bronchodilator aerosol may be helpful prior to inhaling the medicine.

When to Call Your Doctor

Most people experience few or no side effects from this drug. How-ever, any medicine can sometimes cause unwanted effects. Call your doctor if you develop fever or coughing, dizziness or severe headaches, joint or muscle pain, nausea or vomiting, trouble in swallowing, swollen glands, severe nasal congestion, difficulty in breathing or increased wheezing.

Allergic Reactions

Call your doctor immediately if you think you may be allergic to the medicine or if you develop a skin rash, hives, itching, swelling of the face or difficulty in breathing. If you cannot reach your doctor, phone a hospital emergency department.

Storage

Store the capsules in a cool, dry, dark place. Do not refrigerate the capsules. Do not freeze the solution.

Store INTAL and TILADE INHALERS at room temperature. Do not place in hot water or near radiators, stoves or other sources of heat. Do not puncture, burn or incinerate the container (even when it is empty).

▶ **CROMOGLYCATE SODIUM (NASAL)**
RYNACROM CARTRIDGES, RYNACROM NASAL SOLUTION

Purpose

This nasal medicine is used to help prevent and treat allergic rhinitis. The medicine helps relieve the symptoms of nasal congestion, runny nose, sneezing, difficulty in breathing and postnasal drip.

Allergies/Warnings

If you have ever had an allergic reaction to CROMOGLYCATE, tell your doctor and pharmacist before you take any of this medicine. Tell your doctor and pharmacist if you have nasal polyps. This medicine may not be able to reach the nasal membranes if you have nasal polyps, and may not be effective.

How to Use This Medicine

Time of Administration

It is very important that you take this medicine exactly as your doctor has prescribed. Do not miss any doses during the treatment period and take the medicine even if you feel well. Try to take this medicine at the same time(s) every day so that you will have a constant level of medicine in your nose.

203

How to Administer

For RYNACROM NASAL SOLUTION:

- Assemble the unit according to the special instructions that come with the medicine and use the special RYNACROM device to administer the spray into the nose.
- Do not wash the pump unit before transferring it to the refill bottle.
- Before using the nasal spray, blow the nose gently. This will remove mucous from the nose and make it possible for the medicine to have better contact with the nasal membranes. If your nose is severely congested, your doctor may recommend that you use a nasal decongestant first.
- Insert the tip of the RYNACROM device into the nostril and press the bottle firmly upward with the thumb in order to release 1 dose. One spray releases 1 dose. Sniff gently at the same time.
- If the unit does not spray properly, the outside case may be cleaned with warm water and thoroughly dried in order to remove any material that could clog the spray opening.
- When the bottle is empty, remove it from the plastic case, unscrew the pump and insert a refill.

Be sure to replace the cap on the RYNACROM pump after every use so that dirt cannot get into the solution.

For RYNACROM CARTRIDGES:

- Use the cartridge with the special RYNACROM NASAL INSUFFLATOR tube.
- Follow the instructions that come with the medicine.
- Clean the device carefully following the manufacturer's instructions. Improper cleaning may cause the medicine to be useless.
- It is recommended that the special spray device be replaced every six months.

Special Instructions

Length of Therapy

It may take 1 to 4 weeks before the full benefit is noticed. Seasonal allergic rhinitis (often associated with high pollen counts during certain seasons) will usually respond after 1 week of treatment. Chronic or perennial allergic rhinitis (occurs year-round) may take up to 4 weeks before a response is seen.

Do not stop using this medicine suddenly. It is recommended that the dosage be reduced gradually over at least 7 days.

Protect Yourself from Insect Bites and Stings

Insect bites and stings are not only painful and a nuisance, but they can also be life-threatening to those who are allergic to insect venom. Protect yourself from such bites and stings by taking the following precautions:

- Keep garbage in containers and cover food when picnicking or camping.
- Wear shoes when outdoors, especially when in grass and fields.
- Avoid wearing perfumes, including perfumed deodorants, hairsprays, etc.
- Avoid wearing brightly colored clothes since these attract bees.
- Wear long pants and socks when in areas where ticks are common. Ticks can carry both Rocky Mountain spotted fever and Lyme disease.
- Use an insect repellent when in an area where there are mosquitoes or other biting insects. A highly effective, all-purpose repellent is DEET (N,N-diethyl-m-toluamide), *but do not use this for children under the age of two because of the risk of central nervous system toxicity.* Always read the product cautions when using insect repellents on young children.

If you are allergic to insect bites or stings:

- Ask your doctor or pharmacist about emergency kits for insect stings available upon prescription.
- Seek medical attention immediately after being bitten or stung.
- Apply ice packs to the sting site as soon as possible to help slow absorption of the insect venom and reduce itching, swelling and pain.
- If the culprit was a bee or wasp, scrape the stinger away gently (you can use a credit card to do this). Do not use tweezers or you may squeeze more venom into the wound.

Pregnancy/Breastfeeding

Women who are pregnant, breastfeeding or planning to become pregnant should tell their doctor before taking this medicine.

Special Precautions

Some patients may experience nasal stinging or sneezing immediately after using the medicine. This is not unusual. Call your doctor if the stinging or sneezing becomes severe.

You may also experience an occasional headache, cough and/or unpleasant taste in the mouth. This is not unusual. Call your doctor if they become bothersome.

When to Call Your Doctor

Most people experience few or no side effects from this drug. However, any medicine can sometimes cause unwanted effects. Call your doctor if your symptoms do not improve or get worse, or if you develop nosebleeds, coughing, a rash, trouble swallowing, wheezing or difficulty breathing, increased sneezing or severe burning in the nose.

Allergic Reactions

Call your doctor immediately if you think you may be allergic to the medicine or if you develop a skin rash, hives, itching, swelling of the face or difficulty in breathing. If you cannot reach your doctor, phone a hospital emergency department.

Storage

Store the cartridges at room temperature and in a cool, dry, place. Storage in a damp area may make the medicine unusable.

▶ **CROMOGLYCATE SODIUM (OPHTHALMIC)**
OPTICROM, VISTACROM

Purpose

This medicine is used to treat seasonal allergic disorders of the eye.

Allergies/Warnings

If you have ever had an allergic reaction to CROMOGLYCATE, tell your doctor and pharmacist before you take any of this medicine.

How to Use This Medicine

Time of Administration

It is very important that you use this medicine exactly as your doctor has prescribed. Do not miss any doses. Try to use the medicine at the same time(s) every day so that you will have a constant level of the medicine in your eye.

How to Administer
For eye drops:
- *See* Eye Drops (page 24).

For eye ointment:
- *See* Eye Ointments (page 26).

Special Instructions

Length of Therapy
Decreased itching, tearing, redness and discharge are usually evident within a few days of treatment. Treatment may be required for up to 6 weeks.

Pregnancy/Breastfeeding
Women who are pregnant, breastfeeding or planning to become pregnant should tell their doctor before taking this medicine.

Special Precautions
For eye drops:
- The manufacturer recommends that people who wear soft (hydrophilic) contact lenses should not wear them during treatment.

For eye ointment:
- The eye ointment should not be used when hard or soft contact lenses are being worn.

This medicine may cause a mild stinging or burning sensation. This is not unusual.

Do not share this eye medicine with other people. Any germs or infections could be transferred.

Vision may be blurred for a few seconds after you apply the ointment. Do not drive a car or operate dangerous machinery until your vision has cleared.

When to Call Your Doctor
Most people experience few or no side effects from this drug. However, any medicine can sometimes cause unwanted effects. Call your doctor if you develop severe swelling of the eye, unexplained burning or stinging, or if the condition does not improve.

Allergic Reactions

Call your doctor immediately if you think you may be allergic to the medicine or if you develop a skin rash, hives, itching, swelling of the face or difficulty in breathing. If you cannot reach your doctor, phone a hospital emergency department.

Storage

Store in a cool, dark place.

Discard any unused medicine 4 weeks after opening the bottle or tube or sooner if the label indicates an earlier expiration date.

▶ CYCLOBENZAPRINE (ORAL)

FLEXERIL

Purpose

This medicine is used to relax muscles and to help relieve muscle pain and stiffness.

Allergies/Warnings

If you have ever had an allergic reaction to any medicine or if you have glaucoma, an enlarged prostate, difficulty urinating, hyperthyroidism, heart condition or any other medical condition, tell your doctor and pharmacist before you take any of this medicine.

How to Use This Medicine

Time of Administration

This medicine may be taken with food or a glass of water.

Special Instructions

Length of Therapy

This medicine should only be used for short periods of time (generally up to 2 or 3 weeks).

Do not take any more of this medicine than your doctor has prescribed and do not stop taking this medicine suddenly without the approval of your doctor. It may be necessary for your doctor to reduce your dose slowly since your body may need time to adjust. If you suddenly stop taking the medicine, you may develop nausea, headache or tiredness.

Pregnancy/Breastfeeding

Women who are pregnant, breastfeeding or planning to become pregnant should tell their doctor before taking this medicine.

Drug Interactions

It is important that you obtain the advice of your doctor or pharmacist before taking any other prescription or nonprescription medicines including pain relievers, sleeping pills, tranquilizers, medicine for seizures, muscle relaxants, anesthetics, medicines for depression or medicines for allergies or colds, or sinus products. Combining this medicine with some of these drugs could cause drowsiness or dizziness.

There are other drug interactions that can occur. If you are taking any other medicines, be sure to check first with your pharmacist or doctor.

Alcohol

Do not drink alcoholic beverages while taking this drug without the approval of your doctor, because the combination could cause severe drowsiness.

Special Precautions

If your mouth becomes dry, drink water, suck ice chips or a hard, sour candy (sugarless) or chew gum (sugarless). Sugarless products are recommended in order to avoid dental problems. You may wish to ask your pharmacist about special solutions, called artificial saliva, that can also be used to help restore moisture in the mouth. It is especially important to brush and floss your teeth regularly if you develop a dry mouth, to help prevent gum problems.

This drug commonly causes dizziness and drowsiness. Do not drive a car, pilot an airplane, operate dangerous machinery or do jobs that require you to be alert until you know how you are going to react to the drug. You should also be careful going up and down stairs. Sit or lie down at the first sign of dizziness. Tell your doctor if the drowsiness or dizziness continues.

This medicine may cause some people to become constipated. To help prevent constipation, try increasing the amount of bulk in your diet (for example, bran, fresh fruits and salads), exercising more often or drinking more fluids (unless otherwise directed). Call your doctor if the constipation continues.

When to Call Your Doctor

Most people experience few or no side effects from this drug. However, any medicine can sometimes cause unwanted effects. Call your

doctor if you develop fast or irregular heartbeats, difficulty breathing, numbness of the hands or feet, stomach pain or constipation, trembling, difficulty in urinating (passing your water), eye pain, unusual sweating, seizures, unusual nervousness, or if you become confused or depressed.

Allergic Reactions

Call your doctor immediately if you think you may be allergic to the medicine or if you develop a skin rash, hives, itching, swelling of the face or difficulty in breathing. If you cannot reach your doctor, phone a hospital emergency department.

Brushing with Tartar Control Toothpaste?

Do you have burning or itching around your mouth? If you do, it may be caused by the tartar control toothpaste you are using.

Dermatologists at the University of Maryland Hospital conducted a study in which patients brushed with tartar control toothpaste 3 times a day. The skin around the patients' mouths and at the corners became red, scaly and cracked. Shortly after they stopped brushing with the tartar control toothpaste, the patients' rashes cleared up. The rash reappeared when the patients were retested.

The researchers concluded that certain compounds in tartar control toothpaste may irritate the mucous membranes and other sensitive tissues around the mouth.

▶ CYPROHEPTADINE HCl (ORAL)
PERIACTIN

Purpose

This medicine is often used to help relieve symptoms (such as itching) of certain types of allergic conditions. This drug has several other uses (such as increasing the appetite and promoting weight gain) and the reason it was prescribed depends upon your condition. Check with your doctor if you do not understand why you are taking it.

Allergies/Warnings

If you have ever had an allergic reaction to any medicine or if you have asthma, glaucoma, an enlarged prostate, urinary retention (a type of bladder problem), high blood pressure or diabetes, tell your doctor and pharmacist before you take any of this medicine.

This medicine is not recommended for children under 2 years of age.

How to Use This Medicine

Time of Administration

It is best to take this medicine with food to help prevent stomach upset.

For syrup:
• *See* Oral Liquid Medicines (page 17).

Special Instructions

Length of Therapy

Do not take this medicine more often or longer than recommended by your doctor. To do so may increase your chance of developing side effects.

Pregnancy/Breastfeeding

Women who are pregnant, breastfeeding or planning to become pregnant should tell their doctor before taking this medicine. Safe use during pregnancy has not been established.

Drug Interactions

It is important that you obtain the advice of your doctor or pharmacist before taking any other prescription or nonprescription medicines including pain relievers, sleeping pills, tranquilizers, medicine for seizures, muscle relaxants, anesthetics, medicines for depression or other medicines for allergies. Combining this medicine with some of these drugs could cause drowsiness or dizziness.

There are other drug interactions that can occur. If you are taking any other medicines, be sure to check first with your pharmacist or doctor.

Alcohol

Do not drink alcoholic beverages while taking this drug without the approval of your doctor because the combination could cause drowsiness. One drink may have the same effect that 2 or 3 drinks normally would have.

Special Precautions

In some people, this drug may initially cause dizziness or drowsiness. Do not drive a car, pilot an airplane, operate dangerous machinery or do jobs that require you to be alert until you know how you are going to react to the drug. If you become dizzy or drowsy, you should be careful going up and down stairs. Sit or lie down at the first sign of dizziness. Tell your doctor if the dizziness or drowsiness continues.

People over 65 years of age may be more sensitive to these side effects.

If your mouth becomes dry, drink water, suck ice chips or a hard, sour candy (sugarless) or chew gum (sugarless). Sugarless products are recommended in order to avoid dental problems. You may wish to ask your pharmacist about special solutions, called artificial saliva, that can also be used to help restore moisture in the mouth. It is especially important to brush and floss your teeth regularly if you develop a dry mouth, to help prevent gum problems.

When to Call Your Doctor

Most people experience few or no side effects from this drug. However, any medicine can sometimes cause unwanted effects. Call your doctor if you develop a skin rash, fast or irregular heartbeats, blurred vision, stomach pain, unexplained weakness or tiredness, unexplained sore throat, fever or mouth sores, unusual bruising or bleeding, unexplained nervousness, restlessness or irritability (especially in children), trouble sleeping or difficulty in urinating (passing your water), or if mucous (lung secretions) becomes thicker than usual.

Storage

If you were prescribed PERIACTIN SYRUP:

* Do not freeze the medicine.

▶ **(ORAL):**

DICLOFENAC SODIUM

APO-DICLO, NOVODIFENAC, VOLTAREN, VOLTAREN S.R.

FENOPROFEN CALCIUM

NALFON

FLURBIPROFEN
ANSAID, FROBEN

IBUPROFEN
ACTIPROFEN, ADVIL, AMERSOL, APO-IBUPROFEN, MEDIPREN, MOTRIN, MOTRIN IB, NOVOPROFEN

KETOPROFEN
APO-KETO, APO-KETO-E, ORUDIS, ORUDIS E-50, ORUDIS E-100, ORUDIS SR, RHODIS, RHODIS E-50, RHODIS E-100

NAPROXEN
APO-NAPROXEN, NAPROSYN, NAPROSYN SR, NAXEN, NOVONAPROX

NAPROXEN SODIUM
ANAPROX, APO-NAPRO-NA, NOVONAPROX SODIUM, SYNFLEX

PIROXICAM
APO-PIROXICAM, FELDENE, NOVOPIROCAM

SULINDAC
APO-SULIN, CLINORIL, NOVOSUNDAC

TIAPROFENIC ACID
SURGAM

TOLMETIN SODIUM
TOLECTIN

(RECTAL):
DICLOFENAC
VOLTAREN SUPPOSITORIES

KETOPROFEN
ORUDIS SUPPOSITORIES, RHODIS SUPPOSITORIES

NAPROXEN
NAPROSYN SUPPOSITORIES, NAXEN SUPPOSITORIES

PIROXICAM
FELDENE SUPPOSITORIES

Purpose

This medicine is used to help relieve pain. Some of the medicines are to help relieve inflammation, stiffness, swelling and joint pain in certain kinds of arthritis or rheumatism. Some of the products are used to relieve menstrual cramps, dental pain and the symptoms of gout, bursitis, tendinitis, muscle sprains or strains.

Allergies/Warnings

If you have ever had an allergic reaction to ASA (acetylsalicylic acid) or any other medicine or if you suffer from hay fever, asthma, nasal polyps, ulcers or stomach problems (such as heartburn), heart, kidney or liver problems or high blood pressure, tell your doctor and pharmacist before you take any of this medicine.

Tell your doctor if you take diuretics (water pills).

How to Use This Medicine

Time of Administration
For tablets and capsules containing FENOPROFEN, FLURBIPROFEN, IBUPROFEN, KETOPROFEN (ORUDIS CAPSULES), NAPROXEN, PIROXICAM, TIAPROFENIC ACID *and* TOLMETIN:

• This medicine will work whether or not you take it with food. To help lessen stomach upset, your doctor may recommend that you take this medicine with some food, after a meal or with a glass of milk. Always take the medicine with a full glass of water, unless otherwise directed. It also may be helpful *not* to lie down for 15 minutes after taking the medicine so that the medicine can reach the stomach. Call your doctor if you develop stomach upset (indigestion, nausea, vomiting, stomach pain) that does not go away.

If you were prescribed APO-DICLO, APO-KETO-E, NOVODIFENAC, ORUDIS E-50, ORUDIS E-100, RHODIS E-50, RHODIS E-100, VOLTAREN:

• It is best to take this medicine with a glass of water—not with milk or antacids. Milk or antacids can interfere with the special coating on this medicine.

For tablets containing DICLOFENAC or SULINDAC:

• Always take this medicine with food or immediately after meals to help prevent stomach upset. If you develop persistent stomach pain, nausea, vomiting or indigestion, contact your doctor.

If you were prescribed APO-KETO-E, NAPROSYN SR, ORUDIS E-50, ORUDIS E-100, ORUDIS SR, RHODIS E-50, RHODIS E-100, VOLTAREN *or* VOLTAREN S.R.:

• This medicine must be swallowed whole. Do not crush, chew or break tablets into pieces.

For suppositories:
- *See* Rectal Suppositories (page 39).

If you were prescribed NAPROSYN LIQUID:
- Shake the liquid well before pouring so that an accurate dose can be measured. It is recommended that you use a medicine spoon or oral liquid syringe to measure the dose. *See* How to Use Medicine Spoon (page 22) *or* Oral Liquid Syringe (page 17).

Special Instructions

Length of Therapy

This medicine will not cure arthritis but it can help control inflammation that can increase damage to your joints. It is very important that you take this medicine regularly and that you *do not miss any doses.* If you miss a dose, the level of the medicine in your body will fall and the drug will not be as effective. Only if the drug is at the right level will it be able to decrease the inflammation and swelling in your joints and help prevent further damage.

If you are taking this medicine for a joint or bone problem, you may have to take the drug for a few weeks before you feel its full benefits. Long-term therapy is often required in arthritis.

This medicine does not replace any exercise or rest programs or use of heat/cold treatments your doctor may have prescribed.

Pregnancy/Breastfeeding

Women who are pregnant, breastfeeding or planning to become pregnant should tell their doctor before taking this medicine. Use of this medicine during pregnancy, especially the last three months, and during breastfeeding is not recommended.

Drug Interactions

Do not take any other medicines containing ASA (acetylsalicylic acid), or salicylates or other prescription medicines used to treat arthritis, while you are taking this medicine without contacting your doctor.

It is usually safe to take ACETAMINOPHEN for fever or the occasional headache. Check with your pharmacist.

Do not take TOLMETIN with antacids containing sodium bicarbonate (baking soda) because you might take too much sodium.

Beekeepers Lose Immunity to Bee Stings

Beekeepers should think twice before taking some anti-inflammatory drugs. It appears that some medicines may reverse their immunity to bee stings.

During the last few years, several new nonsteroidal anti-inflammatory drugs have been developed to relieve pain and reduce stiffness, swelling and joint pain associated with inflammation. Such drugs include IBUPROFEN, FENOPROFEN, NAPROXEN, KETOPROFEN, SULINDAC, PIROXICAM and TOLMETIN.

It is well known that beekeepers develop an immunity to bee stings. It has even been reported that some people get temporary relief from the pain of arthritis if they sustain several bee stings. The *British Medical Journal* reported that two people with an immunity to bee stings taking a nonsteroidal anti-inflammatory drug had suffered serious allergic reactions to bee and wasp stings:

A 66-year-old beekeeper had developed an immunity to bee stings over 6 years. She was prescribed a nonsteroidal anti-inflammatory drug for osteoarthrosis. A few months after taking the drug, she was stung on the wrists while working around the beehives and within 15 minutes developed heart palpitations, a rash and swelling of the mouth and tongue, making it difficult for her to breathe. She stopped taking the drug. When she was stung again 48 hours later, she did not develop a reaction.

Another report described the 48-year-old wife of a beekeeper who had been taking a nonsteroidal anti-inflammatory drug for five months for osteoarthritis. Previously she had only skin reactions to wasp stings but one day she developed widespread swelling; red, itchy rash; heart palpitations and shortness of breath within 2 minutes of being stung by a wasp. Hospitalization was necessary.

Until more is learned about the reason for these reactions, beekeepers should be aware of the potential hazard associated with these drugs and bee stings.

Alcohol

Do not drink alcoholic beverages while taking this drug without the approval of your doctor because the combination could cause stomach problems.

Special Precautions

In some people, this drug may cause dizziness or blurred vision. Do not drive a car, pilot an airplane, operate dangerous machinery or do jobs that require you to be alert until you know how you are going to react to this drug. If you become dizzy, you should be careful going up and down stairs. Sit or lie down at the first sign of dizziness. Tell your doctor if you have been dizzy. Call your doctor if you develop blurred vision.

This medicine may cause some people to become constipated. To help prevent constipation, try increasing the amount of bulk in your diet (for example, bran, fresh fruits and salads), exercising more often or drinking more fluids (unless otherwise directed). Call your doctor if the constipation continues.

When to Call Your Doctor

Most people experience few or no side effects from this drug. However, any medicine can sometimes cause unwanted effects. Call your doctor if you develop a skin rash, sore throat or fever, chills, flulike symptoms, ringing or buzzing in the ears, hearing problems, a feeling of fullness in the ears, fast heartbeats, shortness of breath, wheezing or tightness in the chest, swelling of the legs or ankles or sudden weight gain, blurred vision or changes in your eyesight, hearing loss or ear pain, bloody or black stools, severe stomach pain, vomiting of blood, yellow color to the skin or eyes, unusual bruising or bleeding, unusual tiredness or weakness, depression, confusion, difficulty in urinating (passing your water), decrease in the amount of urine, blood in the urine or a persistent headache.

Allergic Reactions

Call your doctor immediately if you think you may be allergic to the medicine or if you develop a skin rash, hives, itching, fast or irregular heartbeats, fainting, swelling of the face or difficulty in breathing. If you cannot reach your doctor, phone a hospital emergency department.

Storage

For tablets and capsules:
• Store the medicine in a cool, dry, dark place.

217

For suppositories:
• *See* Rectal Suppositories (page 39).

Refills

Do not stop taking this medicine without your doctor's approval and do not go without medicine between prescription refills. Call your pharmacist for a refill 2 or 3 days before you will run out of the medicine.

Discuss with your pharmacist the implications of dispensing all your refills for this medicine with the same manufacturer's product. (*See* Generic Drugs, page 13.)

Miscellaneous

Carry an identification card in your wallet or wear a medical alert bracelet indicating that you are taking this medicine, as well as the names and phone numbers of your doctors. If you do not already carry such a card, complete the Medicine Card in this book. Always tell your dentist, pharmacist and other doctors who are treating you that you are taking this medicine.

▶ DICYCLOMINE HCl (ORAL)
BENTYLOL, BENTYLOL DOSPAN, FORMULEX, LOMINE, PROTYLOL, SPASMOBAN

DICYCLOMINE HCl-PHENOBARBITAL
DICLOPHEN, SPASMOBAN-PH

Purpose
This medicine is used to help relax muscles and to help relieve cramps and spasms of the stomach and bowels. It is also used in infants (over 6 months of age) to treat infant colic.

Allergies/Warnings
If you have ever had an allergic reaction to ATROPINE, a barbiturate or any other drug used to relax the stomach or bowels, or if you have glaucoma, enlarged prostate, difficulty urinating (passing your water) or any other medical condition, tell your doctor and pharmacist before you take any of this medicine.

How to Use This Medicine

Time of Administration

Take this medicine approximately 30 minutes before a meal unless otherwise directed.

If this medicine is prescribed for an infant, it should be given 15 minutes before feeding.

How to Administer

If you were prescribed BENTYLOL DOSPAN TABLETS:
- These tablets are long-acting and must be swallowed whole. Do not crush or chew the tablets.

For infants (over 6 months of age):
- If the syrup form of the drug has been prescribed for a baby, the syrup should be mixed with an equal amount of water.
- Measure the dose very carefully for the baby. If a spoon is used to measure the dose, it is recommended that you use a medicine spoon or an oral liquid syringe that you can obtain from your pharmacist. These are more accurate than the average household teaspoon. *See* Oral Liquid Syringe (page 17) and Medicine Spoon (page 22).

Special Instructions

Length of Therapy

Do not take this medicine more often or longer than recommended by your doctor. To do so may increase your chance of developing side effects.

If you were prescribed DICLOPHEN *or* SPASMOBAN-PH:
- Do not stop taking this medicine suddenly without the approval of your doctor. It may be necessary for your doctor to reduce your dose slowly since your body may need time to adjust.
- Check with your doctor if you develop any of the following while you are slowly stopping the medicine: nausea or vomiting, feeling faint, trembling, seizures, changes in vision or trouble sleeping.

Pregnancy/Breastfeeding

Women who are pregnant or planning to become pregnant should tell their doctor before taking this medicine.

Women who are breastfeeding should tell their doctor before taking this medicine. This drug may decrease the amount of breast milk produced and may appear in the breast milk.

Drug Interactions

It is important that you obtain the advice of your doctor or pharmacist before taking any other prescription or nonprescription medicines including pain relievers, sleeping pills, tranquilizers, medicine for seizures, muscle relaxants, anesthetics, medicines for depression or medicines for allergies, colds or sinus conditions. Combining this medicine with some of these drugs could cause drowsiness or dizziness.

Do not take this medicine at the same time as an antacid or an antidiarrhea medicine. Try to space them at least 1 hour apart.

There are other drug interactions that can occur. If you are taking any other medicines, be sure to check first with your pharmacist or doctor.

Alcohol

Do not drink alcoholic beverages while taking this drug without the approval of your doctor because the combination could cause severe drowsiness or dizziness. One drink may have the same effect that 2 or 3 drinks normally would have.

Special Precautions

If your mouth becomes dry, drink water, suck ice chips or a hard, sour candy (sugarless) or chew gum (sugarless). Sugarless products are recommended in order to avoid dental problems. You may wish to ask your pharmacist about special solutions, called artificial saliva, that can also be used to help restore moisture in the mouth. It is especially important to brush and floss your teeth regularly if you develop a dry mouth, to help prevent gum problems.

In some people, this drug may cause dizziness, drowsiness or blurred vision. Do not drive a car, pilot an airplane, operate dangerous machinery or do jobs that require you to be alert if you are dizzy or drowsy. You should also be careful going up and down stairs. Sit or lie down at the first sign of dizziness. Tell your doctor if these problems continue.

An urge to urinate (pass your water) with an inability to do so sometimes occurs with this drug. Urinating before taking the drug each time may help relieve this problem. Tell your doctor if you are having this problem.

You may become more sensitive to heat because your body may perspire less while you are taking this drug. Be careful not to become overheated during exercise or in hot weather. Try to avoid strenuous exercise, standing for long periods of time (especially in hot weather), hot showers, hot baths, saunas or Jacuzzis while taking this medicine.

If your eyes become more sensitive to sunlight, it may help to wear sunglasses.

This medicine may cause some people to become constipated. To help prevent constipation, try increasing the amount of bulk in your diet (for example, bran, fresh fruits and salads), exercising more often or drinking more fluids (unless otherwise directed). Call your doctor if the constipation continues.

Medicines for Children

Do not give any medicine to a child less than 1 year of age unless the medicine has been prescribed by your doctor.

Do not give any nonprescription drugs to children between 1 and 12 years of age unless the doses for the different age groups or weights are listed on the package container.

If you have any questions, check with your pharmacist.

When to Call Your Doctor

Most people experience few or no side effects from this drug. However, any medicine can sometimes cause unwanted effects. Call your doctor if you develop a skin rash, diarrhea or constipation, difficulty urinating (passing your water), unusual restlessness or confusion, flushing, blurred vision, eye pain or fast heartbeats.

If you were prescribed DICLOPHEN *or* SPASMOBAN-PH:
• Also call your doctor if you develop a sore throat, fever, mouth sores, a staggering walk, a yellow color to the skin or eyes, unusual bruising or bleeding, slow heartbeats or shortness of breath, bothersome sleepiness or tiredness during the day, unusual nervousness, confusion or depression, hallucinations, trouble sleeping, nightmares or slurred speech.

Allergic Reactions

Call your doctor immediately if you think you may be allergic to the medicine or if you develop a skin rash, hives, itching, swelling of the face or difficulty in breathing. If you cannot reach your doctor, phone a hospital emergency department.

Effect of Diarrhea on Drugs

If a person has diarrhea, some medicines may be absorbed poorly:

If a medicine is normally absorbed in the intestines, diarrhea can cause the medicine to move too quickly through the intestines for complete absorption to occur.

The same problem can occur if a person develops diarrhea after taking strong, irritating laxatives.

▶ **DIFLUNISAL (ORAL)**
DOLOBID

Purpose

This medicine is used to help relieve pain. It is also used to help relieve inflammation, stiffness, swelling and joint pain in certain kinds of arthritis.

Allergies/Warnings

If you have ever had an allergic reaction to ASA or any other medicine or if you suffer from hay fever, asthma, nasal polyps, ulcers or other medical problems, tell your doctor and pharmacist before you take any of this medicine.

How to Use This Medicine

Time of Administration

This medicine will work whether or not you take it with food. However, if you develop stomach upset after taking the drug, take it with some food or a glass of milk. If the stomach upset continues, check with your doctor.

How to Administer

Swallow the tablets whole with a full glass of water. Do not crush, chew or break them into pieces.

Special Instructions

Length of Therapy

This medicine will not cure arthritis but it can help control inflammation that may damage your joints. It is very important that you take this medicine regularly and that you *do not miss any doses*. If you miss a dose, the level of the medicine in your body will fall and the drug will not be as effective. Only if the drug is at the right level will it be able to decrease the inflammation and swelling in your joints and help prevent further damage.

It may take up to 1 or 2 weeks before you feel the full benefit of the medicine.

Pregnancy/Breastfeeding

Women who are pregnant, breastfeeding or planning to become pregnant should tell their doctor before taking this medicine. Use of this medicine during pregnancy, especially the last 3 months, is not recommended.

Drug Interactions

Check with your doctor or pharmacist before taking any other medicines containing ASA, ACETAMINOPHEN or salicylates or other medicines used to treat arthritis while you are taking this medicine.

Do not take antacids on a regular basis while you are taking this medicine because the antacids may decrease the effect of this medicine. Occasional doses of antacids may not interfere with your therapy. Check with your pharmacist or doctor.

Alcohol

Do not drink alcoholic beverages while taking this drug without the approval of your doctor because the combination could cause stomach problems.

Special Precautions

In some people, this medicine may cause dizziness. Do not drive a car, pilot an airplane, operate dangerous machinery or do jobs that require you to be alert until you know how you are going to react to this drug. If you become dizzy, you should be careful going up and down stairs. Sit or lie down at the first sign of dizziness. Tell your doctor if you have been dizzy.

When to Call Your Doctor

Most people experience few or no side effects from this drug. However, any medicine can sometimes cause unwanted effects. Call your doctor if you develop a skin rash, sore throat or fever, ringing or buzzing in the ears, a feeling of fullness in the ears, swelling of the legs or ankles or sudden weight gain, bloody or black stools, severe stomach pain, vomiting of blood, yellow color to the skin or eyes, unusual bruising or bleeding, sudden decrease in urination (passing of water), unusual tiredness or weakness or confusion.

Allergic Reactions

Call your doctor immediately if you think you may be allergic to the medicine or if you develop a skin rash, hives, itching, swelling of the face or difficulty in breathing. If you cannot reach your doctor, phone a hospital emergency department.

Refills

Do not stop taking this medicine without your doctor's approval and do not go without medicine between prescription refills. Call your pharmacist for a refill 2 or 3 days before you will run out of the medicine.

Miscellaneous

Carry an identification card in your wallet or wear a medical alert bracelet indicating that you are taking this medicine, as well as the names and phone numbers of your doctors. If you do not already carry such a card, complete the Medicine Card in this book. Always tell your dentist, pharmacist and other doctors who are treating you that you are taking this medicine.

▶ DIGOXIN (ORAL)
LANOXIN, LANOXIN PEDIATRIC ELIXIR

Purpose

This medicine is used to help make the heartbeat strong and steady. This can also help improve blood circulation.

Allergies/Warnings

Be sure to tell your doctor and pharmacist if you are allergic to any medicine.

How to Use This Medicine

Time of Administration

Take the medicine at the time recommended by your physician.

How to Administer

Take the medicine with a full glass of water.

If you were prescribed LANOXIN PEDIATRIC ELIXIR:
- A dropper is used to measure the dose. If you do not fully understand how to use the dropper to measure an accurate dose, *see* Medicine Dropper (page 21).

Special Instructions

Length of Therapy
It is very important that you take this medicine exactly as your doctor has prescribed. Do not miss any doses and take the medicine even if you feel well. Try to take this medicine at the same time(s) every day so that you will have a constant level of medicine in your body. Do not take extra tablets without your doctor's approval. Note: Some people may only need to take the medicine every second or third day.

Pregnancy/Breastfeeding
Women who are pregnant, breastfeeding or planning to become pregnant should tell their doctor before taking this medicine.

Drug Interactions
Some nonprescription drugs can interfere with this medicine or aggravate your heart condition. Do not take any of the following without the approval of your doctor or pharmacist: antacids; laxatives; cough, cold or sinus products; antidiarrhea products; asthma or allergy products.

There are other drug interactions that can occur. If you are taking any other medicines, be sure to check with your pharmacist or doctor.

Special Precautions
It is recommended that you learn how to check your pulse rate. Ask your doctor or nurse to teach you. Check your pulse regularly while you are taking this medicine. If your pulse becomes much slower than usual (or if it is less than 50 beats per minute) or if the rhythm and force of your pulse change, check with your doctor. The dose of your medicine may have to be adjusted. A pulse rate that is too slow may cause circulation problems.

When to Call Your Doctor
Most people experience few or no side effects from this drug. However, any medicine can sometimes cause unwanted effects. Call your doctor immediately if you develop nausea, vomiting, diarrhea, loss of appetite, blurred vision, changes in color vision (such as yellow or

green vision or halos around objects), depression, confusion, bothersome headaches, unusual tiredness or weakness, skin rash or hives, or
if your pulse rate becomes slower than normal or changes in rhythm
or force.

Refills

Do not stop taking this medicine without your doctor's approval
and do not go without medicine between prescription refills. Call your
pharmacist for a refill 2 or 3 days before you will run out of the
medicine.

Miscellaneous

Carry an identification card in your wallet or wear a medical alert
bracelet indicating that you are taking this medicine, as well as the
names and phone numbers of your doctors. If you do not already carry
such a card, complete the Medicine Card in this book. Always tell your
dentist, pharmacist and other doctors who are treating you that you
are taking this medicine.

Yellow Dyes in Medicines Causing Allergies

Many Canadian pharmaceutical manufacturers are removing tartrazine dye (FD&C Yellow No. 5) from their medications. The
reason is that some people are hypersensitive to tartrazine and
will develop asthma, itching of the skin, swelling and runny nose.
Tartrazine hypersensitivity is frequently seen in patients who are
also hypersensitive to ASA.

Many questions about tartrazine hypersensitivity remain unan-
swered. In the meantime, sensitive patients should avoid foods
and drugs containing this yellow dye. It is not sufficient to avoid
yellow-colored foods or drugs since the dye is often included in
many other color blends, such as turquoise, green or maroon.

If you think you are allergic to tartrazine, discuss this with your
doctor and tell your pharmacist. Your pharmacist can tell you if
your medications are tartrazine-free.

▶ **DILTIAZEM (ORAL)**
Apo-Diltiaz, Cardizem, Cardizem SR

NIFEDIPINE
Adalat, Adalat FT, Adalat P.A. 10, Adalat P.A. 20, Apo-Nifed, Novo-Nifedin

VERAPAMIL
Apo-Verap, Isoptin, Isoptin SR, Novoveramil

Purpose

This medicine is a type of drug called a calcium channel blocker and is used to help relieve and control angina attacks (chest pains). It does this by improving the supply of blood and oxygen to the heart. It eases the work of the heart and relaxes and widens narrowed blood vessels in the heart. It will not relieve an angina attack that has already started because it starts to work too slowly.

These medicines are also used to treat high blood pressure and a number of other conditions. Check with your doctor if you do not know why it has been prescribed.

Allergies/Warnings

Be sure to tell your doctor and pharmacist if you are allergic to any medicine.

How to Use This Medicine

Time of Administration

If you were prescribed DILTIAZEM or NIFEDIPINE:

- This medicine can be taken with a little fluid during or after meals. It may also be taken with a glass of water on an empty stomach at least 1 hour before (or 2 hours after) eating food.
- If dizziness, flushing, or swelling of the feet occurs (more common with NIFEDIPINE), it may help to take the medicine with some food.

If you were prescribed VERAPAMIL:

- Take this medicine with food.

How to Administer

If you were prescribed ADALAT P.A. 10, ADALAT P.A. 20, CARDIZEM SR, ISOPTIN SR:

- These medicines are long-acting and must be swallowed whole. Do not crush, chew or break them into pieces.

If you were prescribed ADALAT FT:
- These tablets must be swallowed whole.

Special Instructions

Length of Therapy

Do not take any more of this medicine than your doctor has pre-scribed and do not stop taking this medicine suddenly without the approval of your doctor. It may be necessary for your doctor to reduce your dose slowly since your body will need time to adjust. It could be harmful and could cause an angina attack if you suddenly stopped taking the medicine.

Pregnancy/Breastfeeding

Women who are pregnant, breastfeeding or planning to become pregnant should not take DILTIAZEM or NIFEDIPINE, and should tell their doctor before taking VERAPAMIL.

Drug Interactions

Some nonprescription drugs can aggravate your heart condition. Do not take any of the following without the approval of your doctor or pharmacist: cough, cold or sinus products; asthma or allergy products. Read the label of the product to see if there is a warning. If there is, check with your doctor or pharmacist before using the product.

Alcohol

Do not drink alcoholic beverages after taking this medicine because the combination may cause a serious drop in blood pressure, dizziness and/or fainting.

Special Precautions

During the first few days of taking NIFEDIPINE, you may experience a headache. It may be relieved by taking the capsules with some food or, if your doctor agrees, by taking ASA or ACETAMINOPHEN. This is a normal side effect and it usually disappears within a few days. Call your doctor if it continues.

If this medicine causes dizziness, lightheadedness or fainting, you should be careful going up and down stairs and you should not change positions too rapidly. Sit or lie down at the first sign of dizziness. Do not drive a car, pilot an airplane or operate machinery if you experience dizziness.

Keep a record of the number of angina attacks you have as well as a list of the possible causes of the attacks. This information will help your physician give you the best treatment. Be sure to tell your doctor if you have an increase in the number, length or severity of attacks.

Cigarette smoking can aggravate angina and is a special risk for people who have heart conditions.

Check with your doctor about the amount of exercise that is safe for you. This medicine can reduce chest pain resulting from too much exercise and make it difficult to tell when a person has exercised just the right amount.

This medicine may cause some people to become constipated. To help prevent constipation, try increasing the amount of bulk in your diet (for example, bran, fresh fruits and salads), exercising more often or drinking more fluids (unless otherwise directed). Call your doctor if the constipation continues.

For NIFEDIPINE:
- If you have diabetes, your diabetes medication may have to be adjusted.
- If you think your blood sugar is not normal or harder to control, call your doctor.

For DILTIAZEM *or* VERAPAMIL:
- Ask your doctor how to check your pulse rate. Check your pulse regularly while you are taking this medicine. If your pulse becomes much slower than usual or if it is less than 50 beats per minute, check with your doctor about taking the drug that day. The dose of your medicine may have to be adjusted. A pulse rate that is too slow may cause circulation problems.

When to Call Your Doctor

Most people experience few or no side effects from this drug. However, any medicine can sometimes cause unwanted effects.

For NIFEDIPINE:
- Call your doctor if you develop fainting spells, a skin rash, swelling of the ankles, legs or feet, difficulty in breathing, coughing, swelling or soreness of the gums, unusually fast heartbeats, or if your chest pain is not relieved.

For DILTIAZEM:
- Call your doctor if you develop fainting spells, a skin rash, unusually slow heartbeats, swelling of the ankles, legs or feet, or if your chest pain is not relieved.

For VERAPAMIL:
- Call your doctor if you develop fainting spells, a skin rash, difficulty in breathing, coughing, unusually fast or slow heartbeats, swelling of the ankles, legs or feet, or if your chest pain is not relieved.

Allergic Reactions
Call your doctor immediately if you think you may be allergic to the medicine or if you develop a skin rash, hives, itching, swelling of the face or difficulty in breathing. If you cannot reach your doctor, phone a hospital emergency department.

Storage
ADALAT capsules and tablets are sensitive to light. Therefore, keep the medicine in the container in which they were dispensed.

Traveling Overseas? Don't Forget Your Medicines

If you are planning a trip to a foreign country, here are some practical tips about your medicines:

- Be sure to take enough of your regular medicines with you on the trip. If you do not have enough medicine to last for the entire trip, ask your doctor to prescribe an additional quantity of the medicine.

- If your doctor gives you a new prescription, get it filled at a pharmacy *before* you leave home. Foreign pharmacies will not accept prescriptions from Canadian physicians.

- Carry your medicines with you in your hand luggage. Do *not* put them in your suitcases because:
  - Luggage can get lost.
  - Luggage is often exposed to hot and cold temperatures at airports and in the baggage area of the plane. This can lower the potency of the medicines.

- Carry a list of your medicines with you. This list should include the generic name of the medicine, the brand name of the medicine, the strength, the manufacturer, the prescription number and the phone number of your pharmacy at home.

  In foreign countries, the same brand name of a drug may contain a different dose of the medicine or may even contain a different drug!

- If you are taking a narcotic or a habit-forming drug, it is a good idea to get a letter from your doctor stating that you must take this medicine. This will help avoid any problems when suspicious customs agents ask you about the narcotics. Always keep the medicines in the original prescription containers with the prescription label attached.

- If any of your medicines can make you more sensitive to the sun, take along sunglasses and a sunscreen agent and try not to stay in the sun for long periods of time.

- If you become ill in a foreign country and must take a foreign drug, be sure to get the foreign doctor to write down the name, dosage and manufacturer of the drug he or she is prescribing. Your doctor at home will need this information.

Refills
Do not stop taking this medicine without your doctor's approval and do not go without medicine between prescription refills. Call your pharmacist for a refill 2 or 3 days before you will run out of the medicine.

Discuss with your pharmacist the implications of dispensing all your refills for this medicine with the same manufacturer's product. (*See* Generic Drugs, page 13.)

Miscellaneous
Carry an identification card in your wallet or wear a medical alert bracelet indicating that you are taking this medicine, as well as the names and phone numbers of your doctors. If you do not already carry such a card, complete the Medicine Card in this book. Always tell your dentist, pharmacist and other doctors who are treating you that you are taking this medicine.

▶ **DIPYRIDAMOLE (ORAL)**
Apo-Dipyridamole, Novodipiradol, Persantine

DIPYRIDAMOLE-ASA
Asasantine

Purpose

This medicine is used to help prevent angina attacks (chest pains). It will not relieve an angina attack that has already started because it starts to work too slowly.

It is also used alone or combined with other drugs, such as ASA, after a heart attack to lessen the risk of another heart attack, and after some types of blood vessel surgery to prevent clotting of the blood.

It may also be used to treat some other conditions. Check with your doctor if you do not know why the drug has been prescribed.

Aging and the Color of Medicines

As a person gets older, the lens of the eye tends to yellow. This makes vision less clear, glare becomes more of a problem and it is more difficult to distinguish between blue and green, and white and yellow.

If a person has difficulty distinguishing between these colors and if he or she is taking medicines that are white and yellow (or blue and green), there is a chance that he or she will get the medicines mixed up and not take them correctly.

It is important to distinguish the white from the yellow tablets (or the blue from the green tablets) in some way. One way is to ask the pharmacist to dispense the drugs in different size containers and to label the vials clearly with large lettering.

How to Use This Medicine

Time of Administration

Take this medicine with a glass of water on an empty stomach at least 1 hour before (or 2 hours after) eating food. The drug may be taken with a light snack or a glass of milk if it upsets your stomach.

Special Instructions

Length of Therapy

It may be necessary to take this medicine for 2 or 3 months before you feel its full benefit.

If you are taking this medicine for angina, do not stop taking it suddenly without the approval of your doctor. It will be necessary for your doctor to reduce your dose slowly since your body will need time to adjust. It could be harmful and make your condition worse if you suddenly stopped taking the medicine.

Pregnancy/Breastfeeding

Women who are pregnant, breastfeeding or planning to become pregnant should tell their doctor before taking this medicine.

Drug Interactions

Some nonprescription drugs can aggravate your condition. Do not take any of the following without the approval of your doctor or pharmacist: cough, cold or sinus products; asthma or allergy products. Read the label of the product to see if there is a warning. If there is, check with your doctor or pharmacist before using the product.

Alcohol

Do not drink alcoholic beverages without the approval of your doctor while you are taking this medicine as the combination may make you feel dizzy or faint.

Special Precautions

If you become dizzy or feel faint, sit or lie down until these effects pass. Always get up slowly after you have been sitting or lying down. Get out of bed slowly in the morning and dangle your feet over the edge of the bed for a few minutes before standing up. Do not drive a car, pilot an airplane, operate dangerous machinery or do jobs that require you to be alert if you are dizzy.

When you first start taking this drug, you may get a headache or flushing. These are common side effects and will usually disappear within a few days. Call your doctor if they continue.

Cigarette smoking can aggravate angina and is a special risk for people who have heart conditions.

When to Call Your Doctor

Most people experience few or no side effects from this drug. However, any medicine can sometimes cause unwanted effects. Call your

doctor if you develop a skin rash, chest pain, fainting spells, nausea or vomiting, severe headaches or persistent stomach cramps.

Refills

Do not stop taking this medicine without your doctor's approval and do not go without medicine between prescription refills. Call your pharmacist for a refill 2 or 3 days before you will run out of the medicine.

Discuss with your pharmacist the implications of dispensing all your refills for this medicine with the same manufacturer's product. (*See* Generic Drugs, page 13.)

Miscellaneous

Carry an identification card in your wallet or wear a medical alert bracelet indicating that you are taking this medicine, as well as the names and phone numbers of your doctors. If you do not already carry such a card, complete the Medicine Card in this book. Always tell your dentist, pharmacist and other doctors who are treating you that you are taking this medicine.

Do Not Swallow Topical Pain Killers

If you are applying a topical anesthetic (pain killer) to the inside of the mouth or gums, you should spit out the medicine and not swallow it. The anesthetic could cause side effects if you swallowed it and it passed into your bloodstream.

This is why topical anesthetics (for example, LIDOCAINE) should not be prescribed for the relief of teething discomfort in infants. Infants do not know how to spit out the medicines.

There is a report in *Clinical Pediatrics* of an 11-month-old infant who developed seizures after being treated with a topical lidocaine 2% solution. The mother had applied the solution to the infant's gum with her finger 5 or 6 times a day for seven days. Approximately 80 mL of the solution had been used. It was not possible to determine whether the toxic lidocaine blood level was due to absorption of the drug from the infant's gums or from the infant swallowing the anesthetic.

▶ DISOPYRAMIDE (ORAL)
NORPACE, NORPACE CR, RYTHMODAN, RYTHMODAN-LA

Purpose
This medicine is used to help make the heart beat at a regular, normal rate and rhythm.

Allergies/Warnings
Be sure to tell your doctor and pharmacist if you are allergic to any medicine or if you have glaucoma, diabetes, congestive heart failure, a prostate problem, difficulty urinating or any other medical condition.

How to Use This Medicine

Time of Administration
It is best to take this medicine with a glass of water on an empty stomach. However, if you develop stomach upset after taking the drug, take it with some food. Call your doctor if you continue to have an upset stomach.

How to Administer
Take the medicine with a full glass of water unless otherwise directed.

If you were prescribed NORPACE CR *or* RYTHMODAN-LA:
- These medicines are long-acting and must be swallowed whole. Do not crush or chew them.

Special Instructions

Length of Therapy
It is very important that you take this medicine exactly as your doctor has prescribed. Do not miss any doses. Take the medicine even if you feel well. Try to take this medicine at the same time(s) every day so that you will have a constant level of medicine in your body. Do not take extra tablets without your doctor's approval.

Do not stop taking this medicine suddenly without the approval of your doctor. It will be necessary for your doctor to reduce your dose slowly since your body will need time to adjust. It could be harmful and make your condition worse if you suddenly stopped taking the medicine.

Pregnancy/Breastfeeding

Women who are pregnant, breastfeeding or planning to become pregnant should tell their doctor before taking this medicine.

Drug Interactions

Some nonprescription drugs can interfere with this medicine or aggravate your heart condition. Do not take any of the following without the approval of your doctor or pharmacist: antacids or baking soda; cough, cold or sinus products; asthma or allergy products.

Alcohol

Do not drink alcoholic beverages while taking this drug without the approval of your doctor because the combination could cause dizziness, fainting or, rarely, low blood sugar.

Special Precautions

If this medicine causes dizziness or lightheadedness, you should be careful going up and down stairs and you should not change positions too rapidly. Lightheadedness is more likely to occur if you stand up suddenly—this is due to blood collecting in the legs and lasts for a few seconds. Therefore, get up from a sitting or lying position more slowly and tighten and relax your leg muscles or wiggle your toes to help promote circulation. In the morning, get out of bed slowly and dangle your feet over the edge of the bed for a few minutes before standing up. Sit or lie down at the first sign of dizziness. Do not drive a car, pilot an airplane, operate dangerous machinery or do jobs that require you to be alert if you have been dizzy.

You may become more sensitive to heat because your body may perspire less while you are taking this drug. Be careful not to become overheated during exercise or in hot weather. Try to avoid strenuous exercise, standing for long periods of time (especially in hot weather), hot showers, hot baths, saunas or Jacuzzis while taking this medicine.

If your mouth becomes dry, drink water, suck ice chips or a hard, sour candy (sugarless) or chew gum (sugarless). Sugarless products are recommended in order to avoid dental problems. You may wish to ask your pharmacist about special solutions, called artificial saliva, that can also be used to help restore moisture in the mouth. It is especially important to brush and floss your teeth regularly if you develop a dry mouth, to help prevent gum problems.

If your eyes become dry, ask your pharmacist or doctor to recommend a lubricating/wetting solution or artificial tears. This side effect is more common in elderly people.

This medicine may rarely cause the blood sugar to fall in some people. This side effect is more common in patients with congestive heart failure or diabetes. If you develop sweating, shaking, drowsiness, headache, excessive hunger, nausea, nervousness, chills, cold sweats, cool pale skin, confusion, unusual tiredness or weakness, eat or drink a food containing sugar and call your doctor right away.

This medicine may cause some people to become constipated. To help prevent constipation, try increasing the amount of bulk in your diet (for example, bran, fresh fruits and salads), exercising more often or drinking more fluids (unless otherwise directed). Call your doctor if the constipation continues.

When to Call Your Doctor

Most people experience few or no side effects from this drug. However, any medicine can sometimes cause unwanted effects. Call your doctor if you develop a sore throat, fever, mouth sores, fainting, difficulty urinating (passing your water), shortness of breath, chest pains, unusually slow or fast heartbeats, confusion or depression, unusual nervousness, a yellow color to the skin or eyes, eye pain, swelling of the legs or ankles, sudden weight gain of 5 pounds (2.5 kg) or more or muscle weakness.

Allergic Reactions

Call your doctor immediately if you think you may be allergic to the medicine or if you develop a skin rash, hives, itching, swelling of the face or difficulty in breathing. If you cannot reach your doctor, phone a hospital emergency department.

Refills

Do not stop taking this medicine without your doctor's approval and do not go without medicine between prescription refills. Call your pharmacist for a refill 2 or 3 days before you will run out of the medicine.

Discuss with your pharmacist the implications of dispensing all your refills for this medicine with the same manufacturer's product. (*See* Generic Drugs, page 13.) The long-acting medicines (NORPACE CR and RYTHMODAN-LA) are not interchangeable.

Miscellaneous

Carry an identification card in your wallet or wear a medical alert bracelet indicating that you are taking this medicine, as well as the names and phone numbers of your doctors. If you do not already carry such a card, complete the Medicine Card in this book. Always tell your dentist, pharmacist and other doctors who are treating you that you are taking this medicine.

▶ **DIVALPROEX SODIUM (ORAL)**
EPIVAL

VALPROIC ACID
DEPAKENE

Purpose

This medicine is used to help control seizures. It is commonly used in the treatment of epilepsy.

Allergies/Warnings

If you have ever had an allergic reaction to an anticonvulsant or seizure medicine, tell your doctor and pharmacist before you take any of this medicine. Also tell your doctor if you have any liver problems.

How to Use This Medicine

Time of Administration

It is very important that you take this medicine exactly as your doctor has prescribed. Do not miss any doses and take the medicine even if you feel well. Try to take this medicine at the same time(s) every day so that you will have a constant level of medicine in your body. This is the only way that you can receive the full benefit of the medicine. If you forget to take this medicine, the amount of medicine in your blood will decrease and you may have seizures.

How to Administer

Take this medicine after food if it upsets your stomach. Call your doctor if you continue to have stomach upset or if you develop nausea, vomiting, diarrhea or constipation.

For DEPAKENE 500 mg CAPSULES *and* EPIVAL TABLETS:
- This medicine has a special coating and should be swallowed whole. Do not chew or break the tablets or capsules open.

For DEPAKENE SYRUP:
- If a dropper, oral liquid syringe or special measuring spoon is used to measure the dose and you do not fully understand how to use

it, *see* Medicine Dropper (page 21), Oral Liquid Syringe (page 17) and Medicine Spoon (page 22).

Special Instructions

Length of Therapy

Do not stop taking this medicine suddenly without the approval of your doctor. It usually will be necessary for your doctor to slowly reduce your dose since your body will need time to adjust. You could develop seizures if you suddenly stopped taking the medicine.

Pregnancy/Breastfeeding

Women who are pregnant or planning to become pregnant should tell their doctor before taking this medicine.

Women should not breastfeed without their doctor's approval. This medicine can pass into the breast milk and cause side effects in the infant.

Drug Interactions

It is important that you obtain the advice of your doctor or pharmacist before taking any other prescription and nonprescription medicines including pain relievers, sleeping pills, tranquilizers, medicine for seizures, muscle relaxants, anesthetics, anticoagulants (blood thinners), medicines for depression or medicines for allergies. Combining this medicine with some of these drugs could cause drowsiness or dizziness.

There are other drug interactions that can occur. If you are taking any other medicines, be sure to check first with your pharmacist or doctor.

Alcohol

Do not drink alcoholic beverages while taking this drug without the approval of your doctor because the combination could cause drowsiness. One drink may have the same effect that 2 or 3 drinks normally would have.

Special Precautions

Be sure to keep your doctor's appointments so that your doctor can check your progress. This is especially important during the first few months of therapy, when the doctor will decide the best dose of this medicine for your condition.

This medicine may cause dizziness, drowsiness or blurred vision in some people. If you become dizzy, you should be careful going up and down stairs. Sit or lie down at the first sign of dizziness. Do not drive a car, use a sewing machine, operate dangerous machinery or do jobs that require you to be alert until you know how you are going to react to the drug. Tell your doctor if you are dizzy or drowsy or have blurred vision.

If this medicine is for a child, do not let him or her ride a bike, climb trees, etc. until you can determine how he or she is going to react to this medicine. Children could hurt themselves if they participated in these activities when they were dizzy.

Avoid swimming alone or taking part in high-risk sports in which a sudden seizure could cause injury.

This medicine can cause weight gain and, less frequently, hair loss.

For patients with diabetes:
• This medicine can cause the test for urinary ketones to be falsely high. Check with your doctor.

When to Call Your Doctor
Most people experience few or no side effects from this drug. However, any medicine can sometimes cause unwanted effects. Call your doctor if you develop a sore throat, fever, or mouth sores, skin rash and itching, swollen glands, unusual bruising or bleeding, changes in vision, fast eye movements, muscle or joint pain, menstrual irregularity (in women), swelling of the hands or feet, loss of appetite, vomiting, tremors or shaking, light-colored stools or yellow color to the skin or eyes, or if you become "hyper," confused or depressed.

Call your doctor if you have an increase in the frequency of seizures.

Allergic Reactions
Allergic reactions to this medicine are very uncommon. Call your doctor immediately if you think you may be allergic to the medicine or if you develop a skin rash, hives, itching, swelling of the face or difficulty in breathing. If you cannot reach your doctor, phone a hospital emergency department.

Refills
Do not stop taking this medicine without your doctor's approval and do not go without medicine between prescription refills. Call your pharmacist for a refill 2 or 3 days before you will run out of the medicine.

Miscellaneous

Carry an identification card in your wallet or wear a medical alert bracelet indicating that you are taking this medicine, as well as the names and phone numbers of your doctors. If you do not already carry such a card, complete the Medicine Card in this book. Always tell your dentist, pharmacist and other doctors who are treating you that you are taking this medicine.

▶ **DOMPERIDONE (ORAL)**
MOTILIUM

METOCLOPRAMIDE
APO-METOCLOP, EMEX, MAXERAN, REGLAN

Purpose

This medicine is used to treat certain types of stomach and intestinal disorders in which there is nausea, vomiting and a persistent feeling of fullness after eating. DOMPERIDONE may also be used to prevent similar symptoms from certain medicines used to treat Parkinson's Disease.

Allergies/Warnings

If you have ever had an allergic reaction to any medicine or if you have seizures or any other medical condition, tell your doctor and pharmacist before you take any of this medicine.

How to Use This Medicine

Time of Administration

Take this medicine 15 to 30 minutes *before* meals unless otherwise directed. If your physician prescribes a dose at bedtime, be sure to eat a snack 15 to 30 minutes *after* taking the medicine.

Relief of nausea should occur after the first few doses.

How to Administer
For liquid medicines:
• If a spoon is used to measure the dose, it is recommended that you use a medicine spoon or an oral liquid syringe, which you can obtain from your pharmacist. *See* Medicine Spoon (page 22) and Oral Liquid Syringe (page 17).

Special Instructions

Length of Therapy

Do not take this medicine more often or longer than recommended by your doctor. You may increase your chance of developing side effects.

Pregnancy/Breastfeeding

Women who are pregnant, breastfeeding or planning to become pregnant should tell their doctor before taking this medicine.

Drug Interactions

Check with your pharmacist or doctor before purchasing any pain relievers, nonprescription drugs, sleeping pills, tranquilizers, medicine for seizures, muscle relaxants, anesthetics, medicines for diarrhea, glaucoma, depression or allergies without the permission of your doctor. Combining this medicine with some of these drugs could cause significant drowsiness or dizziness.

There are other drug interactions that can occur. If you are taking any other medicines, be sure to check first with your pharmacist or doctor.

Alcohol

Do not drink alcoholic beverages while taking this drug because it may make the drowsiness worse.

Special Precautions

If you become dizzy, you should be careful going up and down stairs. Do not drive a car, pilot an airplane, operate dangerous machinery or do jobs that require you to be alert until you know how you are going to react to the drug. Sit or lie down at the first sign of dizziness. Tell your doctor if the dizziness continues.

When to Call Your Doctor

Most people experience few or no side effects from this drug. However, any medicine can sometimes cause unwanted effects. Call your doctor immediately if you develop unusual movements of the face, tongue, hands or eyes, trembling, shuffling walk, unusual muscle stiffness, stiff neck, depression or severe drowsiness.

Rarely, some people taking this medicine may notice a slight increase in the size of their breasts or some breast soreness. Women may notice changes in their menstrual periods. If you develop any of these problems, stop the medicine and consult your doctor immediately.

Allergic Reactions

Call your doctor immediately if you think you may be allergic to the medicine or if you develop a skin rash, hives, itching, swelling of the face or difficulty in breathing. If you cannot reach your doctor, phone a hospital emergency department.

Storage

Store the medicine at room temperature away from heat and light.

▶ DOXYCYCLINE (ORAL)
APO-DOXY, DOXYCIN, NOVODOXYLIN, VIBRA-TABS, VIBRAMYCIN, VIBRA-TABS C-PAK

MINOCYCLINE
MINOCIN

Purpose

This medicine is an antibiotic used to treat certain types of infections. Your doctor has prescribed this antibiotic for your present infection only. Do not use it for other infections or give it to other people. This medicine is also used to treat acne.

Allergies/Warnings

If you have ever had an allergic reaction to TETRACYCLINE or any other medicine, tell your doctor and pharmacist before you take any of this medicine.

If you have ever had allergies, asthma, hay fever, or hives, tell your doctor or pharmacist before taking any of this medicine.

This medicine should not be given to children under 12 years of age unless directed by your doctor. The medicine may permanently discolor the child's teeth and slow down the growth of the teeth and bones.

How to Use This Medicine

Time of Administration

This medicine should be taken with food. This will help prevent stomach upset. Call your doctor if you develop stomach upset.

Space your doses of the medicine around the clock (throughout the entire day of 24 hours). For example, if you are to take 2 doses each day, space the doses 12 hours apart. This will keep a constant level of the medicine in your body.

How to Administer

For tablets and capsules:

- Take the tablets and capsules with a full glass (8 oz or 240 mL) of water. This will help prevent irritation of the stomach and esophagus.

For APO-DOXY, NOVODOXYLIN, VIBRAMYCIN *and* VIBRA-TABS:

- Sit up or stand up when you take each dose in order to help prevent "heartburn" or irritation of the esophagus. It is also best to take the evening dose at least 1 hour before going to bed.

Special Instructions

Length of Therapy

It is important to take all of this medicine plus any refills that your doctor told you to take. Do not stop taking this medicine earlier than your doctor has recommended even if you begin to feel better. If you stop taking the medicine too soon, the infection may return.

This is especially important if you are taking the medicine to cure a strep infection because, if the infection is not completely cleared up, serious heart problems could develop later. After treatment for a strep infection, your doctor may want to do a test to make sure that the infection is gone.

Pregnancy/Breastfeeding

Women who are pregnant or planning to become pregnant should tell their doctor before taking this medicine.

This medicine is not recommended during pregnancy since it may cause permanent discoloration of the infant's teeth and may slow down the normal growth and development of the infant's teeth and bones.

Women who are breastfeeding should tell their doctor before taking this medicine. This medicine may pass into the breast milk and cause discoloration of the infant's teeth and may slow down the normal growth and development of the infant's teeth and bones.

Drug Interactions

Some antacids and laxatives can make this medicine less effective if they are taken at the same time. This includes products which contain aluminum, magnesium, bismuth, Epsom salt or sodium bicarbonate (baking soda). In addition, if you are taking MINOCYCLINE, products containing calcium can make this drug less effective.

Check with your pharmacist before you purchase any antacids or laxatives. If you must take antacids or laxatives, they should be taken at least 2 hours before or after this medicine.

Iron pills or vitamins containing minerals can also make this medicine less effective. In addition, products containing zinc can make this drug less effective. If you must take these products, take them 3 hours before (or 2 hours after) this medicine.

There have been some reports that oral contraceptives (birth control pills) may not work as well while you are taking this medicine. Unplanned pregnancies may occur. Ask your doctor about using another form of birth control while you are taking these antibiotics. Also call your doctor if you develop spotting or breakthrough bleeding since these can be signs of decreased birth control effect.

Special Precautions

This medicine may make some people more sensitive to sunlight and some tanning lamps. When you begin taking this medicine, try to avoid too much sun until you see how you are going to react. If your skin does become more sensitive to sunlight, tell your doctor and try not to stay in direct sunlight for extended periods of time. While in the sun, wear protective clothing and sunglasses. You may wish to ask your pharmacist about suitable sunscreen products. Call your doctor if you become sunburned.

It has been reported that MINOCYCLINE may cause dizziness or lightheadedness. Do not drive a car, pilot an airplane, operate dangerous machinery or do jobs that require you to be alert until you know how you are going to react to the drug. If you become dizzy or drowsy, you should be careful going up and down stairs. Sit or lie down at the first sign of dizziness. Tell your doctor if the dizziness continues.

When to Call Your Doctor

Call your doctor if your symptoms do not improve within a few days (or a few weeks or months if you are taking the medicine for acne) or if they become worse.

Any medicine can sometimes cause unwanted effects. Call your doctor if you develop severe cramps or burning of the stomach, vomiting, severe watery diarrhea, skin rash, dark-colored tongue, sore mouth or tongue, itching of the rectal or genital areas or, in women, a vaginal discharge that was not present before you started the medicine.

Allergic Reactions

Call your doctor immediately if you think you may be allergic to the medicine or if you develop a skin rash, hives, itching, swelling of the face or difficulty in breathing. If you cannot reach your doctor, phone a hospital emergency department.

Storage

Store the medicine in a cool, dark place and keep the bottle tightly closed.

If for some reason you cannot take all of the medicine, take the unused portion back to your pharmacist. You should discuss why you cannot finish the medicine with your pharmacist. Do not take any unused medicine after the discard (expiration) date on the bottle.

Refills

Do not go without medicine between prescription refills. Call your pharmacist for a refill 2 or 3 days before you will run out of the medicine.

Avoiding Drug Interactions

Some drug interactions can be avoided by spacing the 2 drugs far enough apart so that they are not in the stomach at the same time.

For example, the antibiotic effect of TETRACYCLINE can be decreased if a person takes an iron supplement at the same time. The iron binds with the TETRACYCLINE and prevents some of the TETRACYCLINE from being absorbed from the stomach.

With this interaction, it is not necessary for the person to stop taking either of the medicines. The drug interaction can be *avoided* by simply taking the iron supplement at least 3 hours before or 2 hours after the TETRACYCLINE. A long-acting iron supplement must not be used, because the drug interaction can still occur.

This interaction also applies to other drugs related to TETRACYCLINE such as DEMECLOCYCLINE, DOXYCYCLINE and MINOCYCLINE.

▶ **ERYTHROMYCIN BASE (ORAL and TOPICAL)**
APO-ERYTHRO BASE, APO-ERYTHRO E-C, E-MYCIN, ERYC,
ERYTHROMID, NOVORYTHRO BASE, PCE

ERYTHROMYCIN ESTOLATE
ILOSONE, NOVORYTHRO ESTOLATE

ERYTHROMYCIN ETHYLSUCCINATE
APO-ERYTHRO-ES, EES 200, EES 400, EES 600

ERYTHROMYCIN STEARATE
APO-ERYTHRO-S, ERYTHROCIN, NOVORYTHRO STEARATE

Purpose

This medicine is an antibiotic used to treat certain types of infections.
Your doctor has prescribed this antibiotic for your present infection.
Do not use it for other infections or give it to other people. This
medicine is also used to help control acne.

Allergies/Warnings

If you have ever had an allergic reaction to ERYTHROMYCIN or
any other medicine or if you have liver problems, tell your doctor and
pharmacist before you take any of this medicine.

How to Use This Medicine

Time of Administration

The time you take your medicine depends on the brand of medicine
your doctor prescribed. Take your medicine according to the following
instructions:

If you were prescribed APO-ERYTHRO BASE, APO-ERYTHRO-S,
ERYTHROCIN, ERYC, ERYTHROMID, NOVORYTHRO BASE,
NOVORYTHRO STEARATE, PCE:
- It is best to take this medicine with a glass of water on an empty
  stomach at least 1 hour before (or 2 hours after) eating food. Do
  not drink acidic fruit juices (such as orange or grapefruit juice) within
  1 hour of taking this medicine. Take the medicine at the proper
  time even if you skip a meal. If you develop stomach upset after
  taking the drug, take it with some food. Call your doctor if you
  continue to have an upset stomach.

If you were prescribed APO-ERYTHRO-ES *or* EES:
- Take the medicine *immediately after* meals.

247

If you were prescribed ILOSONE *or* NOVORYTHRO ESTOLATE CAPSULES *or* LIQUID:
- The medicine may be taken without regard to meals, either on an empty stomach or with food.

How to Administer
- Take the medicine with a full glass of water unless otherwise directed.

If you were prescribed EES CHEWABLE:
- Chew the tablets well before swallowing. Do not swallow the tablets whole. After you have chewed and swallowed the small pieces of the tablet, you may wish to drink some water.

If you were prescribed APO-ERYTHRO E-C *or* E-MYCIN:
- This medicine has a special coating and must be swallowed whole. Do not crush, chew or break it into pieces.
- Take it with a glass of water on an empty stomach 1 hour before or 2 hours after food.

If you or your child were prescribed ERYC 125:
- These capsules may be swallowed whole.
- Patients who have difficulty swallowing capsules may sprinkle the contents on food:
- Hold the capsule with the clear end down and the orange end up. Gently twist off the orange cap to open.
- Sprinkle ALL the medicine inside the capsule on a small amount (e.g., a spoonful) of applesauce, fruit jam or jelly, or ice cream.
- Swallow the spoonful of food containing the medicine. Do not crush or chew any of the pellets.
- Then drink a full glass of water to make sure all the pellets are swallowed.
- NOTE: If you accidentally spill the medicine, start over with a new capsule to make sure a full dose is taken.

For liquid medicines:
- If you were prescribed a suspension, shake the bottle well each time before pouring so that you can measure an accurate dose.
- If a spoon is used to measure the dose, it is recommended that you use a medicine spoon or an oral liquid syringe, which you can obtain from your pharmacist. These are more accurate than the average household teaspoon. *See* Oral Liquid Syringe (page 17) and Medicine Spoon (page 22).

If you were prescribed the topical solution:
- *See* Creams, Ointments, Gels, Solutions and Lotions (page 36).

Special Instructions

Length of Therapy

It is important to take all of this medicine plus any refills that your doctor told you to take. Do not stop taking this medicine earlier than your doctor has recommended even if you begin to feel better. If you stop taking the medicine too soon, the infection may return. This is especially important if you are taking the medicine to cure a strep infection, because if the infection is not completely cleared up, serious heart problems could develop later. After treatment for a strep infection, your doctor may want to do a test to make sure that the infection is gone.

Pregnancy/Breastfeeding

Women who are pregnant, breastfeeding or planning to become pregnant should tell their doctor before taking this medicine.

Special Precautions

This medicine sometimes causes diarrhea. Call your doctor if the diarrhea becomes severe and watery or does not go away after a few days. Do not try to treat the diarrhea yourself without first discussing it with your doctor.

When to Call Your Doctor

Call your doctor if your symptoms do not improve within a few days or if they become worse.

For oral medications:
- Most people experience few or no side effects from this drug. However, any medicine can sometimes cause unwanted effects. Call your doctor if you develop an unexplained fever, chills, sore mouth or tongue, severe stomach cramps, dark-colored urine, unusual weakness or tiredness, severe nausea or vomiting, pale-colored stools or a yellow color of the skin or eyes, rectal or genital itching or, in women, a vaginal discharge that was not present before you started taking the medicine.

For skin preparations:
- Call your doctor if your condition does not improve or if you develop redness, burning, tenderness or scaling of the skin.

Allergic Reactions

Call your doctor immediately if you think you may be allergic to the medicine or if you develop a skin rash, hives, itching, swelling of the face or difficulty in breathing. If you cannot reach your doctor, phone a hospital emergency department.

Storage

Some liquid forms of ERYTHROMYCIN should be kept in the refrigerator. Do not freeze. Follow the directions on the container.

If for some reason you cannot take all of the medicine, take the unused portion back to your pharmacist. You should discuss why you cannot finish the medicine with your pharmacist. Do not take any unused medicine after the discard (expiration) date on the bottle.

Refills

Do not go without medicine between prescription refills. Call your pharmacist for a refill 2 or 3 days before you will run out of the medicine.

Miscellaneous

For topical preparations:

- This medicine is for external use only. Do not swallow it. Keep it away from the eyes, mouth and nostrils.

▶ ERYTHROMYCIN ETHYLSUCCINATE-SULFISOXAZOLE (ORAL)

PEDIAZOLE

Purpose

This medicine contains two antibiotics and is used to treat middle-ear infections (acute otitis media) in children.

Your doctor has prescribed this antibiotic for the present infection. Do not use it for other infections or give it to other people.

Allergies/Warnings

If the child has ever had an allergic reaction to ERYTHROMYCIN or sulfa drugs or any other medicine (including diabetes medicines) or if the child has any liver problems, tell your doctor and pharmacist before you give any of this medicine.

This medicine should not be used in infants less than 2 months of age.

What Can You Do If Your Child Refuses to Take a Medicine?

If a parent is having difficulty administering a medicine to a child, it may be easier to gain the cooperation of the child if a positive approach is used. For example, children love to imitate and may be more cooperative if the parent says, "Here is your medicine. Drink it and I will give you some special medicine for your teddy bear."

It may also help to let children choose which of their medicines they would like first and let them choose whether they want to take it on your lap or in their favorite chair.

It often helps to let the child handle the oral liquid syringe or the medicine spoon before it is filled with the medicine. This gives the child an opportunity to become familiar with the device so that he or she is not frightened.

When you know that a medicine does not taste good, be honest with the child. Don't try to trick the child by telling him or her that the medicine tastes good. The child will soon find out that you have tricked him or her and will be less cooperative the next time.

After the child has taken the medicine, a flavored drink or a glass of water may help to remove any aftertaste of the medicine. Ask your pharmacist if there are any fruit juices that should not be given immediately after administering the medicine. Some medicines are destroyed by fruit juices.

If you are administering a liquid medicine by means of an oral liquid syringe, point the tip of the syringe to the inside of the cheek or the back side of the mouth. This will help prevent drooling or choking. *Slowly* squirt the medicine into the mouth and allow the child to swallow naturally.

How to Use This Medicine

Time of Administration

This medicine may be taken without regard to meals but it is best to take it *immediately* after meals.

Try to space the medicine throughout the day in equally spaced intervals. Try to space the doses "around the clock" (throughout the entire day of 24 hours). For example, if the child is to receive 4 doses each day, space the doses as close to 6 hours apart as possible. This will keep a constant level of the medicine in the body.

Do not forget to give the child any doses. Arrange a schedule so that the child will also be able to receive necessary doses at school.

How to Administer

This medicine should be taken with a full glass of water with or without food. The medicine has a strawberry-banana flavor.

Shake the bottle well each time before pouring so that an accurate dose can be measured.

If a spoon is used to measure the dose, it is recommended that you use a medicine spoon or an oral liquid syringe, which you can obtain from your pharmacist. These are more accurate than the average household teaspoon. If you are using an oral liquid syringe, wash it thoroughly with warm water after each use. *See* How to Use Oral Liquid Syringe (page 17).

Special Instructions

Length of Therapy

It is important to give the child all of this medicine plus any refills that your doctor told you to give. Do not stop this medicine earlier than your doctor has recommended even if the child starts to feel better. If you stop giving the medicine too soon, the infection may return.

Pregnancy/Breastfeeding

This medicine should not be used in the last stages of pregnancy and/or during breastfeeding.

Special Precautions

This medicine sometimes causes diarrhea. Call your doctor if the diarrhea becomes severe and watery or does not go away after a few days. Do not try to treat the diarrhea yourself without first discussing it with your doctor.

This medicine may make some people more sensitive to sunlight and some tanning lamps. When your child begins taking this medicine, try to have the child avoid too much sun until you see how he or she is going to react. If the skin does become more sensitive to sunlight, tell your doctor and try to keep the child out of direct sunlight for extended periods of time. While in the sun, he or she should wear protective clothing and sunglasses. You may wish to ask your pharmacist about suitable sunscreen products. Call your doctor if the child becomes sunburned.

Since this medicine contains a "sulfa" drug, it is important that the child drink an adequate amount of water or other liquids in order to prevent kidney problems.

If the child becomes dizzy, warn him/her to be careful going up and down stairs. The child should sit or lie down at the first sign of dizziness. Tell your doctor if the dizziness continues.

When to Call Your Doctor

Call your doctor if the symptoms do not improve within a few days or if they become worse.

Most people experience few or no side effects from this drug. However, any medicine can sometimes cause unwanted effects. Call your doctor if your child develops an unexplained fever, chills, sore throat, mouth sores, severe stomach cramps, dark-colored urine, unusual weakness or tiredness, severe nausea or vomiting, unusual pale skin, unusual bruising or bleeding, swelling of the front part of the neck or eyes, difficulty in swallowing, hearing loss, unusual joint or lower back pain, blood in the urine, pain while urinating (passing water), redness, blistering, peeling or loosening of the skin, pale-colored stools, a yellow color of the skin or eyes or rectal or genital itching.

Allergic Reactions

Call your doctor immediately if you think your child may be allergic to the medicine or if he or she develops a skin rash, hives, itching, swelling of the face or difficulty in breathing. If you cannot reach your doctor, phone a hospital emergency department.

Storage

Some liquid forms of ERYTHROMYCIN should be kept in the refrigerator. Do not freeze. Follow the directions on the container.

If for some reason you cannot give all of the medicine, take the unused portion back to your pharmacist. You should discuss why you cannot finish the medicine with your pharmacist. Do not give any unused medicine after the discard (expiration) date on the bottle.

Refills

Do not go without medicine between prescription refills. Call your pharmacist for a refill 2 or 3 days before you will run out of the medicine.

▶ **ETHACRYNIC ACID (ORAL)**
EDECRIN

FUROSEMIDE
APO-FUROSEMIDE, LASIX, NOVOSEMIDE, URITOL

Purpose

This medicine is used to help the body get rid of excess fluids and to decrease swelling in several types of medical conditions. The medicine does this by increasing the amount of urine and is commonly called a water pill or fluid pill. FUROSEMIDE is also used to treat high blood pressure.

Allergies/Warnings

Be sure to tell your doctor or pharmacist if you are allergic to sulfa drugs, thiazide diuretics or any medicine or if you have any medical conditions.

How to Use This Medicine

Time of Administration

Try to take this medicine at the same time(s) every day so that you have a constant level of the medicine in your body.

When you first start taking this medicine, you will probably urinate (pass your water) more often and in larger amounts than usual. Therefore, if you are to take 1 dose each day, take it in the morning after breakfast. Do not initially take a dose at bedtime or you may have to get up during the night to go to the bathroom.

If you are to take more than 1 dose each day, take the last dose approximately 6 hours before bedtime so that you will not have to get up during the night to go to the bathroom. This effect will usually lessen after you have taken the drug for a while.

How to Administer

Take this medicine with food, meals or milk if it upsets your stomach.

For LASIX SOLUTION:

• Measure the dose carefully using the dropper or the special spoon that comes with the medicine. For more information, *see* Medicine Dropper (page 21) and Medicine Spoon (page 22).

Special Instructions

Length of Therapy
For patients with high blood pressure:
- High blood pressure (hypertension) is a long-term condition and it will probably be necessary for you to take the drug for a long time even if you feel better. If high blood pressure is not treated, it can lead to serious problems such as heart failure, strokes, blood vessel problems or kidney problems.

It is very important that you take this medicine as your doctor has directed and that you do not miss any doses. Otherwise, you cannot expect the drug to keep your blood pressure down or remove excess fluid.

Pregnancy/Breastfeeding
Women who are pregnant or planning to become pregnant should tell their doctor before taking this medicine.

This medicine passes into the breast milk and breastfeeding should be stopped.

Drug Interactions
Some nonprescription drugs can aggravate high blood pressure. Do not take any of the following without the approval of your doctor or pharmacist: cough, cold or sinus products; asthma or allergy products, since they may increase your blood pressure. Read the label of the nonprescription drug product to see if there is a warning. If there is, check with your doctor or pharmacist before using the product.

Do not take large doses of ASA or products containing ASA without the approval of your pharmacist.

Alcohol
Be careful drinking alcoholic beverages while taking this medicine because it could make the possible side effect of dizziness worse.

Special Precautions
This medicine normally causes your body to lose potassium. The body has warning signs to let you know if too much potassium is being lost. Call your doctor if you become unusually thirsty or if you develop leg cramps, unusual weakness, fatigue, vomiting, confusion or an irregular pulse. Since these symptoms may not be present in all patients, your doctor may wish to check your blood occasionally to see if it is low in potassium. Depending upon your dose, your doctor may pre-

scribe some medicine to replace the potassium or he or she may recommend that you regularly eat foods that contain a lot of potassium (see Appendix A). *Do not change your diet unless your doctor tells you to.*

If this medicine causes dizziness or lightheadedness, you should be careful going up and down stairs and you should not change positions too rapidly. Lightheadedness is more likely to occur if you stand up suddenly—this is due to blood collecting in the legs and lasts for a few seconds. Therefore, get up from a sitting or lying position more slowly and tighten and relax your leg muscles or wiggle your toes to help promote circulation. In the morning, get out of bed slowly and dangle your feet over the edge of the bed for a few minutes before standing up. Sit or lie down at the first sign of dizziness. Do not drive a car, pilot an airplane, operate dangerous machinery or do jobs that require you to be alert if you are dizzy. Tell your doctor if you have been dizzy.

In order to help prevent dizziness or fainting, your doctor may also recommend that you avoid strenuous exercise, standing for long periods of time (especially in hot weather), hot showers, Jacuzzis, hot baths or saunas.

People more than 65 years of age may be more sensitive to the side effects of dizziness and potassium loss.

For FUROSEMIDE *only:*
• This medicine may make some people more sensitive to sunlight and some tanning lamps. When you begin taking this medicine, try to avoid too much sun until you see how you are going to react. If your skin does become more sensitive to sunlight, tell your doctor and try not to stay in direct sunlight for extended periods of time. While in the sun, wear protective clothing and sunglasses. You may wish to ask your pharmacist about suitable sunscreen products. Call your doctor if you become sunburned.

For patients with diabetes:
• This medicine may cause your blood sugar to rise. Carefully test your blood or urine for sugar while you are taking this medicine. Call your doctor if you think your blood sugar is higher than normal or harder to control.

When to Call Your Doctor
Most people experience few or no side effects from this drug. However, any medicine can sometimes cause unwanted effects. Call your

doctor if you develop an unexplained sore throat, chills or fever, ringing or buzzing or a feeling of fullness in the ears, any loss of hearing, sharp stomach pain, chest pain, sharp joint pain, severe muscle or leg cramps, unusual fatigue, unusual sweating, mental confusion, headache, fainting, unusual bruising or bleeding, a yellow color to the skin or eyes or a sudden weight gain of 5 pounds (2.5 kg) or more. Also call your doctor if you feel sick or develop vomiting or diarrhea.

For ETHACRYNIC ACID:
- Stop taking the medicine and call your doctor immediately if you develop severe, watery diarrhea.
- Also call your doctor if you develop red or black stools.

Allergic Reactions

Call your doctor immediately if you think you may be allergic to the medicine or if you develop a skin rash, hives, itching, swelling of the face or difficulty in breathing. If you cannot reach your doctor, phone a hospital emergency department.

Refills

Do not stop taking this medicine without your doctor's approval and do not go without medicine between prescription refills. Call your pharmacist for a refill 2 or 3 days before you will run out of the medicine.

Discuss with your pharmacist the implications of dispensing all your refills for this medicine with the same manufacturer's product. (*See* Generic Drugs, page 13.)

▶ **ETHOSUXIMIDE (ORAL)**
ZARONTIN

METHSUXIMIDE
CELONTIN

Purpose

This medicine is used to help control seizures. It is commonly used in the treatment of epilepsy.

Allergies/Warnings

If you have ever had an allergic reaction to an anticonvulsant or seizure medicine, tell your doctor and pharmacist before you take any of this medicine.

How to Use This Medicine

Time of Administration

It is very important that you take this medicine exactly as your doctor has prescribed. Do not miss any doses and take the medicine even if you feel well. Try to take this medicine at the same time(s) every day so that you will have a constant level of medicine in your body. This is the only way that you can receive the full benefit of the medicine. If you forget to take this medicine, the amount of medicine in your blood will decrease and you may have seizures.

How to Administer

Take this medicine with food if it upsets your stomach. Call your doctor if you continue to have stomach upset.

For ZARONTIN SYRUP:

- If a dropper, oral liquid syringe or special measuring spoon is used to measure the dose and you do not fully understand how to use it, *see* Medicine Dropper (page 21) and Medicine Spoon (page 22).

Special Instructions

Length of Therapy

Do not stop taking this medicine suddenly without the approval of your doctor. It usually will be necessary for your doctor to slowly reduce your dose since your body will need time to adjust. You could develop seizures if you suddenly stopped taking the medicine.

Pregnancy/Breastfeeding

Women who are pregnant or planning to become pregnant should tell their doctor before taking this medicine.

Women should not breastfeed without their doctor's approval. This medicine can pass into the breast milk and cause side effects in the infant.

Drug Interactions

It is important that you obtain the advice of your doctor or pharmacist before taking any other prescription or nonprescription medicines including pain relievers, sleeping pills, tranquilizers, medicine for seizures, muscle relaxants, anesthetics, medicines for depression or medicines for allergies. Combining this medicine with some of these drugs could cause drowsiness or dizziness.

There are other drug interactions that can occur. If you are taking any other medicines, be sure to check first with your pharmacist or doctor.

Alcohol

Do not drink alcoholic beverages while taking this drug without the approval of your doctor because the combination could cause drowsiness or an increase in the frequency of your seizures. One drink may have the same effect that 2 or 3 drinks normally would have.

Special Precautions

Be sure to keep your doctor's appointments so that your doctor can check your progress. This is especially important during the first few months of therapy, when the doctor will decide the best dose of this medicine for your condition. To make sure that your dose is correct, your doctor may wish to take a blood sample periodically to measure the amount of medicine in it.

This medicine may cause dizziness, drowsiness or blurred vision in some people. If you become dizzy, you should be careful going up and down stairs. Sit or lie down at the first sign of dizziness. Do not drive a car, do not pilot an airplane, use a sewing machine, operate dangerous machinery or do jobs that require you to be alert until you know how you are going to react to the drug. Tell your doctor if you are dizzy, drowsy or have blurred vision. It may be necessary to lower your dose.

If this medicine is for a child, do not let him or her ride a bike, climb trees, etc. until you can determine how he or she is going to react to this medicine. Children could hurt themselves if they participated in these activities when they were dizzy.

Avoid swimming alone or taking part in high-risk sports in which a sudden seizure could cause injury.

When to Call Your Doctor

Most people experience few or no side effects from this drug. However, any medicine can sometimes cause unwanted effects. Call your doctor if you develop a sore throat, fever or mouth sores, skin rash and itching, swollen glands, persistent hiccups, unusual bruising or bleeding, or if you become confused or depressed.

Call your doctor if you have an increase in the frequency of seizures.

Allergic Reactions

Call your doctor immediately if you think you may be allergic to the medicine or if you develop a skin rash, hives, itching, swelling of the face or difficulty in breathing. If you cannot reach your doctor, phone a hospital emergency department.

Refills

Do not stop taking this medicine without your doctor's approval and do not go without medicine between prescription refills. Call your pharmacist for a refill 2 or 3 days before you will run out of the medicine.

Miscellaneous

Carry an identification card in your wallet or wear a medical alert bracelet indicating that you are taking this medicine, as well as the names and phone numbers of your doctors. If you do not already carry such a card, complete the Medicine Card in this book. Always tell your dentist, pharmacist and other doctors who are treating you that you are taking this medicine.

▶ **FLOCTAFENINE (ORAL)**
IDARAC

Purpose

This medicine is used to help relieve pain.

Allergies/Warnings

If you have ever had an allergic reaction to FLOCTAFENINE, or if you have ever had bowel inflammation (such as Crohn's disease or ulcerative colitis), a stomach ulcer or kidney disease, or if you are taking "blood thinners," tell your doctor, dentist or pharmacist.

How to Use This Medicine

How to Administer

Take this medicine with a glass of water.

Special Instructions

Pregnancy/Breastfeeding

Women who are pregnant, breastfeeding or planning to become pregnant should tell their doctor before taking this medicine. Generally, this medication should not be used during pregnancy and is not recommended during breastfeeding.

Be Aware of "Quack Cures"

Millions of dollars are spent annually on quack cures.

Quack cures cost us more than just money. They can cost us our lives. Quackery is health fraud and is the promotion of medical remedies which are ineffective or have not been proven to be effective.

Most people think that the government screens all health product advertising *before* it is released. This is not true except for those drugs and medical devices that require premarket approval by the Health Protection Branch. The only way that law enforcement authorities can take action is after the advertisements have appeared. Often this is too late.

Many quacks sell their products through post office boxes and are "fly-by-night" operators. They have usually moved to another location by the time refund requests come in. They do this in order to avoid law enforcement officials.

There are some things you can do to protect yourself:

- Be wary of any "special," "secret" or "ancient" formulas that are only available through the mail from one supplier.
- Be wary of testimonials from satisfied users or famous people. You want scientific proof about a product's efficacy.
- Be wary of claims that one product can cure several types of ailments.
- Be wary of claims that the product will "cure" a condition.
- Be wary of door-to-door salesmen or people who sell their products at public lectures who use high pressure sales tactics.
- Do not give your credit card number or send an order through the mail until you have assurance that the product is not a quack product. Check with your doctor or pharmacist.

Special Precautions

In some people, this drug may cause dizziness or drowsiness. Do not drive a car, pilot an airplane, operate dangerous machinery or do jobs that require you to be alert, if you are drowsy or dizzy. You should also be careful going up and down stairs. Sit or lie down at the first sign of dizziness. Tell your doctor if the dizziness or drowsiness continues.

Length of Therapy

This medicine should not be used longer than recommended by your doctor.

When to Call Your Doctor

Call your doctor if the medicine does not relieve your symptoms or if they get worse.

Most people experience few or no side effects from this drug. However, any medicine can cause unwanted effects. Call your doctor if you develop burning or pain on urination (passing your water), increased frequency of urination, strong smelling urine, nausea, stomach upset or abdominal pain, black or tarry stools.

Allergic Reactions

Call your doctor immediately if you think you may be allergic to the medicine or if you develop a skin rash, hives, swelling of the face or difficulty breathing. If you cannot reach your doctor, phone a hospital emergency department.

▶ FLUOXETINE HCL (ORAL)
PROZAC

Purpose

This medicine is used to help relieve the symptoms of depression.

Allergies/Warnings

If you have ever had an allergic reaction to any medicine, tell your doctor or pharmacist before taking this medicine.

Before taking this medicine, tell your doctor about any other medical conditions (for example, liver disease or seizures) which you may have had or currently have.

How to Use This Medicine

Time of Administration

This medicine should be taken in the morning. It may be taken without regard to meals. Take it either with food or on an empty stomach. If you develop mild nausea, it can often be relieved by taking the medicine with food.

Special Instructions

Length of Therapy

It is important that you take the medicine regularly and that you do not miss any doses. The full effect of the medicine may not be noticed immediately, but usually takes several weeks. Early signs of improvement are better sleep, increased energy and improved mood. Do not stop taking the medicine when you first feel better or you may feel worse later.

Since the medicine does not have an immediate effect on your mood, do not attempt to adjust the dose according to your moods. Continue to take the dose prescribed for you. Do not take an extra dose if you are having a bad day.

Do not stop taking this medicine suddenly without the approval of your doctor. It will be necessary for your doctor to reduce your dose slowly since your body will need time to adjust. It could make your condition worse if you suddenly stopped taking the medicine.

Pregnancy/Breastfeeding

Women who are pregnant, breastfeeding or planning to become pregnant should not use this medicine without their doctor's approval.

Drug Interactions

This medicine may interact with other medicines. Therefore, do not take any prescription or nonprescription medicine without first checking with your doctor or pharmacist.

Also, do not stop taking any other medicines you may be taking without checking first with your doctor or pharmacist.

Even after you have stopped taking this medicine, it will stay in your body for several weeks. Therefore, be sure to check with your doctor or pharmacist before taking any other medicine during the several weeks after you have stopped taking this medicine.

Alcohol

It is recommended that you avoid alcohol while taking this drug.

Special Precautions

Any medicine has a few unwanted side effects. Many of these side effects are annoying, but you should try to keep taking the medicine unless your doctor tells you to stop it. Because this medicine takes a few weeks to work, the side effects show the doctor that the drug is starting to work. This medicine commonly causes nervousness, anxiety, insomnia, headaches, sweating, nausea, loss of appetite and fatigue, which usually decreases as the treatment is continued. If these effects continue or are very bothersome, contact your physician.

Make sure you know how you are going to react to this medicine and whether it will make you dizzy or drowsy. Do not drive a car, pilot an airplane, operate dangerous machinery or do jobs that require you to be alert if you are dizzy or drowsy.

For Patients with Diabetes:
- This drug may cause your blood sugar to *fall*. Carefully test your blood sugar while you are taking this medicine, and be aware of symptoms of low blood sugar. Talk to your doctor about the need to adjust your insulin or diabetes medicine.
- Several weeks after you stop taking this medicine, you may find that your blood sugar will *rise*. Carefully test your blood or urine for sugar. Call your doctor if you think your blood sugar is higher than normal or more difficult to control.

When to Call Your Doctor

Any medicine can sometimes cause unwanted side effects. Some adverse effects tend to decrease with time. Make sure your doctor is aware of persistent loss of appetite, nausea, muscle or joint pain, diarrhea, headaches, nervousness, shakiness, dizziness or excessive sweating. Call your doctor if you develop unusual hostile feelings or suicidal thoughts (rare).

Allergic Reactions

Call your doctor immediately if you think you may be allergic to the medicine or if you develop a skin rash, hives, swelling of the face or difficulty breathing. If you cannot reach your doctor, phone a hospital emergency department.

Miscellaneous

Carry an identification card in your wallet or wear a medical alert bracelet indicating that you are taking this medicine, as well as the names and phone numbers of your doctors. If you do not already carry such a card, complete the Medicine Card in this book. Always tell your dentist, pharmacist and other doctors who are treating you that you are taking this medicine.

▶ **FLURAZEPAM (ORAL)**
APO-FLURAZEPAM, DALMANE, NOVOFLUPAM, PMS FLURAZEPAM, SOMNOL

TEMAZEPAM
RESTORIL

TRIAZOLAM
APO-TRIAZO, HALCION

Purpose
This medicine is used to treat some types of sleep disorders.

Allergies/Warnings
If you have ever had an allergic reaction to any medicine or if you have depression or any medical problem, tell your doctor and pharmacist before you take any of this medicine.

How to Use This Medicine

Time of Administration
Take this medicine at least 20 to 30 minutes before you want to fall asleep. Go to bed after you have taken the medicine. Do not smoke in bed after you have taken it because you could fall asleep and cause a fire.

How to Administer
This medicine may be taken either with food or on an empty stomach.

Special Instructions

Length of Therapy
Sleeping medicines are only useful for a short time. If used for too long, they lose their effectiveness. Do not take any more of this medicine than your doctor has prescribed.

Do not stop taking this medicine suddenly without the approval of your doctor. It may be necessary for your doctor to reduce your dose slowly since your body may need time to adjust.

Check with your doctor if you develop any of the following while you are slowly stopping the medicine: nausea or vomiting, trembling, seizures, muscle cramps, stomach cramps, unusual sweating, fast heartbeats or trouble sleeping, or if you become confused, irritable or nervous.

Pregnancy/Breastfeeding

Women who are pregnant, breastfeeding or planning to become pregnant should tell their doctor before taking this medicine. This medicine should generally not be used during pregnancy and is not generally recommended during breastfeeding.

Drug Interactions

It is important that you obtain the advice of your doctor or pharmacist before taking any other prescription or nonprescription medicines, including pain relievers, sleeping pills, tranquilizers or medicines for depression, cough, cold or allergy medicines. Excessive drowsiness or confusion may occur when some of these drugs are taken together.

There are other drug interactions that can occur. If you are taking any other medicines, be sure to check first with your pharmacist or doctor.

Alcohol

Do not drink alcoholic beverages while taking this drug or for a few days after you have stopped taking the drug without the approval of your doctor. The combination could cause drowsiness. One drink (even during the day) may have the same effect that 2 or 3 drinks normally would have.

Special Precautions

Be careful if you have to get up during the night while taking this medicine. You may not feel as alert as usual.

If you have problems sleeping, you should avoid caffeinated beverages, certain cold decongestants and strenuous exercise in the evenings as they make it more difficult to fall asleep. There are other drug interactions that can occur. If you are taking any other medicines, be sure to check with your pharmacist or doctor.

If this medicine causes dizziness or drowsiness the next day after you take it, do not drive a car, pilot an airplane, operate dangerous machinery or do jobs that require you to be alert. You should also be careful going up and down stairs. Sit or lie down at the first sign of dizziness.

If this hangover drowsiness becomes bothersome, call your doctor.

If you do not fall asleep after taking the prescribed amount, do *not* take an additional dose unless advised by your doctor.

You may experience a sleep problem (insomnia) on the first night or two after stopping the drug. This is not a reason for restarting the medicine and your sleep should gradually return to normal.

When to Call Your Doctor

Most people experience few or no side effects from this drug. However, any medicine can sometimes cause unwanted effects. Call your doctor if you develop a sore throat, fever, mouth sores, a staggering walk, a yellow color to the skin or eyes, slow heartbeats or shortness of breath, unusual tiredness or nervousness, stomach pain, confusion or depression, seizures, hallucinations, trouble sleeping, slurred speech, severe drowsiness, ringing or buzzing in the ears or numbness or tingling of the hands or feet.

Allergic Reactions

Call your doctor immediately if you think you may be allergic to the medicine or if you develop a skin rash, hives, itching, swelling of the face or difficulty in breathing. If you cannot reach your doctor, phone a hospital emergency department.

▶ FLUVOXAMINE (ORAL)
Luvox

Purpose
This medicine is used to help relieve the symptoms of depression.

Allergies/Warnings
If you have ever had an allergic reaction to any medicine, tell your doctor or pharmacist before taking this medicine.

Before taking this medicine, tell your doctor about any other medical conditions (e.g., liver disease or seizures) which you may have had or currently have.

How to Use This Medicine

Time of Administration
This medicine should be taken at bedtime unless otherwise directed by your doctor.

How to Administer
This medicine should be swallowed whole with a glassful of water.

Special Instructions

Length of Therapy

It is important that you take the medicine regularly and that you do not miss any doses. The full effect of the medicine may not be noticed immediately, but usually takes 10 days or up to several weeks. Early signs of improvement are better sleep, increased energy and improved mood. Do not stop taking the medicine when you first feel better or you may feel worse in 3 or 4 days.

Since the medicine does not have an immediate effect on your mood, do not attempt to adjust the dose according to your moods, but continue to take the dose prescribed for you. Do not take an extra dose if you are having a bad day.

Do not stop taking this medicine suddenly without the approval of your doctor. It will be necessary for your doctor to reduce your dose slowly since your body will need time to adjust. It could make your condition worse if you suddenly stopped taking the medicine.

Pregnancy/Breastfeeding

Women who are pregnant, breastfeeding or planning to become pregnant should not use this medicine without their doctor's approval.

Drug Interactions

This medicine may interact with other medicines. Therefore, do not take any prescription or nonprescription medicine without first checking with your doctor or pharmacist.

Also, do not stop taking any other medicines you may be taking without checking first with your doctor or pharmacist.

Alcohol

Do not drink alcoholic beverages while taking this medicine or for several days after you have stopped taking this drug, without the approval of your doctor. The combination could cause severe drowsiness. One drink may have the same effect as 2 or 3 drinks normally would have.

Special Precautions

Any medicine has a few unwanted side effects. Many of these side effects are annoying, but you should try to keep taking the medicine unless your doctor tells you to stop it. Because this medicine takes a few weeks to work, the side effects show the doctor that the drug is starting to work. Most of these side effects will go away as your body adjusts to the medicine but some may not.

Make sure you know how you are going to react to this medicine and whether it will make you dizzy or drowsy. Do not drive a car, pilot an airplane, operate dangerous machinery or do jobs that require you to be alert if you are dizzy or drowsy. The drowsiness may decrease over time.

If your mouth becomes dry, drink water, suck ice chips or a hard sour candy (sugarless) or chew gum (sugarless). Sugarless products are recommended to avoid dental problems. You may wish to ask your pharmacist about special solutions, called artificial saliva, that can also be used to help restore moisture in the mouth. Call your doctor if your mouth becomes extremely dry.

This medicine may cause some people to become constipated. To help prevent constipation, try increasing the amount of bulk in your diet (for example, bran, fresh fruits and salads), exercising more often or drinking more fluids (unless otherwise directed). Call your doctor if the constipation continues.

When to Call Your Doctor

This medicine rarely has been associated with convulsions. Stop taking this medicine if you have a seizure and inform your doctor as soon as possible.

Many adverse effects tend to decrease with time. Make sure you let your doctor know if you have persistent nausea, vomiting, shakiness, changes in appetite, headache, nervousness, difficulty sleeping, weakness, drowsiness, excessive sweating, blurred vision or suicidal thoughts.

Allergic Reactions

Call your doctor immediately if you think you may be allergic to the medicine or if you have a skin rash or itching.

Refills

Do not stop taking this medicine without your doctor's approval and do not go without medicine between prescription refills. Call your pharmacist for a refill 2 or 3 days before you will run out of the medicine.

Miscellaneous

Carry an identification card in your wallet or wear a medical alert bracelet indicating that you are taking this medicine, as well as the names and phone numbers of your doctors. If you do not already carry such a card, complete the Medicine Card in this book. Always tell your dentist, pharmacist and other doctors who are treating you that you are taking this medicine.

▶ GEMFIBROZIL
LOPID

Purpose
This medicine is used to lower cholesterol and lipids in the blood.

Allergies/Warnings
If you have ever had an allergic reaction to any medicine or if you are taking an anticoagulant ("blood thinner") or other medicines to lower cholesterol, tell your doctor and pharmacist before you take any of this medicine.

How to Use This Medicine
Time of Administration
This medicine is usually taken twice a day. Take it 30 minutes before the morning and evening meal unless otherwise directed.

Special Instructions
Length of Therapy
It is very important to take this medicine exactly as your doctor has prescribed. Otherwise you cannot expect the medicine to control your condition.

Pregnancy/Breastfeeding
Women who are pregnant, breastfeeding or planning to become pregnant should not take this medicine.

Special Precautions
Your doctor may prescribe a special diet while you are taking this medicine. Be sure to follow the diet closely as this will help to control your condition also.

It is important that you go to have any blood tests which your doctor may recommend while you are taking this medicine.

Drug Interactions
This medicine can interact with "blood thinners" and certain other medicines. Do not start or stop taking other medicines without checking with your doctor.

When to Call Your Doctor
This medicine may cause mild stomach upset, abdominal pain, nausea, constipation or diarrhea. These usually disappear after you have

taken the medicine for a while. If these side effects persist, call your doctor. Also call your doctor if you develop pain in the big toe.

Allergic Reactions

Call your doctor immediately if you think you may be allergic to the medicine or if you develop a skin rash, hives, itching, swelling of the face or difficulty in breathing. If you cannot reach your doctor, phone a hospital emergency department.

▶ **HALOPERIDOL (ORAL)**
APO-HALOPERIDOL, HALDOL, NOVOPERIDOL, PERIDOL, PMS HALOPERIDOL

Purpose

This medicine has many uses and the reason it was prescribed depends upon your condition. Check with your doctor if you do not fully understand why you are taking it.

Allergies/Warnings

If you have ever had an allergic reaction to any medicine or if you have high blood pressure, seizures, heart problems, enlarged prostate, difficulty urinating (passing your water), Parkinson's disease, glaucoma or any other medical problem, tell your doctor and pharmacist before you take any of this medicine.

Also tell your doctor if you are hypersensitive to tartrazine (a yellow dye). HALDOL 1mg, 5mg and 10mg contain tartrazine.

How to Use This Medicine

How to Administer

Take this medicine with food or immediately after meals to help prevent stomach upset unless otherwise directed.

For liquid medicine:
- The liquid medicine may be mixed with milk, food or water. Do *not* mix it with tea or coffee or some juices because this may decrease the effect of the medicine.
- A dropper is used to measure the dose. If you do not fully understand how to use it, *see* Medicine Dropper (page 21).
- Do not get the liquid on your skin or clothing.

Special Instructions

Length of Therapy

It is important that you take the medicine regularly and that you do not miss any doses. The full benefit of the medicine may not be noticed immediately, but may take from a few days to a few weeks.

Do not stop taking this medicine suddenly without the approval of your doctor. It will be necessary for your doctor to reduce your dose slowly since your body will need time to adjust. It could make your condition worse if you suddenly stopped taking the medicine. After you have stopped taking this medicine, you must observe the following precautions (*see* Alcohol, below) for 1 to 2 weeks since some of the medicine will still be in your body.

Pregnancy/Breastfeeding

Women who are pregnant, breastfeeding or planning to become pregnant should tell their doctor before taking this medicine.

Drug Interactions

It is important that you obtain the advice of your doctor or pharmacist before taking any other prescription or nonprescription medicines, including pain relievers, sleeping pills, other tranquilizers or medicines for depression, cough, cold or allergies.

There are other drug interactions that can occur. If you are taking any other medicines, be sure to check first with your pharmacist or doctor.

Alcohol

Do not drink alcoholic beverages while taking this drug without the approval of your doctor. The combination could irritate your stomach and could cause drowsiness or dizziness. One drink may have the same effect that 2 or 3 drinks normally would have.

If you have been taking this medicine regularly for several days or weeks, it is recommended not to drink alcohol for 2 weeks after you have stopped taking the medicine. Depending on your dose, it may take this long for the drug to be eliminated from your body.

Special Precautions

If this medicine causes dizziness or lightheadedness, you should be careful going up and down stairs and you should not change positions too rapidly. Lightheadedness is more likely to occur if you stand up suddenly—this is due to blood collecting in the legs and lasts for a few seconds. Therefore, get up from a sitting or lying position more slowly and tighten and relax your leg muscles or wiggle your toes to help promote circulation. In the morning, get out of bed slowly and dangle your feet over the edge of the bed for a few minutes before standing up. Sit or lie down at the first sign of dizziness. Tell your doctor if you have been dizzy.

In some people, this drug may cause drowsiness, especially after any increase in your dose. Do not drive a car, pilot an airplane, operate dangerous machinery or do jobs that require you to be alert until you know how you are going to react to this drug.

If your mouth becomes dry, drink water, suck ice chips or a hard, sour candy (sugarless) or chew gum (sugarless). Sugarless products are recommended in order to avoid dental problems. You may wish to ask your pharmacist about special solutions, called artificial saliva, that can also be used to help restore moisture in the mouth. It is especially important to brush and floss your teeth regularly if you develop a dry mouth, to help prevent gum problems.

This medicine may cause some people to become constipated. To help prevent constipation, try increasing the amount of bulk in your diet (for example, bran, fresh fruits and salads), exercising more often or drinking more fluids (unless otherwise directed). Call your doctor if the constipation continues.

You may become more sensitive to heat because your body may perspire less while you are taking this drug. Be careful not to become overheated during exercise or in hot weather. Try to avoid strenuous exercise, standing for long periods of time (especially in hot weather), hot showers, hot baths, saunas or Jacuzzis while taking this medicine.

Some patients may also become more sensitive to cold and should dress warmly during cold weather and limit exposure to cold temperatures.

This medicine often makes some people more sensitive to sunlight and some tanning lamps. When you begin taking this medicine, try to avoid too much sun until you see how you are going to react. If your skin does become more sensitive to sunlight, tell your doctor and try not to stay in direct sunlight for extended periods of time. While in the sun, wear protective clothing and sunglasses. You may wish to ask your pharmacist about suitable sunscreen products. Call your doctor if you become sunburned.

When to Call Your Doctor

Any medicine can cause unwanted effects. Call your doctor if you develop a sore throat, fever, mouth sores, changes in vision, difficulty in urinating (passing your water), decreased sexual ability, a yellow color in the skin or eyes, fast heartbeats, a skin rash, nausea or vomiting, fainting spells or seizures.

Call your doctor if you become restless or unable to sit still or sleep or if you develop drooling, confusion, menstrual irregularities, difficulty breathing, speaking or swallowing, disturbed gait or shuffling walk, tremors, shakiness or unusual movements of the face, tongue or hands or stiffness of the face or body.

If you develop painful muscle spasms, call your doctor or go to the hospital emergency room, since treatment can be given to provide rapid relief of this problem.

Chronic Hallucinations from Nose Drops

There are now 2 reports in the medical literature suggesting that heavy use of decongestant nose drops may cause psychoses (bizarre behavior) in some patients.

A 61-year-old man had been using a variety of nasal decongestant drops and sprays for a sinus condition since the early 1940s. After several years, he used the products every 30 minutes because of an impending feeling of suffocation. He reported heavy threatening voices and frightening visual imagery, usually at night, for the last 20 years.

When the nose drops and sprays were stopped and appropriate treatment started, the nasal obstruction gradually decreased and the symptoms of psychoses and anxiety disappeared. The symptoms reappeared when the patient had the flu and started taking decongestants at high doses. The hallucinations and delusions once again stopped when the doctor stopped the decongestants.

The *Journal of the American Medical Association* reported that 4 months later, the patient had no nasal congestion and had sustained relief from hallucinations for the first time in 20 years.

As a general rule, never use nasal decongestant drops or sprays for more than a few days. The symptoms of nasal congestion that you are treating can also become a side effect of the decongestants. Rebound congestion can occur if the nasal decongestant drops or sprays are used too long.

Storage

Store the liquid medicine in a cool, dark place.

Refills

Do not stop taking this medicine without your doctor's approval and do not go without medicine between prescription refills. Call your pharmacist for a refill 2 or 3 days before you will run out of the medicine.

Discuss with your pharmacist the implications of dispensing all your refills for this medicine with the same manufacturer's product. (*See* Generic Drugs, page 13.)

Miscellaneous

Carry an identification card in your wallet or wear a medical alert bracelet indicating that you are taking this medicine, as well as the names and phone numbers of your doctors. If you do not already carry such a card, complete the Medicine Card in this book. Always tell your dentist, pharmacist and other doctors who are treating you that you are taking this medicine.

► HYDRALAZINE (ORAL)
APRESOLINE, NOVO-HYALAZIN

Purpose

This medicine is used to treat high blood pressure.

Allergies/Warnings

If you have ever had an allergic reaction to any medicine, tell your doctor and pharmacist before you take any of this medicine.

How to Use This Medicine

Time of Administration

Try to take the medicine at the same time(s) every day so that you have a constant level of the medicine in your body.

How to Administer

It is best to take this medicine with food because food helps the body to absorb more of the drug.

Special Instructions

Length of Therapy

High blood pressure (hypertension) is a long-term condition and it will probably be necessary for you to take the drug for a long time in spite of the fact that you feel better. If high blood pressure is not treated, it can lead to serious problems such as heart failure, strokes, blood vessel problems or kidney problems. It is very important that you take this medicine as your doctor has directed and that you do not miss any doses. Otherwise, you cannot expect the drug to keep your blood pressure down.

Do not take any more of this medicine than your doctor has prescribed and *do not stop taking this medicine suddenly without the approval of your doctor.* It will be necessary for your doctor to reduce your dose slowly since your body will need time to adjust. It could be harmful and make your condition worse if you suddenly stopped taking the medicine.

Pregnancy/Breastfeeding

Women who are pregnant, breastfeeding or planning to become pregnant should tell their doctor before taking this medicine.

Drug Interactions

Some nonprescription drugs can aggravate your condition. Do not take any of the following without the approval of your doctor or pharmacist: cough, cold or sinus products; asthma, allergy or hay fever products, since they could increase your blood pressure. Read the label of the product to see if there is a warning. If there is, check with your doctor or pharmacist before using the product.

This medicine may lower vitamin B_6 levels in the body. Signs of low vitamin B_6 (pyroxidine) include numbness or tingling of the fingers or toes, and shakiness. Call your doctor if this occurs—he may want to consider vitamin B_6 supplements.

Alcohol

Do not drink alcoholic beverages while taking this drug without the approval of your doctor because the combination could make the possible side effect of dizziness worse.

Special Precautions

If this medicine causes dizziness or lightheadedness, you should be careful going up and down stairs and you should not change positions too rapidly. Lightheadedness is more likely to occur if you stand up suddenly—this is due to blood collecting in the legs and lasts for a few seconds. Therefore, get up from a sitting or lying position more slowly and tighten and relax your leg muscles or wiggle your toes to help promote circulation. In the morning, get out of bed slowly and dangle your feet over the edge of the bed for a few minutes before standing up. Sit or lie down at the first sign of dizziness. Tell your doctor you have been dizzy. In order to help prevent dizziness or fainting, your doctor may also recommend that you avoid strenuous exercise, standing for long periods of time (especially in hot weather), hot showers, hot baths, Jacuzzis or saunas.

If you become dizzy, you should not drive a car, pilot an airplane, operate dangerous machinery or do jobs that require you to be alert.

Follow any special diet your doctor may have ordered. He or she may want you to limit the amount of salt in your diet.

Headaches may occur during the first few days of therapy, but they usually disappear within the first week. If they continue, call your doctor.

When to Call Your Doctor

Most people experience few or no side effects from this drug. However, any medicine can sometimes cause unwanted effects. Call your doctor if you develop a sore throat, itching, fast heartbeats, swelling of the legs or ankles, sudden weight gain of 5 pounds (2.5 kg) or more, swelling of the glands in the neck or armpits or numbness or tingling in the hands or feet.

Stop taking this medicine and call your doctor immediately if you develop joint or muscle pain, a skin rash, fever, chest pains, unusual tiredness or weakness or other unexplained symptoms.

Refills

Do not stop taking this medicine without your doctor's approval and do not go without medicine between prescription refills. Call your pharmacist for a refill 2 or 3 days before you will run out of the medicine.

Discuss with your pharmacist the implications of dispensing all your refills for this medicine with the same manufacturer's product. (*See* Generic Drugs, page 13.)

Miscellaneous

Carry an identification card in your wallet or wear a medical alert bracelet indicating that you are taking this medicine, as well as the names and phone numbers of your doctors. If you do not already carry such a card, complete the Medicine Card in this book. Always tell your dentist, pharmacist and other doctors who are treating you that you are taking this medicine.

> # Stomach Acid during the Night
>
> Stomach acid secretions are highest during the night.
>
> Stomach acid secretion reaches a peak during the night between 10 P.M. and 2 A.M. The lowest point is during late morning just before lunch. Anti-ulcer drugs that block the secretion of stomach acids may have their greatest effect during the sleeping hours.

▶ # HYDROCODONE - PHENYLTOLOXAMINE (ORAL)
TUSSIONEX

Purpose
This is a strong cough medicine used to help relieve dry irritating coughs that have not responded to other cough medicines.

Allergies/Warnings
If you have ever had an allergic reaction to HYDROCODONE or CODEINE medicine or if you have asthma, glaucoma, an enlarged prostate or difficulty urinating (passing your water), tell your doctor before you take any of this medicine.

This medicine should not be used in children under the age of 1 year or weighing less than 9 kg (20 pounds).

How to Use This Medicine

Time of Administration
This medicine may be taken without regard to meals. Take it either with food or on an empty stomach. If stomach upset occurs, take it with some food or a glass of milk.

How to Administer
For tablets:
• Take with a glass of water or with food.

For liquid medicine:
• Shake the bottle well each time before pouring so that you can measure an accurate dose.
• Since a spoon is used to measure the dose, it is recommended that you use a medicine spoon or an oral liquid syringe, which you can

obtain from your pharmacist. These are more accurate than the average household teaspoon. *See* Oral Liquid Syringe (page 17) and Medicine Dropper (page 21).

- Do *not* dilute the liquid medicine or mix with other liquid medicines. This could change the way the medicine acts and could result in an overdose. Try not to drink other liquids immediately after taking this medicine so that the medicine will work properly.

Important Dosage Information for Asians

Asians need lower dosages of certain medicines than Caucasians, due to their slower metabolic rate.

The effects on Asians and Caucasians of a single dose of an antidepressant medicine were compared in a recent study*. The researchers found that it took Asian patients 4 hours longer than Caucasians to reach maximum blood levels of the medicine. It also took Asian patients longer to eliminate the medicine from their bodies. The reason is that Asian people metabolized the drug at a slower rate and the drug stayed in their bodies for a longer period of time.

This study shows that Asian patients may need lower dosages of some medicines.

*The study was conducted in July 1990 at the Los Angeles County/ University of Southern California Medical Center.

Special Instructions

Length of Therapy
Do not use this medicine for more than 1 week without the advice of your doctor. When used for a long period of time, the drug can become less effective. Also, when used in large doses for a long period of time, the drug can become habit-forming.

If you have had to take this medicine for more than a few weeks, do not stop taking this medicine suddenly without the approval of your doctor. It may be necessary for your doctor to reduce your dose slowly since your body will need time to adjust. It could be harmful and make your condition worse if you suddenly did not receive the medicine.

Pregnancy/Breastfeeding

Women who are pregnant, breastfeeding or planning to become pregnant should not take this medicine.

Drug Interactions

It is important that you obtain the advice of your doctor or pharmacist before taking any other prescription or nonprescription medicines including pain relievers, sleeping pills, tranquilizers, medicine for seizures, muscle relaxants, anesthetics, medicines for depression or medicines for allergies. Combining this medicine with some of these drugs could cause drowsiness or dizziness.

There are other drug interactions that can occur. If you are taking any other medicines, be sure to check first with your pharmacist or doctor.

Alcohol

Do not drink alcoholic beverages while taking this drug without the approval of your doctor because the combination could cause drowsiness or dizziness. One drink may have the same effect that 2 or 3 drinks normally would have.

Special Precautions

If you feel nauseated or sick to your stomach when you first start taking this medicine, it may help to lie down for a few minutes. Lying down may also help any dizziness go away.

In some people, this drug may initially cause dizziness or drowsiness. Do not drive a car, pilot an airplane, operate dangerous machinery or do jobs that require you to be alert until you know how you are going to react to the drug. If you have been dizzy, tell your doctor at your next visit. Your dose may have to be adjusted.

If this medicine causes dizziness or lightheadedness, you should be careful going up and down stairs and you should not change positions too rapidly. Lightheadedness is more likely to occur if you stand up suddenly—this is due to blood collecting in the legs and lasts for a few seconds. Therefore, get up from a sitting or lying position more slowly and tighten and relax your leg muscles or wiggle your toes to help promote circulation. In the morning, get out of bed slowly and dangle your feet over the edge of the bed for a few minutes before standing up. Sit or lie down at the first sign of dizziness. Tell your doctor if you have been dizzy.

In order to help prevent dizziness or fainting, your doctor may also recommend that you avoid strenuous exercise, standing for long periods of time (especially in hot weather), hot showers, hot baths, Jacuzzis or saunas.

If your mouth becomes dry, drink water, suck ice chips or a hard, sour candy (sugarless) or chew gum (sugarless). Sugarless products are recommended in order to avoid dental problems. You may wish to ask your pharmacist about special solutions, called artificial saliva, that can also be used to help restore moisture in the mouth. It is especially important to brush and floss your teeth regularly if you develop a dry mouth, to help prevent gum problems.

This medicine may cause some people to become constipated. To help prevent constipation, try increasing the amount of bulk in your diet (for example, bran, fresh fruits and salads), exercising more often or drinking more fluids (unless otherwise directed). Call your doctor if the constipation continues.

Trouble Swallowing Pills?

Do you have trouble swallowing tablets and capsules? Try this technique the next time you have to swallow a medication.

Place a small piece of bread (or another piece of soft food) on your tongue. Place the tablet or capsule next to the piece of bread. Take a drink of water and swallow the bread.

Guess what? The chances are very high that you swallowed the medicine too!

Every day we swallow many pieces of food which are much larger than any of the tablets or capsules you will ever have to take. Many of the problems people have swallowing tablets and capsules are psychological and this simple technique has helped many people to overcome this problem.

When to Call Your Doctor

Call your doctor if the cough lasts longer than 1 week or if you develop a fever, skin rash or constant headache.

Most people experience few or no side effects from this drug. However, any medicine can sometimes cause unwanted effects. Call your doctor if you develop a skin rash, fast or slow heartbeats, unexplained nervousness, restlessness or irritability, trouble sleeping, shortness of breath, fainting, confusion, hallucinations or depression, seizures, ringing or buzzing in the ears, difficulty in urinating (passing your water), or if mucous (lung secretions) becomes thicker than normal.

People over 65 years of age may be more sensitive to these side effects.

Children may be more sensitive to the breathing problems. Therefore, this medicine should not be used in children under 1 year of age.

Allergic Reactions

Call your doctor immediately if you think you may be allergic to the medicine or if you develop a skin rash, hives, itching, swelling of the face or difficulty in breathing. If you cannot reach your doctor, phone a hospital emergency department.

▶ HYDROXYZINE HCl (ORAL)
Apo-Hydroxyzine, Atarax, Multipax, Novohydroxyzin, PMS Hydroxyzine

Purpose
This medicine is used to help relieve the symptoms of anxiety and tension and certain types of emotional problems, allergic conditions and skin rashes. This drug has several other uses and the reason it was prescribed depends upon your condition. Check with your doctor if you do not fully understand why you are taking it.

Allergies/Warnings
If you have ever had an allergic reaction to any medicine, tell your doctor and pharmacist before you take any of this medicine.

How to Use This Medicine

How to Administer
For capsules:
• Take the medicine with food or a full glass of water unless otherwise directed.

For liquid medicine:
• It is recommended that you use a medicine spoon or an oral liquid syringe, which you can obtain from your pharmacist. These are more accurate than the average household teaspoon. See Oral Liquid Syringe (page 17) and Medicine Spoon (page 22).

Does Half a Tablet Contain Half the Dose?

Not always!

When a tablet is manufactured, the drug is mixed with several inactive ingredients. If the drug is not mixed exactly evenly, one side of the tablet may contain more of the drug than the other side.

In one study reported in a leading medical journal, researchers evaluated whether tablets broke evenly into 2 halves of equivalent and accurate doses. The tablets were broken along the score lines (indentations) and each half-tablet was weighed. A tablet was classified as excellent if 95% of the halves were within 5% of the expected weight.

Of the 13 brands of antihypertensive medications tested, only 2 brands were rated as excellent and contained equal doses in each half of the tablets. Eight brands were classed as moderate (within 5 to 10% of the expected weight) and 3 brands showed more than a 10% error in weight.

This is not critical with most drugs. However, if the drug is very potent, uneven distribution of the medicine in a tablet could be important. Ask your doctor if you have any questions.

Special Instructions

Pregnancy/Breastfeeding
Women who are pregnant, breastfeeding or planning to become pregnant should tell their doctor before taking this medicine.

Drug Interactions
It is important that you obtain the advice of your doctor or pharmacist before taking any other prescription or nonprescription medicines, including pain relievers, sleeping pills, tranquilizers or medicines for depression, cough, cold or allergies. Excessive drowsiness may occur in some people.

There are other drug interactions that can occur. If you are taking any other medicines, be sure to check first with your pharmacist or doctor.

Attention Breastfeeding Women!

Topical application of lanolin or vitamin E is a popular treatment for sore nipples when a woman begins breastfeeding. As with the use of any drugs during breastfeeding, there are important considerations that should be taken into account.

Women who are breastfeeding and allergic to wool should not apply lanolin to their nipples. Lanolin is made from the wool of sheep and the woman could experience an allergic reaction.

Vitamin E oil applied to the nipples of breastfeeding women has been reported to be absorbed by babies and to cause high vitamin E levels in the babies' blood. It is not known whether the infants directly ingested and absorbed the vitamin E or whether the vitamin E was absorbed by the mother and transferred to the infant through the breast milk. The risk of the elevated vitamin E levels in the infants has not been established.

Alcohol

Do not drink alcoholic beverages while taking this drug or for a few days after stopping the drug without the approval of your doctor because the combination could cause drowsiness. One drink may have the same effect that 2 or 3 drinks normally would have.

Special Precautions

In some people, this drug may cause dizziness or drowsiness. Do not drive a car, pilot an airplane, operate dangerous machinery or do jobs that require you to be alert if you are dizzy or drowsy. You should also be careful going up and down stairs. Tell your doctor if the dizziness continues.

If your mouth becomes dry, drink water, suck ice chips or a hard, sour candy (sugarless) or chew gum (sugarless). Sugarless products are recommended in order to avoid dental problems. You may wish to ask your pharmacist about special solutions, called artificial saliva, that can also be used to help restore moisture in the mouth. It is especially important to brush and floss your teeth regularly if you develop a dry mouth, to help prevent gum problems.

When to Call Your Doctor

Most people experience few or no side effects from this drug. However, any medicine can sometimes cause unwanted effects. Call your doctor if you develop a skin rash, sore throat, fever, mouth sores, fainting, trembling, difficulty urinating (passing your water), shakiness or seizures.

Allergic Reactions

Call your doctor immediately if you think you may be allergic to the medicine or if you develop a skin rash, hives, itching, swelling of the face or difficulty in breathing. If you cannot reach your doctor, phone a hospital emergency department.

Do Not Double the Next Dose

You should *not* double your next dose if you forget to take a previous one, without checking with your doctor or pharmacist.

All medications are slightly different. In some cases, doubling the next dose will be advisable and will not cause any problems. However, with other drugs, doubling the next dose could put too much drug into the bloodstream and cause serious toxic effects.

Examples of some drugs that should *not* be doubled are:

WARFARIN (a blood thinner)
THYROID medicines
DIGOXIN (medicine for the heart) and
PHENYTOIN (medicine for epilepsy)

The best advice is to try to keep track of your doses and do your best not to miss any doses. There are several aids available in pharmacies and you can prepare your own reminder list on a calendar. If you do miss a dose, call your doctor or pharmacist for advice.

▶ **INDOMETHACIN (ORAL)**
APO-INDOMETHACIN, INDOCID, INDOCID SR, NOVOMETHACIN

INDOMETHACIN (RECTAL)
INDOCID SUPPOSITORIES

Purpose

This medicine is used to help relieve certain types of pain. It is also used to help relieve inflammation, stiffness, swelling and joint pain in certain kinds of arthritis and gout.

The sustained-release (INDOCID SR) capsules are not meant to treat gout.

Allergies/Warnings

If you have ever had an allergic reaction to ASA (acetylsalicylic acid) or any other medicine or if you suffer from hay fever, asthma, nasal polyps, ulcers or any other medical problems, tell your doctor and pharmacist before you take any of this medicine.

How to Use This Medicine

Time of Administration

Always take this medicine with food or a glass of milk or immediately after meals to help prevent stomach upset (indigestion, nausea, vomiting, stomach pain). It is recommended that you do not lie down within 15 minutes after taking the medicine so that the capsule can reach the stomach. If you develop persistent stomach pain, contact your doctor.

How to Administer

If you were prescribed INDOCID SR:
- These capsules must be swallowed whole. Do not crush or break them open.

If you were prescribed INDOCID SUPPOSITORIES:
- *See* Rectal Suppositories (page 39).

Special Instructions

Length of Therapy

This medicine will not cure arthritis but it can help control inflammation that can increase damage to your joints. It is very important that you take this medicine regularly and that you *do not miss any doses.* If you miss a dose, the level of the medicine in your body will fall and the drug will not be as effective. Only if the drug is at the right level will it be able to decrease the inflammation and swelling in your joints and help prevent further damage.

If you are taking this medicine for a joint or bone problem, you may have to take the drug from a few days to 4 weeks before you feel its full benefits. Long-term therapy is often required in arthritis.

This medicine does not replace any exercise or rest programs or use of heat/cold treatments your doctor may have prescribed.

Pregnancy/Breastfeeding

Women who are pregnant, breastfeeding or planning to become pregnant should tell their doctor before taking this medicine. Use of this medicine during pregnancy, especially the last 3 months, and during breastfeeding is not recommended.

Drug Interactions

Do not take any other medicines containing ASA (acetylsalicylic acid) or salicylates while you are taking this medicine without the approval of your doctor. The combination could cause stomach problems.

It is usually safe to take ACETAMINOPHEN for fever or the occasional headache. Check first with your pharmacist.

Alcohol

Do not drink alcoholic beverages while taking this drug without the approval of your doctor because the combination could cause stomach problems.

Special Precautions

In some people, this drug may cause dizziness or drowsiness. Do not drive a car, pilot an airplane, operate dangerous machinery or do jobs that require you to be alert until you know how you are going to react to this drug. If you become dizzy, you should be careful going up and down stairs. Sit or lie down at the first sign of dizziness. Tell your doctor if you have been dizzy.

This medicine may cause some people to become constipated. To help prevent constipation, try increasing the amount of bulk in your diet (for example, bran, fresh fruits and salads), exercising more often or drinking more fluids (unless otherwise directed). Call your doctor if the constipation continues.

When to Call Your Doctor

Most people experience few or no side effects from this drug. However, any medicine can sometimes cause unwanted effects. Call your doctor if you develop a skin rash, sore throat or fever, chills, ringing or buzzing in the ears, any loss of hearing, fast heartbeats, swelling of the legs or ankles or sudden weight gain, blurred vision or changes in your eyesight, bloody or black stools, severe stomach pain, vomiting, diarrhea (loose bowel movements), a yellow color to the skin or eyes, unusual bruising or bleeding, unusual tiredness or weakness, confusion or depression, seizures, blood in the urine or a persistent headache.

Allergic Reactions

Call your doctor immediately if you think you may be allergic to the medicine or if you develop a skin rash, hives, itching, swelling of the face or difficulty in breathing. If you cannot reach your doctor, phone a hospital emergency department.

Storage

For tablets and capsules:
- Store in a cool, dry, dark place.

For suppositories:
- *See* Rectal Suppositories (page 39).

Refills

Do not stop taking this medicine without your doctor's approval and do not go without medicine between prescription refills. Call your pharmacist for a refill 2 or 3 days before you will run out of the medicine.

Laxatives

Laxatives should not be used for longer than 1 week unless directed by your doctor.

Laxatives are not designed for long-term use. Chronic overuse of harsh stimulant laxatives can lead to a lazy colon—and constipation—and the person may be unable to have a bowel movement without taking a laxative. Excessive use of some laxatives can also result in serious diarrhea, liver disease and electrolyte imbalance.

If you self-medicate with a laxative longer than 1 week and there has been no improvement in your condition, consult your doctor. In addition, pay special attention to your diet and eat foods containing a high amount of fiber, drink adequate amounts of liquids and get the proper amount of exercise.

Miscellaneous

Carry an identification card in your wallet or wear a medical alert bracelet indicating that you are taking this medicine, as well as the names and phone numbers of your doctors. If you do not already carry such a card, complete the Medicine Card in this book. Always tell your dentist, pharmacist and other doctors who are treating you that you are taking this medicine.

▶ IPRATROPIUM BROMIDE (INHALATION)
ATROVENT

Purpose

This medicine is used to help open the bronchioles (air passages in the lungs), make breathing easier and relieve wheezing and shortness of breath. It is used in the treatment of bronchial asthma and chronic bronchitis.

The medicine is not usually used alone to treat an acute asthma attack. Be sure you know how to treat an asthma attack should one occur. Check with your doctor.

Allergies/Warnings

If you have ever had an allergic reaction to any medicine or if you have glaucoma, enlarged prostate (men), difficulty in urinating (passing your water) or any other medical condition, tell your doctor or pharmacist before taking this medicine.

How to Use the Medicine

How to Administer
For aerosol inhaler:
- *See* Inhalers (page 31).
- Follow the special instructions that come with the inhaler.
- Shake the inhaler well each time before use.
- The mouthpiece of the inhaler should be kept clean and dry. The metal canister must be fully and firmly positioned in the outer "shell" and rotated occasionally.
- Do not inhale the medicine more often than directed by your doctor. If your doctor has prescribed a second puff, wait at least 1 to 2 minutes before shaking the container again and repeating the procedure.

- If difficulty in breathing persists or if relief is not obtained with your usual dosage, call your doctor immediately.
- The mouthpiece should be washed in warm water once a week.

Special Instructions

Length of Therapy

Do not use this medicine more often or longer than recommended by your doctor.

Pregnancy/Breastfeeding

Women who are pregnant, breastfeeding or planning to become pregnant should tell their doctor before taking this medicine.

Drug Interactions

Some nonprescription drugs can aggravate your condition. Do not take any of the following without the approval of your doctor or pharmacist: cough, cold, sinus products, ASA-containing products, asthma or allergy products. Read the label of all nonprescription drug products to see if there is a warning. If there is, check with your doctor or pharmacist before purchasing the product.

Do not take other inhaled medicines unless they have been prescribed by your doctor while you are taking this medicine.

It is important that you obtain the advice of your doctor or pharmacist before taking any other prescription medicines, including sleeping pills, tranquilizers, and medicines to treat depression, heart disease or diarrhea.

Special Precautions

Avoid accidentally spraying the contents of the inhaler into your eyes. If you do get the spray in your eyes, rinse them immediately with cool water.

In some people, this drug may cause dizziness or blurred vision. Do not drive a car, pilot an airplane, operate dangerous machinery or do jobs that require you to be alert and have good vision if you are dizzy or have blurred vision.

If dryness of the mouth or throat occurs after you use this medicine, rinsing or gargling with warm water after inhaling the medicine may help.

In some people, this medicine may cause a bad taste in the mouth. This is only temporary and will go away after you have stopped using the medicine.

An urge to urinate (pass your water) with an inability to do so sometimes occurs with the medicine. Urinating before taking the drug each time may help relieve the problem. Tell your doctor if you are having this problem.

When to Call Your Doctor

Call your doctor if this medicine does not relieve your breathing problems.

Most people experience few or no side effects from this drug. However, any medicine can sometimes cause unwanted effects. Call your doctor if you develop rapid or irregular heartbeats, muscle tremors, severe dizziness or blurred vision.

Storage

Store the inhaler at room temperature. Do not place it in hot water or near radiators, stoves, or other sources of heat. Do not puncture, burn or incinerate the container (even when it is empty).

► ISOCARBOXAZID (ORAL)
MARPLAN

PHENELZINE
NARDIL

TRANYLCYPROMINE
PARNATE

Purpose

This medicine is used to help relieve the symptoms of depression and other conditions. It belongs to a group of medicines called Monoamine Oxidase Inhibitors, or "MAO Inhibitors."

Allergies/Warnings

If you have ever had an allergic reaction to any medicine or if you have high blood pressure, seizures, heart problems or glaucoma or any other medical condition, tell your doctor and pharmacist before you take any of this medicine.

Before you take this medicine, be sure to tell your doctor if you have taken *any other medicines* (either prescription or nonprescription drugs) within the last 2 weeks.

How to Use This Medicine

How to Administer
Take this medicine with a glass of water.

Special Instructions

Length of Therapy
It is important that you take the medicine regularly and that you do not miss any doses. The full effect of the medicine will not be noticed immediately, but may take from a few days to several weeks. Early signs of improvement are increased appetite, better sleep, increased energy and improved mood. *Do not stop taking the medicine* when you first feel better or you may feel worse in 3 or 4 days.

Do not stop taking this medicine suddenly without the approval of your doctor. It will be necessary for your doctor to reduce your dose slowly since your body will need time to adjust. It could be harmful and make your condition worse if you suddenly stopped taking the medicine. After you have stopped taking this medicine, you must continue to observe the following precautions (*see* Special Precautions, below) for 2 weeks since some of the medicine will still be in your body.

Pregnancy/Breastfeeding
Women who are pregnant, breastfeeding or planning to become pregnant should tell their doctor before taking this medicine.

Drug Interactions
It is very important that you obtain the advice of your doctor or pharmacist before taking any other prescription or nonprescription medicines, including pain relievers, sleeping pills, tranquilizers or medicines for depression, cough or cold, sinus, hay fever or allergy medicines, because the combination could cause drowsiness, high blood pressure or other complications. Also check the label to see if there is any warning about taking the product with Monoamine Oxidase Inhibitors or MAO Inhibitors.

Do not drink excessive amounts of caffeine (coffee, tea, colas, etc.) or take nonprescription medicines containing caffeine. Check with your pharmacist if you do not know if a product contains caffeine.

There are other drug interactions that can occur. If you are taking any other medicines, be sure to check first with your pharmacist or doctor.

Alcohol

Do not drink alcoholic beverages while taking this drug because the combination could cause a serious reaction.

Special Precautions

When you are taking this medicine and for *at least 2 weeks after* your treatment ends, you must be very careful about your diet. Eating some of the following foods (usually aged, fermented or smoked foods) or beverages could cause a very unpleasant reaction (severe headache, nausea, vomiting or chest pains) in some people:

Cheese and Dairy Products

Foods to Avoid:
- Aged and natural cheeses (for example, cheddar, blue, Camembert, Stilton, Gruyère, Brie, Swiss and Emmenthaler).
- In general, avoid foods in which aging is used to increase the flavor.
- Lasagna, pizza, and other foods containing cheese.

Foods Allowed:
- All milk products except those listed to avoid.
- Cream cheese, processed cheese, ricotta cheese and cottage cheese are safe to eat.
- Sour cream or yogurt when used before the "Best Before" date on the carton.

Meat and Fish

Foods to Avoid:
- Game meat (such as duck and goose).
- Chicken livers or beef livers.
- Dry fermented sausage (such as fermented bolognas and salamis, pepperoni and summer sausage).
- Smoked or pickled fish.
- Pickled or kippered herring.
- Bouillon and commercial gravies in large amounts.
- Caviar (controversial).

Foods Allowed:
- All meats except those listed to avoid.
- Eat fresh meats promptly or freeze until ready to use.

Fruits and Vegetables

Foods to Avoid:
- Canned figs, raisins (controversial).
- The pods of broad beans (also called fava beans, Italian beans).
- Avocados (particularly if overripe).
- Bananas (particularly if overripe).
- Overripe or decaying food.

Foods Allowed:
- All fruits and vegetables except those listed to avoid.

Foods and Medicines Containing Yeast

Foods to Avoid:
- Yeast extracts (such as Marmite, Bovril, brewer's yeast, some packaged soups) or meat extracts.
- Vitamins containing yeast.

Foods Allowed:
- Baker's yeast.

Alcoholic Beverages

Avoid:
- Wines, especially Chianti and other heavy red wines.
- Alcoholic beverages, including sherry and beer and ale. These beverages can also cause flushing of the face and sweating.

Miscellaneous

Foods to Avoid:
- Any foods which are overripe, fermenting or slightly "off."
- Excessive amounts of chocolate or cocoa (controversial).
- Excessive amounts of caffeine — for example, coffee, tea, cola beverages (controversial).
- Soy sauce (controversial).
- Meat tenderizers (controversial).

Foods Allowed:
- All breads and cereals.

If you took this medicine with any of these substances and nothing happened, do not assume that it will be safe for you to do it again. Foods, beverages and medicines vary greatly in their ability to cause the reaction.

If you feel that you will not be able to follow these dietary restrictions, you should talk with your doctor about alternative treatments.

Any medicine has a few unwanted side effects. Many of these side effects are annoying but you should try to keep taking this medicine unless your doctor tells you to stop it. Because this medicine takes a few weeks to work, the side effects show the doctor that the drug is starting to work. Most of these side effects will go away as your body adjusts to the medicine, but some may not.

If this medicine causes dizziness or lightheadedness, you should be careful going up and down stairs and you should not change positions too rapidly. Lightheadedness is more likely to occur if you stand up suddenly—this is due to blood collecting in the legs and lasts for a few seconds. Therefore, get up from a sitting or lying position more slowly and tighten and relax your leg muscles or wiggle your toes to help promote circulation. In the morning, get out of bed slowly and dangle your feet over the edge of the bed for a few minutes before standing up. Sit or lie down at the first sign of dizziness. Tell your doctor if you have been dizzy. In order to help prevent dizziness or fainting, your doctor may also recommend that you avoid strenuous exercise, standing for long periods of time (especially in hot weather), hot showers, hot baths, Jacuzzis or saunas.

Make sure you know how you are going to react to this medicine and whether it will make you dizzy or drowsy. Do not drive a car, pilot an airplane, operate dangerous machinery or do jobs that require you to be alert if you are dizzy or drowsy.

If your mouth becomes dry, drink water, suck ice chips or a hard, sour candy (sugarless) or chew gum (sugarless). Sugarless products are recommended in order to avoid dental problems. You may wish to ask your pharmacist about special solutions, called artificial saliva, that can also be used to help restore moisture in the mouth. It is especially important to brush and floss your teeth regularly if you develop a dry mouth, to help prevent gum problems.

This medicine may cause some people to become constipated. To help prevent constipation, try increasing the amount of bulk in your diet (for example, bran, fresh fruits and salads), exercising more often or drinking more fluids (unless otherwise directed). Call your doctor if the constipation continues.

For patients with diabetes:
• This medicine may cause your blood sugar to fall and may also mask or hide some of the signs of low blood sugar (such as blood

pressure changes and faster pulse rate). Be alert for the other signs of low blood sugar that are not masked (such as sweating, hunger, tiredness). If you think your blood sugar is lower than normal, call your doctor. It may be necessary to adjust the dose of your diabetes medications.

When to Call Your Doctor

Stop taking this medicine and call your doctor immediately if you develop severe, pounding headaches, chest pains, rapid heartbeats, nausea, vomiting, stiff neck, high fever, unexplained sweating or dilated (larger) pupils. If you cannot reach your doctor, call an emergency medical service or a hospital emergency department.

Call your doctor if you develop a skin rash, fainting, difficulty in urinating (passing your water), swelling of the legs and ankles, eye pain, changes in ability to see red and green colors, dark-colored urine, diarrhea, insomnia, daytime sleepiness, decreased sexual response, hallucinations, unusual excitability or a yellow color to the skin or eyes.

Refills

Do not stop taking this medicine without your doctor's approval and do not go without medicine between prescription refills. Call your pharmacist for a refill 2 or 3 days before you will run out of the medicine.

Miscellaneous

Carry an identification card in your wallet or wear a medical alert bracelet indicating that you are taking this medicine, as well as the names and phone numbers of your doctors. If you do not already carry such a card, complete the Medicine Card in this book. Always tell your dentist, pharmacist and other doctors who are treating you that you are taking this medicine.

▶ **ISOPROPAMIDE (ORAL)**
DARBID

Purpose

This medicine is used to help relieve spasm and cramping by relaxing the muscles of the stomach and bowels, as well as to decrease the amount of acid formed in the stomach. It is also used in the treatment of peptic ulcer.

Foods Can Interact with Some Drugs

If you are taking a prescription medicine, the food you eat may interact with the drug and cause the drug to work faster or more slowly or may even prevent it from working.

- If TETRACYCLINE is taken with a glass of milk, yogurt or some cheese, the calcium in these foods can bind with the antibiotic and prevent it from being fully absorbed. The TETRACYCLINE is made inactive and excreted in the feces.
- Acidic fruit juices, such as grapefruit juice or orange juice, can interact with PENICILLIN G and prevent the drug from working as well.

Some foods must be strictly avoided with some drugs because the combination could cause a dangerous reaction.

- A group of antidepressant drugs, called Monoamine Oxidase Inhibitors, react with foods that contain a high amount of tyramine (such as aged cheeses, Chianti wine, pickled herring and chicken livers) to cause high blood pressure, severe headaches, nausea or vomiting, brain hemorrhage and, in extreme cases, death. These foods must also be avoided for at least 2 weeks after the drug has been stopped since it takes this long for the drug to be excreted from the body.

Some foods help improve the absorption of drugs.

- GRISEOFULVIN, a drug that is used to treat certain types of fungal infections, works much better if the person eats fatty foods before taking the drug. The fat in the food stimulates the release of bile, which helps to dissolve the drug and improve absorption.

As a general rule:
- Be sure you know if your medicine should be taken with or without food.
- Be sure you know if there are certain foods or beverages that should not be taken at the same time as the drug, or should be avoided during the entire time you are taking the medicine.

Allergies/Warnings

If you have ever had an allergic reaction to iodine or any medicine or if you have high blood pressure, glaucoma, enlarged prostate, difficulty urinating (passing your water) or any other medical condition, tell your doctor and pharmacist before you take any of this medicine.

How to Use This Medicine

How to Administer

Take this medicine with a glass of water.

Special Instructions

Pregnancy/Breastfeeding

Women who are pregnant or planning to become pregnant should tell their doctor before taking this medicine.

Women who are breastfeeding should tell their doctor before taking this medicine. This medicine may decrease the amount of breast milk produced.

Drug Interactions

It is important that you obtain the advice of your doctor or pharmacist before taking any other prescription or nonprescription medicines, including pain relievers, sleeping pills, tranquilizers or medicines for depression, cough, cold, sinus or allergies.

Do not take antacids or medicine for diarrhea within 1 hour of taking the medicine as they could make this medicine less effective.

There are other drug interactions that can occur. If you are taking any other medicines, be sure to check first with your pharmacist or doctor.

Special Precautions

You may become more sensitive to heat because your body may perspire less while you are taking this drug. Be careful not to become overheated during exercise or in hot weather. Try to avoid strenuous exercise, standing for long periods of time (especially in hot weather), hot showers, hot baths, saunas or Jacuzzis while taking this medicine.

If your mouth becomes dry, drink water, suck ice chips or a hard, sour candy (sugarless) or chew gum (sugarless). Sugarless products are recommended in order to avoid dental problems. You may wish to ask your pharmacist about special solutions, called artificial saliva, that can also be used to help restore moisture in the mouth. It is especially important to brush and floss your teeth regularly if you develop a dry mouth, to help prevent gum problems.

An urge to urinate (pass your water) with an inability to do so sometimes occurs with this drug. Urinating before taking the drug each time may help relieve this problem. Tell your doctor if you are having this problem.

This medicine may cause some people to become constipated. To help prevent constipation, try increasing the amount of bulk in your diet (for example, bran, fresh fruits and salads), exercising more often or drinking more fluids (unless otherwise directed). Call your doctor if the constipation continues.

If your eyes become more sensitive to sunlight, it may help to wear sunglasses.

When to Call Your Doctor

Any medicine can sometimes cause unwanted effects. Call your doctor if you develop a skin rash, diarrhea, unusual restlessness, flushing, hazy vision, eye pain, drooping of eyelids, weakness in hand muscles, fever or fast heartbeats.

Allergic Reactions

Call your doctor immediately if you think you may be allergic to the medicine or if you develop a skin rash, hives, itching, swelling of the face or difficulty in breathing. If you cannot reach your doctor, phone a hospital emergency department.

▶ ## ISOPROTERENOL (INHALATION)
ISUPREL MISTOMETER, MEDIHALER-ISO INHALER

PROCATEROL
PRO-AIR

ORCIPRENALINE (ORAL and INHALATION)
ALUPENT METERED AEROSOL, ALUPENT SYRUP, ALUPENT TABLETS

SALBUTAMOL
NOVO-SALMOL, VENTODISK, VENTOLIN INHALER, VENTOLIN NEBULES, VENTOLIN ORAL LIQUID, VENTOLIN RESPIRATOR SOLUTION, VENTOLIN ROTACAPS, VENTOLIN TABLETS, VOLMAX

TERBUTALINE
BRICANYL AEROSOL, BRICANYL TABLETS, BRICANYL TURBUHALER

Purpose

This medicine is used to help open the bronchioles (air passages in the lungs) to make breathing easier and to relieve wheezing and shortness of breath. It is used in the treatment of bronchial asthma and other lung conditions.

SALBUTAMOL is also used to help prevent bronchospasm, shortness of breath and wheezing caused by exercise or cold air. It is taken shortly before exercise or exposure to cold air.

Allergies/Warnings

If you have ever had an allergic reaction to any medicine (including any cough/cold, allergy, heart or weight-reducing medicines), tell your doctor and pharmacist before you take any of this medicine. Also tell your doctor and pharmacist if you have any heart problems, high blood pressure, diabetes, thyroid disease or epilepsy.

How to Use This Medicine

How to Administer

For tablets:
- The tablets may be taken with a glass of water or food. Food may help prevent stomach upset.

For VOLMAX SLOW-RELEASE TABLETS:
- These tablets must be swallowed whole. Do not crush, chew or break them in half.

For syrup:
- See Oral Liquid Medicines (page 17).
- If a spoon is used to measure a dose, it is recommended that you use a medicine spoon or an oral liquid syringe, which you can obtain from your pharmacist.

For VENTOLIN ROTACAPS:
- VENTOLIN ROTACAPS must NOT be swallowed. These capsules are to be used with the VENTOLIN ROTAHALER.

For VENTODISK:
- Follow the special instructions that come with the inhaler.
- Each VENTODISK contains 8 blisters filled with a powder. The VENTODISKS must be used with the VENTODISK DISKHALER.
- Do not use the inhaler more often than directed by your doctor.

- If difficulty in breathing persists or if relief is not obtained with your usual dosage, call your doctor immediately.
- *See* Dry Powder Diskhalers (page 35).
- Do not use the dry powder diskhaler more often than your doctor has prescribed. If your breathing is difficult and is not helped by the prescribed dose, contact your doctor immediately or go to the nearest hospital emergency room.

For aerosol inhalers:
- Follow the special instructions that come with the inhaler. Some inhalers must be turned upside down when used. Some inhalers come with their extender device. Also *see* Metered-Dose Inhalers (page 31).
- Shake the inhaler well each time before use.
- The mouthpiece of the inhaler should be kept clean and dry. The metal canister must be fully and firmly positioned in the outer "shell" and rotated occasionally.
- Do not inhale the medicine more often than directed by your doctor. If your doctor has prescribed a second puff, wait at least 1 to 2 minutes before shaking the container again and repeating the procedure.
- If difficulty in breathing persists or if relief is not obtained with your usual dosage, call your doctor immediately.

For nebulizer solutions:
- Be sure to use the type of nebulizer machine recommended by your doctor and learn how to use it correctly. The solution must not be swallowed.

Special Instructions

Length of Therapy
Do not use this medicine more often or longer than recommended by your doctor. To do so may increase your chance of developing side effects such as tremors or rapid heartbeats.

Pregnancy/Breastfeeding
Women who are pregnant, breastfeeding or planning to become pregnant should tell their doctor before taking this medicine.

Drug Interactions
Some nonprescription drugs can aggravate your condition. Do not take any of the following without the approval of your doctor or phar-

macist: cough, cold, or sinus products; ASA-containing products; asthma or allergy products.

Read the label of the nonprescription drug product to see if there is a warning. If there is, check with your doctor or pharmacist before using the product.

If you have been prescribed the inhaler form of this medicine, do not take other inhaled medicines that have not been prescribed by your doctor while you are using this medicine.

Special Precautions

If you are using the inhaler form of this medicine and a steroid inhaler (such as BECLOMETHASONE or FLUNISOLIDE), use this medicine approximately 10 to 15 minutes before using the steroid inhaler as directed by your doctor. This medicine will help open up the air passages in the lungs and increase the action of the steroid medicine.

In some people, this drug may cause dizziness or drowsiness. Do not drive a car, pilot an airplane, operate dangerous machinery or do jobs that require you to be alert if you are dizzy or drowsy. You should also be careful going up and down stairs. Sit or lie down at the first sign of dizziness. Tell your doctor if the dizziness continues or becomes severe.

People over 60 years of age are more sensitive to the side effects of this medicine. Do not take more of the medicine than prescribed by your doctor.

In some people this medicine may cause a bad taste in the mouth. This is only temporary and will go away after you have finished the medicine.

If dryness of the mouth or throat occurs after you use the inhalation form of the medicine, rinsing or gargling with warm water after inhaling the medicine may help.

For ISOPROTERENOL:

- This medicine may cause the saliva to turn pink to red in color. This is not unusual.
- Do not use the solution if it has turned pink or brown in color or if it contains a sediment.
- It is not unusual for mild flushing of the face or a slightly faster heartbeat to occur just after taking the medicine. This should not last long. If it does, call your doctor.

When to Call Your Doctor

Call your doctor if the medicine does not relieve your breathing problems, or if your sputum turns yellow or green in color.

Most people experience few or no side effects from this drug. However, any medicine can sometimes cause unwanted effects. Call your doctor if you develop chest pain, rapid or irregular heartbeats, continuing nausea or vomiting, muscle cramps, severe headaches, muscle tremors, coughing, flushing, unexplained nervousness, insomnia, severe dizziness or drowsiness.

Allergic Reactions

Call your doctor immediately if you think you may be allergic to the medicine or if you develop a skin rash, hives, itching, swelling of the face or difficulty in breathing. If you cannot reach your doctor, phone a hospital emergency department.

Storage

For VOLMAX TABLETS:
- Keep the tablets in the original blister package and store in a cool place. Do *not* remove the tablets from the package until just before you take the medicine. If these tablets are not stored properly, they will be less effective.

For inhaler:
- *See* Metered-Dose Inhalers (page 31).
- Store these inhalers in a dry (not humid) place away from heat.

For BRICANYL TURBUHALER:
- Never wash the mouthpiece. Use a dry tissue only.

For nebulizer solutions:
- Protect nebulizer solutions from heat and light. Do not use nebulizer solutions if they turn brown or contain a precipitate (sediment) at the bottom of the bottle. Do not use after the discard (expiration) date.

Refills

Discuss with your pharmacist the implications of dispensing all your refills for this medicine with the same manufacturer's product. (*See* Generic Drugs, page 13.)

Drug Timing and Cancer Treatment

Drug timing may be critical in the treatment of cancer.

Researchers at the University of Minnesota have found that the time of administration of certain cancer drugs has a profound effect on their toxicity and complications. Patients who were receiving DOXORUBICIN in the morning and CISPLATIN in the evening had fewer dosage changes, treatment delays and complications than patients who were receiving the two drugs at opposite times of the day.

▶ **ISOSORBIDE DINITRATE (ORAL)**
APO-ISDN, CEDOCARD-SR, CORADUR, CORONEX, ISORDIL, NOVOSORBIDE

ISOSORBIDE DINITRATE (SUBLINGUAL)
APO-ISDN, CORONEX, ISORDIL

Purpose
This medicine is used to help prevent angina (chest pains). It does this by decreasing the demand by the heart for oxygen.

Allergies/Warnings
Be sure to tell your doctor and pharmacist if you are allergic to any medicine. Also tell your doctor if you have glaucoma or kidney disease.

How to Use This Medicine

Time of Administration
For tablets to be placed under the tongue (APO-ISDN, CORONEX *and* ISORDIL SUBLINGUAL TABLETS):
- Carry this medicine with you all the time.
- This medicine should be used at the *first* sign of an attack of angina (chest pains or tightness or squeezing in the chest). Do not wait until the pain becomes severe. *Sit down* as soon as you feel an attack of angina coming on.
- If your doctor recommends, you may help prevent angina by placing a tablet under the tongue 5 or 10 minutes before stressful activities such as strenuous exercise, sexual activity, emotional stress, a heavy

meal, high altitudes or exposure to cold. Let your doctor know what things usually cause your angina so that he or she can advise about preventing attacks.

For medicine to be swallowed (APO-ISDN, CEDOCARD-SR, CORADUR, CORONEX, ISORDIL, NOVOSORBIDE ORAL TABLETS):
- It is best to take this medicine with a glass of water on an empty stomach at least 1 hour before (or 2 hours after) eating food.

How to Administer
The sublingual tablets work faster than the tablets that are swallowed.

For tablets to be placed under the tongue (APO-ISDN, CORONEX *and* ISORDIL SUBLINGUAL TABLETS):
- Sit down.
- Place a tablet *under your tongue* and let it dissolve completely.
- *Do not swallow or chew* the tablet since this drug works faster when it is absorbed through the lining of the mouth.
- Try not to swallow until the tablet is dissolved and do not rinse your mouth for a few minutes afterwards. Do not eat, drink or smoke while the tablet is dissolving.
- This tablet usually has an effect in 2 to 5 minutes. If your angina is not relieved within 5 to 10 minutes, you may dissolve a second tablet under your tongue. If the angina continues for another 5 to 10 minutes, you may dissolve a third tablet. If 3 doses do not relieve your chest pains, call your doctor or nearest emergency medical service immediately or go to the nearest hospital emergency department.
- Try to relax for 15 to 20 minutes after taking the drug and remain calm since this will also help to relieve the attack sooner. If you become dizzy or feel faint, breathe deeply and bend forward with your head between your knees. Always get up slowly after you have been sitting or lying down.

For long-acting medicine (CEDOCARD-SR, CORADUR):
- This medicine must be swallowed whole. Do not crush or chew it.

Special Instructions

Length of Therapy
If you are taking this medicine daily, do not stop taking this medicine suddenly without the approval of your doctor. It will be necessary

for your doctor to reduce your dose slowly since your body will need time to adjust. It could be harmful and cause an angina attack if you suddenly stopped taking the medicine.

Pregnancy/Breastfeeding

Women who are pregnant, breastfeeding or planning to become pregnant should tell their doctor before taking this medicine.

Drug Interactions

Some nonprescription drugs can aggravate your heart condition. Do not take any of the following without the approval of your doctor or pharmacist: cough, cold or sinus products; asthma or allergy products. Read the label of the product to see if there is a warning. If there is, check with your doctor or pharmacist before using the product.

Alcohol

Do not drink alcoholic beverages too soon after taking this medicine as the combination may cause a serious drop in blood pressure, dizziness and/or fainting.

Special Precautions

The first few doses of this medicine may cause dizziness, flushing or headache. This is normal and will usually disappear after you have taken the drug a few times. Sit or lie down until these effects pass. Breathe deeply and bend forward with your head between your knees if you feel faint. Get up slowly after you have been sitting or lying down. It may help to relieve the headache if you take the medicine with some food or, if your doctor agrees, with ASA or acetaminophen. However, if the dizziness or the headaches do not go away, tell your doctor. Your dose may have to be adjusted.

If you become dizzy, you should be careful going up and down stairs. Do not drive a car, pilot an airplane, operate dangerous machinery or do jobs that require you to be alert.

Keep a record of the number of angina attacks and possible causes of the attacks. This information will help your physician give you the best treatment. Be sure to tell your doctor if you have an increase in number, length or severity of attacks.

Cigarette smoking can aggravate angina and is a special risk for people who have heart conditions.

When to Call Your Doctor

Most people experience few or no side effects from this drug. However, any medicine can sometimes cause unwanted effects. Call your

doctor if you develop a skin rash, fainting, nausea or vomiting, a fast pulse or persistent or severe headaches.

Storage
Store in a cool, dry place but not in the refrigerator.

Refills
Do not stop taking this medicine without your doctor's approval and do not go without medicine between prescription refills. Call your pharmacist for a refill 2 or 3 days before you will run out of the medicine.

Discuss with your pharmacist the implications of dispensing all your refills for this medicine with the same manufacturer's product. (*See* Generic Drugs, page 13.)

Miscellaneous
Carry an identification card in your wallet or wear a medical alert bracelet indicating that you are taking this medicine, as well as the names and phone numbers of your doctors. If you do not already carry such a card, complete the Medicine Card in this book. Always tell your dentist, pharmacist and other doctors who are treating you that you are taking this medicine.

▶ **ISOTRETINOIN (ORAL)**
ACCUTANE ROCHE

Purpose
This medicine is used in the treatment of certain types of severe acne that have not responded to the usual acne treatments. It should not be used in mild cases of acne.

Allergies/Warnings
Be sure to tell your doctor and pharmacist if you are allergic to oral vitamin A or any medicine or have any other medical condition.

Also tell your doctor if you are hypersensitive to parabens. ACCUTANE contains parabens as a preservative.

Be sure to tell your doctor if you have diabetes, or if there is a history of diabetes in your family. It may be necessary to test your blood for sugar while you are taking this medicine.

Also tell your doctor if you have epilepsy, are taking any medicines for seizures or have a history of high blood cholesterol or triglycerides.

How to Use This Medicine

Time of Administration

This medicine is usually given one or two times a day, usually for 15 to 20 weeks, unless otherwise directed by your doctor.

How to Administer

Take the medicine with food or meals.

Be sure to read your prescription label carefully and be sure to take the right amount of medicine. Your dose may change when the prescription is refilled.

Special Instructions

Length of Therapy

It is important not to miss any doses. Try to take the medicine at the same time(s) every day so that you have a constant level of medicine in your body. Do *not* take any more of this medicine than your doctor has prescribed because it will increase the chance of developing side effects.

It may take 1 to 2 months before you see a benefit from this medicine.

Pregnancy/Breastfeeding

Women must not become pregnant during therapy or for at least 1 month after stopping the medicine because severe birth defects have occurred in the babies of women who took ACCUTANE *during pregnancy.*

Women *must not* take this medicine until they are sure they are not pregnant. It is strongly recommended that a pregnancy test be done 2 weeks *before* starting the drug. An effective form of birth control must be used at least 1 month *before* starting this medicine and throughout ACCUTANE therapy and for at least 1 month after stopping the drug or until a normal menstrual period has occurred.

If you think you are pregnant after you have started taking the drug or within 1 month after you have stopped the medicine, STOP taking the drug immediately and call your doctor. This medicine can cause serious birth defects.

Women taking this medicine should *not* breastfeed infants.

Drug Interactions

This medicine is related to vitamin A. Therefore, vitamin products and health food supplements containing vitamin A must be avoided while you are receiving this medicine. This is because the vitamin A in these products may add to the unwanted effects of ACCUTANE. If you have any questions about the contents of a vitamin preparation, check with your pharmacist.

While taking this medicine, avoid eating foods that contain very high amounts of vitamin A, such as liver. Foods containing moderate amounts of vitamin A should not cause any problem.

Alcohol

It is best not to drink any alcoholic beverages while taking this medicine.

Special Precautions

During the first few weeks of treatment, your acne may seem to get worse and you may have redness and itching. This usually disappears as you continue to take the medicine. Call your doctor if the redness or itching does not disappear. A late flare-up of acne during the last few weeks of therapy may be seen in some people. It is important to remember that your acne may continue to improve even after you stop the medicine.

Do not give ACCUTANE to anyone else. It has been prescribed for your condition only and may not be suitable for another person.

Because the lipid (fat) levels in the blood can increase while you are taking the medicine, large amounts of foods containing saturated fats (whole milk, cheese, eggs and red meats) should be avoided.

Your doctor will order blood tests when you first begin taking the medicine. These blood tests are usually repeated after 2 weeks and then monthly for the rest of the therapy, or as ordered by your doctor. It is important that you keep your appointments for these blood tests and that you follow any special diet your doctor recommends before the tests. Do not drink any alcoholic beverages for at least 36 hours before the blood tests are done. You must not eat anything for 14 hours before the test. Usually it is requested that you eat supper and then have the blood test the next morning before eating breakfast.

Do not donate blood while you are taking this medicine or for 1 or 2 months after the treatment has been stopped. The medicine will be in your blood and could cause serious effects if a pregnant woman received the blood.

Do not use any skin drying agents or other acne treatments without the approval of your doctor.

Sometimes, skin that was normal (such as hands and feet) may peel. Check with your doctor if this becomes a problem.

If your mouth becomes dry, drink water, suck ice chips or a hard, sour candy (sugarless) or chew gum (sugarless). Sugarless products are recommended in order to avoid dental problems. You may wish to ask your pharmacist about special solutions, called artificial saliva, that can also be used to help restore moisture in the mouth. It is especially important to brush and floss your teeth regularly if you develop a dry mouth, to help prevent gum problems.

Dry lips are a common problem especially during the first 2 weeks of therapy. Petroleum jelly may be helpful. Fruits and vegetables should be cut up and eaten with a fork. Juices should be drunk with a straw. If these simple measures do not relieve the lip tenderness or peeling, call your doctor.

Nosebleeds are also common among people taking ACCUTANE. Petroleum jelly can be gently inserted with a Q-Tip. If nosebleeds persist or become difficult to stop, call your doctor.

Patients wearing contact lenses may notice that they are more sensitive to the lenses during and after treatment. Dry eyes and poor night vision have also been reported. Ask your pharmacist about eye drops, called "artificial tears," to lubricate your eyes. Do not drive a car at night if your night vision becomes poor.

This medicine may make you more sensitive to sunlight and some tanning lamps. When you begin taking the medicine, avoid too much sun until you see how you react. If your skin does become more sensitive, inform your physician and try not to stay in direct sunlight for extended periods of time. While in the sun, wear protective clothing and sunscreens in creamy bases with an SPF of 15 or higher, and proper U-V filtered sunglasses.

This medicine may cause a change in your body's ability to metabolize substances called triglycerides (fats). Your doctor will measure the amount of the substances in your blood in order to determine how your body is responding.

When to Call Your Doctor

This medicine causes side effects that may be noticeable before healing begins. The most common side effects are dry skin and lips, sore, scaly, red, cracked, burning lips, redness, dryness, burning or itching of the eyes, blurred vision or eye pain, hair thinning, rash, peeling of the skin of the palms and soles, muscle, joint or bone aches and pains, dryness of nose, mild nosebleeds and itching. These effects are usually temporary and will usually disappear after you have finished the therapy. Call your doctor if they become bothersome. Your doctor may recommend a dosage change as a precautionary measure or may recommend that you stop taking the medicine.

Call your doctor if your acne becomes extremely tender or if you develop open sores that bleed.

This medicine can also cause some serious side effects. Stop taking the medicine and call your doctor immediately if you develop any unusual symptoms, a skin rash, infection, severe or persistent headache, blurred vision or changes in eyesight, nausea or vomiting, severe stomach pain, diarrhea or rectal bleeding, or if you think you are pregnant.

Storage

ACCUTANE does not have to be refrigerated. However, do not expose the capsules to sunlight or excessive heat.

Keep away from the reach of children.

Miscellaneous

Carry an identification card in your wallet or wear a medical alert bracelet indicating that you are taking this medicine, as well as the names and phone numbers of your doctors. If you do not already carry such a card, complete the Medicine Card in this book. Always tell your dentist, pharmacist and other doctors who are treating you that you are taking this medicine.

Eye Drop Administration

Pressing gently on the bridge of the nose and next to the inner corner of the eyes will help prevent eye drops from being drained away from the eye as quickly.

Tears are constantly drained from the eye through the puncta into the nasolacrimal ducts and then swallowed. Eye drops are drained from the eye in the same manner and this is the reason that eye drops can sometimes be tasted after they are administered.

To slow down the drainage of eye drops, apply gentle pressure on the bridge of the nose for a minute to help block the nasolacrimal duct and keep the medicine in contact with the eye a little bit longer. It also will help to try not to blink more often than usual since blinking will also remove the eye drops from the eye.

▶ **LEVOTHYROXINE SODIUM (ORAL)**
ELTROXIN, SYNTHROID

LIOTHYRONINE
CYTOMEL

THYROGLOBULIN
PROLOID

THYROID (DESICCATED)
THYROID

Purpose

This medicine is a hormone used to treat certain diseases of the thyroid gland and conditions in which the body is not producing enough thyroid hormone. It is also used to treat conditions in which the thyroid gland has been removed.

Allergies/Warnings

If you have ever had an allergic reaction to any medicine or had any other medical condition, tell your doctor and pharmacist before you take any of this medicine.

Also tell your doctor if you are allergic to pork or beef. Some thyroid products are made from pork or beef.

How to Use This Medicine

Time of Administration

It is very important that you take this medicine exactly as your doctor has prescribed. Do not miss any doses and take the medicine even if you feel well. Try to take this medicine at the same time(s) every day so that you will have a constant level of the thyroid hormone in your body. Do not take extra tablets without your doctor's approval.

How to Administer

It is best to take this medicine with some water.

Special Instructions

Length of Therapy

It may take a few days or weeks before you begin to notice any effect from this medicine. Check with your doctor if you continue to have any clumsiness, tiredness, muscle aches, constipation, coldness or weight gain.

It will be several weeks before you will obtain the maximum effect of any dose of this medicine. It may be necessary for your doctor to make several dosage changes and check your blood thyroid level before the best dose is determined.

Depending upon your condition, it may be necessary to take this medicine for the rest of your life, since the body needs thyroid hormone.

Do not stop taking this medicine suddenly without the approval of your doctor.

Pregnancy/Breastfeeding

Women who are breastfeeding should tell their doctor.

Drug Interactions

Some nonprescription drugs can aggravate your condition and cause unnecessary problems. Do not take any of the following without the approval of your doctor or pharmacist: cough, cold, or sinus products; asthma or allergy products. Read the label of the product to see if there is a warning. If there is, check with your doctor or pharmacist before using any of these products.

Special Precautions

It is important to stay in touch with your doctor, especially in the weeks after any dosage change. Blood tests may be needed and the doses of all your medicines may have to be adjusted.

For patients with diabetes:

• This medicine may affect your blood sugar. Carefully test your blood or urine for sugar while you are taking this medicine. Call your doctor if you think your blood sugar is not normal or more difficult to control.

When to Call Your Doctor

Most people experience few or no side effects from this drug. However, any medicine can sometimes cause unwanted effects. Call your doctor if you develop chest pain, shortness of breath, fever, headaches, leg cramps, difficulty sleeping, changes in menstrual periods, fast heartbeats, shakiness, persistent diarrhea, vomiting, unusual nervousness, excessive sweating or sensitivity to heat.

Allergic Reactions

Call your doctor immediately if you think you may be allergic to the medicine or if you develop a skin rash, hives, itching, swelling of the face or difficulty in breathing. If you cannot reach your doctor, phone a hospital emergency department.

Refills

Do not stop taking this medicine without your doctor's approval and do not go without medicine between prescription refills. Call your pharmacist for a refill 2 or 3 days before you will run out of the medicine.

Do not change brands of this medicine without consulting your doctor and pharmacist. Your dosage requirements may vary from one product to another.

Miscellaneous

Carry an identification card in your wallet or wear a medical alert bracelet indicating that you are taking this medicine, as well as the names and phone numbers of your doctors. If you do not already carry such a card, complete the Medicine Card in this book. Always tell your dentist, pharmacist and other doctors who are treating you that you are taking this medicine.

Tip for Ostomy Odors

A very simple method of deodorizing the wastes inside an ostomy pouch is to place a few drops of vanilla extract, peppermint oil or a commercial deodorant on several squares of toilet or facial tissue. The scented tissue can be slipped inside the ostomy pouch where it will deodorize the wastes and can later be flushed down the toilet.

▶ LINDANE (TOPICAL)

GBH, HEXIT, KWELLADA, NCP LINDANE SHAMPOO, PMS LINDANE

Purpose

This medicine is used to treat scabies and lice infestations of the skin or scalp.

Allergies/Warnings

Be sure to tell your doctor and pharmacist if you are allergic to LINDANE or any medicine.

This medicine is pesticidal and potentially toxic. Do not use it without your doctor's or pharmacist's permission.

Carefully read all the package instructions that come with the product you purchased.

How to Use This Medicine

How to Administer

Use plastic disposable gloves or rubber gloves when applying this product to another person.

Instructions for use of lotion or cream in scabies (on the skin):

- If crusts are present, take a warm bath or shower. (Hot water is not recommended because it can cause the blood vessels to dilate and increase the absorption of the product into the bloodstream.) Use a lot of soap to cleanse the skin well and to help remove loose scabs. Clean the tub or shower well after use. Allow the skin to cool before applying the drug.
- Dry the skin well. Shake the lotion well before applying. Then apply a thin layer of the cream or lotion over the entire skin surface. Start at the neck and work down. Rub in well. Do not miss any areas, especially between the fingers and toes, groin and genitals, anal area, as well as the bottom of your feet.
- Leave on for the length of time prescribed by your doctor. Then wash the medicine off the skin completely.
- Put on freshly laundered or dry-cleaned clothing in order to prevent reinfestation.

Instructions for use of lotion or cream in pubic (crab) lice:

- Take a bath or shower that is cool or at room temperature. (Hot water is not recommended because it can cause the blood vessels to dilate and increase the absorption of the product into the bloodstream.) Use a lot of soap to cleanse the skin well and to help remove loose nits. Clean the tub or shower well after use. Allow the skin to cool before applying the drug.
- Dry the skin *thoroughly* and apply a thin layer of the cream or lotion over the affected skin and hair in the pubic area.
- Leave on for the length of time prescribed by your doctor. Then wash the medicine off the skin completely.

- Put on freshly laundered or dry-cleaned clothing in order to prevent reinfestation.
- Your sexual partner should also be treated to prevent spread of the infestation.

Instructions for use of shampoo in head lice:
- Shampoo over the sink. Do not shampoo in the bathtub or shower since this will expose the rest of your body to the product.
- Keep the shampoo out of the eyes. If some does get into the eyes, flush it out with water immediately.
- Apply to dry hair.
- Pour about 1 to 2 tablespoonsful (15 to 30 mL) for short or medium length hair and about 4 tablespoonsful (60 mL) for long hair onto the affected scalp and rub in well for 4 minutes. Be sure to cover all hair areas.
- Then add small quantities of water to form a good lather. Continue to lather and work through the hair vigorously for 4 minutes.
- Rinse the hair thoroughly and rub with a clean, dry towel. Some doctors recommend rinsing the hair with a solution of warm water and vinegar in equal amounts to help remove nits.
- When hair is dry, comb with a fine-tooth comb or use tweezers or scissors to remove any remaining nits (eggs) or nit shells. This is time-consuming but *all nits must be removed.* This will prevent the nits that were not killed by the medicine from hatching into lice later. Combing the hair with a fine-tooth comb soaked in warm vinegar will help remove nits.
- This shampoo should also be used to clean the combs and brushes to prevent spread of the infestation.
- Do not let other members of the family use the comb used to remove the nits.
- The shampoo is *not* to be used as a regular shampoo.

Special Instructions

Length of Therapy

Usually only 1 treatment is necessary. Itching may continue for 1 week after you have applied the medicine. However, if it continues longer than 1 week, call your doctor. You may not have killed all the lice.

Do not use this product more frequently or leave on for a longer period than recommended by your doctor.

Pregnancy/Breastfeeding

Women who are pregnant, breastfeeding or planning to become pregnant should tell their doctor before taking this medicine.

Do not use this product on infants or in children younger than 6 years old without your doctor's permission.

Drug Interactions

If you normally use a hair dressing that has oil in it, shampoo, rinse and dry your hair thoroughly *before* applying the medicated shampoo. This is necessary because the oil on the hair can increase the absorption of the medicated shampoo.

Special Precautions

Disinfect or throw away combs and brushes immediately after using.

Put on freshly laundered clean clothing after each application of the medicine. Use fresh towels and fresh bed sheets after each application. Launder or dry-clean contaminated clothing, since nits can live on clothes for up to 30 days. Clothing that can be washed should be washed in *hot* water and dried on a *hot* setting. Dry-clean the clothes if they cannot stand hot temperatures. This also applies to hats, caps, coats with fur collars or "fake fur" collars. Clothing or pillows that cannot be cleaned can be stored in a sealed bag for 2 weeks.

Carefully vacuum all rugs, upholstered furniture and mattresses to pick up any living lice or nits. Throw away the vacuum bag immediately.

Household pets should be examined for signs of lice and treated by a veterinarian if necessary. Do not use KWELLADA on a cat—you may kill it!

Keep this medicine away from the eyes, mouth, mucous membranes and open wounds such as cuts, scratches or open sores. If some does get into the eyes, flush it away with water immediately.

When to Call Your Doctor

Call your doctor if the condition for which you are using this medicine persists or becomes worse. Also call your doctor if you develop muscle cramps, clumsiness or unsteadiness, seizures, fast heartbeats, vomiting or unusual nervousness.

Storage

Throw away the empty bottle after you have used the medicine and be sure the discarded medicine is out of the reach of children. Do *not* reuse the bottle for anything.

Miscellaneous

This medicine is for external use only. It is poisonous if swallowed.

▶ LITHIUM CARBONATE (ORAL)
CARBOLITH, DURALITH, LITHANE, LITHIZINE

Purpose

This medicine is used to help relieve the symptoms of certain types of mental and emotional conditions. It is also used to help prevent relapses of manic-depressive illness.

Allergies/Warnings

If you have ever had an allergic reaction to any medicine or if you have thyroid problems, diabetes, kidney disease or any other medical condition, tell your doctor and pharmacist before you take any of this medicine.

Be sure to tell your doctor if you are taking *any other medicines* (either prescription or nonprescription drugs).

How to Use This Medicine

How to Administer

Take this medicine with food or milk to help prevent stomach upset.

If you were prescribed DURALITH:
• This medicine must be swallowed whole. Do not crush or chew.

Special Instructions

Length of Therapy

It is important that you take the medicine regularly and that you do not miss any doses. The full effect of the medicine will not be noticed immediately, but may take from 1 week to several weeks. Early signs of improvement include restoration of normal appetite and sleep patterns and return of your mood and energy level to normal. *Do not stop taking* the medicine when you first feel better or you may feel worse in 3 or 4 days.

Since LITHIUM is often used to help prevent relapses of manic episodes and depressive episodes, you may need to take LITHIUM on a prolonged basis. You should discuss the length of your treatment with your doctor.

Pregnancy/Breastfeeding

Women who are pregnant, breastfeeding or planning to become pregnant should not take this medicine without their doctor's approval. Studies have indicated that LITHIUM may cause birth defects, especially if taken during the first three months of pregnancy.

Drug Interactions

It is important that you obtain the advice of your doctor or pharmacist before taking any other prescription or nonprescription medicines, including pain relievers, asthma or allergy medicines, diuretics (water pills), laxatives, sodium bicarbonate (baking soda) or caffeine products.

There are other drug interactions that can occur. If you are taking any other medicines, be sure to check first with your pharmacist or doctor.

Do not drink large quantities of beverages containing caffeine (coffee, tea, colas) while taking this medicine. These beverages can decrease the effect of this medicine and make it less helpful.

Alcohol

Do not drink alcoholic beverages while taking this drug without the approval of your doctor.

Special Precautions

Use a normal amount of table salt in your diet unless otherwise directed. Do not alter your diet or use salt substitutes without first consulting your doctor.

Unless otherwise directed by your doctor, try to drink plenty of water or other liquids (but not beverages containing caffeine) every day while you are taking this medicine. This will help prevent kidney problems.

Keep your regular doctor appointments so that your doctor can check your progress and make sure you are getting the full benefit of this medicine. It is almost always necessary for dosages to be adjusted by the doctor.

It will also be necessary for your doctor to do regular laboratory tests. The *only* time *not* to take your LITHIUM is the morning on the days you have a LITHIUM blood test. Otherwise, your blood test will not give an accurate reading. Always make sure that you have your LITHIUM blood test done as close as possible to 12 hours after your last LITHIUM dose.

Any medicine has a few unwanted side effects. Side effects are annoying but you should try to keep taking the medicine unless your doctor tells you to stop it. Because this medicine takes a few weeks to work, the side effects show the doctor that the drug is starting to work. Some of these side effects will go away as your body adjusts to the medicine but some may not.

A mild hand tremor or shakiness is common when people start taking LITHIUM and it is not harmful. Mild nausea and mild thirst may also occur during the first few days of treatment. These side effects are annoying but usually disappear within a few days. If they persist or become severe, check with your doctor.

If this medicine causes dizziness or lightheadedness, you should be careful going up and down stairs and you should not change positions too rapidly. Sit or lie down at the first sign of dizziness. Tell your doctor if you have been dizzy.

Your doctor may also recommend that you avoid strenuous exercise, standing for long periods of time (especially in hot weather), hot showers, hot baths, Jacuzzis or saunas. You could lose too much water and salt through increased sweating, which can lead to serious side effects.

Do not drive a car, pilot an airplane, operate dangerous machinery or do jobs that require you to be alert if you are dizzy or drowsy.

When to Call Your Doctor

Call your doctor if you develop diarrhea or an increased desire to urinate (pass your water), or pass large amounts of light-colored urine, or develop vomiting, slurred speech, increased trembling of the hands, jerking of the arms or legs, unusual weakness or drowsiness, blurred vision, stomach pains, ringing or buzzing in the ears, swelling of the hands or feet, slow or irregular heartbeats, lack of coordination, convulsions, stiffness of the muscles or confusion.

Check with your doctor if you develop the flu or any other infection that is accompanied by vomiting and/or diarrhea, fever and/or sweating. The loss of too much body water may cause the amount of LITHIUM in your system to increase and your doctor may have to adjust your LITHIUM dose.

Refills

Do not stop taking this medicine without your doctor's approval and do not go without medicine between prescription refills. Call your pharmacist for a refill 2 or 3 days before you will run out of the medicine.

Do not change brands of this medicine without your doctor's approval. The dose you need could be different with different products. Also, do not change from tablets to capsules, or vice versa, unless prescribed by your doctor.

Miscellaneous

Carry an identification card in your wallet or wear a medical alert bracelet indicating that you are taking this medicine, as well as the names and phone numbers of your doctors. If you do not already carry such a card, complete the Medicine Card in this book. Always tell your dentist, pharmacist and other doctors who are treating you that you are taking this medicine.

▶ LOPERAMIDE (ORAL)
IMODIUM

Purpose
This medicine is used in the treatment of diarrhea, including Traveler's Diarrhea. It should not be used to treat diarrhea caused by intestinal toxins from bacteria (e.g., *E.coli*, *Salmonella* or *Shigella*) or diarrhea that develops sometimes from taking some types of antibiotics.

It is also used in the care of ileostomies, colostomies and other types of bowel surgery.

Allergies/Warnings
If you have ever had an allergic reaction to any medicine, tell your doctor and pharmacist before you take any of this medicine.

This medicine should not be given to children under 2 years of age.

How to Use This Medicine

Time of Administration
The medicine should be taken after each unformed stool. Do not take more doses than recommended by your doctor.

How to Administer
For capsules and tablets:
• Take with food or a glass of water.

For liquid medicine:
• *See* Oral Liquid Medicines (page 17).

321

Special Instructions

Length of Therapy

If the diarrhea does not stop or improve after 48 hours, check with your doctor. There are many causes of diarrhea.

Pregnancy/Breastfeeding

Women who are pregnant, breastfeeding or planning to become pregnant should tell their doctor before taking this medicine.

Special Precautions

In some people, this drug may cause dizziness or drowsiness. Do not drive a car, pilot an airplane, operate dangerous machinery or do jobs that require you to be alert if you are dizzy or drowsy. You should also be careful going up and down stairs. Sit or lie down at the first sign of dizziness. Tell your doctor if the dizziness or drowsiness continues.

If your mouth or skin becomes very dry, check with your doctor.

It is important to drink plenty of water or clear fluids when you have diarrhea and while you are taking this medicine.

When to Call Your Doctor

Call your doctor if you develop a fever, abdominal pain, bloating, constipation, nausea, vomiting, irregular heartbeats or severe muscle cramps, if the diarrhea continues or if you have blood in the stools.

Allergic Reactions

Call your doctor immediately if you think you may be allergic to the medicine or if you develop a skin rash, hives, itching, swelling of the face or difficulty in breathing. If you cannot reach your doctor, phone a hospital emergency department.

Preventing Cavities

Children who are taking a medicine in a syrup on a regular basis should brush their teeth or rinse their mouths with water after taking the medicine.

The syrup base of the medicine contains sugar. There is an increased risk of dental cavities in children who are prescribed syrup-based medicines on a frequent dosage schedule for a long period of time.

▶ **LOVASTATIN (ORAL)**
MEVACOR

PRAVASTATIN
PRAVACHOL

SIMVASTATIN
ZOCOR

Purpose

This medicine is used to lower cholesterol and lipids (fat) in the blood.

Allergies/Warnings

If you have ever had liver disease or an allergic reaction to any medicine, or are taking any other medicines to lower cholesterol, tell your doctor and pharmacist before you take any of this medicine.

How to Use This Medicine

Time of Administration
For MEVACOR:
- If you take this medicine once a day, take it with the evening meal. If you take the medicine twice a day, take it with the morning and evening meal unless otherwise directed.

For PRAVACHOL:
- Take this medicine as a single dose at bedtime.

For ZOCOR:
- Take this medicine as a single dose in the evening.

Special Instructions

Length of Therapy
It is very important to take this medicine exactly as your doctor has prescribed. Do not increase or decrease the amount you are taking without first consulting your doctor. Otherwise, you cannot expect the medicine to control your condition.

Pregnancy/Breastfeeding
This medicine should not be taken during pregnancy. Women who are pregnant, breastfeeding or planning to become pregnant should tell their doctor before taking this medicine. Women taking this medicine should not breastfeed (nurse) their infants.

Drug Interactions

This medicine may interact with some blood thinners and other medicines (especially those used to lower cholesterol). Therefore, do not start or stop taking other medicines without calling your doctor first.

Alcohol

Avoid excessive use of alcoholic beverages.

Special Precautions

Your doctor may prescribe a special diet while you are taking this medicine. Be sure to follow the diet closely as this will help to control your condition also.

It is important that you go to have all blood tests and eye tests which your doctor may recommend while you are taking this medicine.

When to Call Your Doctor

Most people experience few or no side effects from this drug. However, any medicine can sometimes cause unwanted effects. Call your doctor if you develop muscle aching, muscle cramps, tiredness, weakness, fever, blurred vision, abdominal pain, constipation or diarrhea, nausea, persistent headache or skin rashes.

▶ MECLIZINE HCI (ORAL)
BONAMINE

Purpose

This medicine is used to help control nausea and vomiting and to help prevent motion sickness. MECLIZINE is also used to treat some types of dizziness.

Allergies/Warnings

If you have ever had an allergic reaction to any medicine or if you have glaucoma, enlarged prostate, difficulty urinating (passing your water), high blood pressure or diabetes, or any other medical condition, tell your doctor and pharmacist before you take any of this medicine.

How to Use This Medicine

Time of Administration

If you are taking this medicine to prevent motion sickness:
- Take this medicine 1 hour before you plan to travel.

If you are taking this medicine to help relieve nausea and vomiting of pregnancy:
- It is best to take the medicine at bedtime.

If you are taking this medicine to help prevent nausea and vomiting caused by radiation treatment:
- Take the medicine 2 to 12 hours before treatment, as directed by your doctor.

How to Administer

These tablets can be chewed, swallowed with water or allowed to dissolve in the mouth.

Special Instructions

Pregnancy/Breastfeeding

Women who are pregnant, breastfeeding or planning to become pregnant should tell their doctor before taking this medicine.

Drug Interactions

It is important that you obtain the advice of your doctor or pharmacist before taking any other prescription or nonprescription medicines, including pain relievers, sleeping pills, tranquilizers or medicines for depression, cough, cold or allergies, because the combination could cause drowsiness.

There are other drug interactions that can occur. If you are taking any other medicines, be sure to check first with your pharmacist or doctor.

Alcohol

Do not drink alcoholic beverages while taking this drug without the approval of your doctor because the combination could cause drowsiness. One drink may have the same effect that 2 or 3 drinks normally would have.

Special Precautions

If your mouth becomes dry, drink water, suck ice chips or a hard, sour candy (sugarless) or chew gum (sugarless). Sugarless products are recommended in order to avoid dental problems. You may wish to ask your pharmacist about special solutions, called artificial saliva, that can also be used to help restore moisture in the mouth. It is especially important to brush and floss your teeth regularly if you develop a dry mouth, to help prevent gum problems.

In some people, this drug may cause drowsiness or blurred vision. Do not drive a car, pilot an airplane, operate dangerous machinery or do jobs that require you to be alert if you are dizzy or drowsy. You should also be careful going up and down stairs. Sit or lie down at the first sign of dizziness. Tell your doctor if these problems continue.

When to Call Your Doctor

Most people experience few or no side effects from this drug. However, any medicine can sometimes cause unwanted effects. Call your doctor if you develop a skin rash, sore throat, fever, mouth sores, difficulty in urinating (passing your water), blurred vision or fast heartbeats.

Allergic Reactions

Call your doctor immediately if you think you may be allergic to the medicine or if you develop a skin rash, hives, itching, swelling of the face or difficulty in breathing. If you cannot reach your doctor, phone a hospital emergency department.

► **MEPHENYTOIN (ORAL)**
MESANTOIN

PHENYTOIN
DILANTIN

Purpose

This medicine is used to help control convulsions and seizures. It is commonly used in the treatment of epilepsy.

Allergies/Warnings

If you have ever had an allergic reaction to an anticonvulsant or seizure medicine, tell your doctor and pharmacist before you take any of this medicine.

How to Use This Medicine

Time of Administration

It is very important that you take this medicine exactly as your doctor has prescribed. Do not miss any doses and take the medicine even if you feel well. Try to take this medicine at the same time(s) every day so that you will have a constant level of medicine in your body. This is the only way that you can receive the full benefit of the medicine. If you forget to take this medicine, the amount of medicine in your blood will decrease and you may have seizures.

In adults, DILANTIN is taken in divided doses throughout the day or once daily. Be sure you know how your doctor wants you to take it.

In children, DILANTIN is given in divided doses throughout the day.

How to Administer

Take this medicine with a full glass of water.

Do not use DILANTIN CAPSULES if they have turned dark in color.

If you were prescribed DILANTIN INFATABS:

• This medicine can either be swallowed whole or chewed well before swallowing.

If you were prescribed DILANTIN SUSPENSION:

• Shake the bottle well each time before pouring so that you can measure an accurate dose.
• If a spoon is used to measure the dose, it is recommended that you use a medicine spoon or an oral liquid syringe, which you can obtain from your pharmacist. *See* Oral Liquid Syringe (page 17) and Medicine Spoon (page 22).

Special Instructions

Length of Therapy

Do not stop taking this medicine suddenly without the approval of your doctor. It usually will be necessary for your doctor to slowly reduce your dose since your body will need time to adjust. You could develop seizures if you suddenly stopped taking the medicine.

Pregnancy/Breastfeeding

Women who are pregnant or planning to become pregnant should tell their doctor before taking this medicine. There have been some reports of birth defects in infants born to women who were taking the medicine during pregnancy.

Women who are breastfeeding should tell their doctor before taking this medicine.

Drug Interactions

Do not take any other medicines without the approval of your doctor or pharmacist. This medicine can interact with several other medicines and cause serious reactions. This includes both prescription and nonprescription medicines, antacids, folic acid, vitamins, sleeping pills, tranquilizers, anticoagulants ("blood thinners"), medicine for seizures, muscle relaxants, anesthetics, medicines for depression and medicines for allergies.

Do not start taking medicines containing calcium (especially calcium supplements and antacids) or foods high in calcium without first checking with your doctor.

There have been some reports that oral contraceptives (birth control pills) may not work as well while you are taking this medicine. Unplanned pregnancies may occur. Ask your doctor about using another form of birth control or adjusting your dose of the birth control pills while you are taking this medicine. Also call your doctor if you develop spotting or breakthrough bleeding since these can be signs of decreased birth control effect.

Alcohol

Do not drink alcoholic beverages while taking this drug without the approval of your doctor because the combination could cause drowsiness or increase the frequency of your seizures. One drink may have the same effect that 2 or 3 drinks normally would have.

Special Precautions

Be sure to keep your doctor's appointments in order that your doctor can check your progress. This is especially important during the first few months of therapy, when the doctor will decide the best dose of this medicine for your condition. To make sure that your dose is correct, your doctor may wish to take a blood sample periodically to measure the amount of medicine in it.

If your doctor decides to switch you from capsules to suspension or tablets (or the other way), he or she will order a blood test to make sure you are getting the correct dose because all the different forms are not equal in strength.

This medicine may cause dizziness in some people. This side effect occurs more commonly with MEPHENYTOIN. If you become dizzy, you should be careful going up and down stairs. Sit or lie down at the first sign of dizziness. Do not drive a car, use a sewing machine, operate dangerous machinery or do jobs that require you to be alert until you know how you are going to react to the drug. Tell your doctor if you are dizzy. If this medicine is for a child, do not let him or her ride a bike, climb trees, etc. until you can determine how he or she is going to react to this medicine. Children can hurt themselves if they participate in these activities when they are dizzy.

While taking this medicine, brush your teeth and massage your gums regularly with a soft toothbrush. Also use dental floss daily. Visit your dentist regularly. The next time you visit your dentist, tell him or her that you are taking this medicine. Call your doctor if your gums become red, tender or swollen. This side effect occurs more commonly in younger patients receiving PHENYTOIN and after 2 to 3 months of therapy.

In some people, the medicine may rarely cause an increase in body and facial hair. If this becomes bothersome, tell your doctor. There are procedures that can be used to remove excessive hair.

For patients with diabetes:
- This medicine may cause your blood sugar to rise. Carefully test your blood or urine for sugar while you are taking this medicine. Call your doctor if you think your blood sugar is higher than normal or harder to control.

When to Call Your Doctor

Any medicine can sometimes cause unwanted effects. Call your doctor if you develop a sore throat, fever or mouth sores, persistent headache, severe nausea or vomiting, changes in vision, slurred speech, joint pain, swollen glands, swollen, tender or bleeding gums, increased facial hair, difficulty in walking, shakiness, easy bruising or bleeding, a yellow color to the skin or eyes, dark-colored urine, confusion or hallucinations, severe dizziness or drowsiness.

Call your doctor immediately if you develop a measles-like skin rash or any other type of rash, or if you develop continuous back-and-forth or rolling eye movements.

Call your doctor if you have an increase in the frequency of seizures.

Allergic Reactions

Call your doctor immediately if you think you may be allergic to the medicine or if you develop a skin rash, hives, itching, swelling of the face or difficulty in breathing. If you cannot reach your doctor, phone a hospital emergency department.

Refills

Do not stop taking this medicine without your doctor's approval and do not go without medicine between prescription refills. Call your pharmacist for a refill 2 or 3 days before you will run out of the medicine.

Miscellaneous

Carry an identification card in your wallet or wear a medical alert bracelet indicating that you are taking this medicine, as well as the names and phone numbers of your doctors. If you do not already carry such a card, complete the Medicine Card in this book. Always tell your dentist, pharmacist and other doctors who are treating you that you are taking this medicine.

▶ METHYLDOPA (ORAL)

ALDOMET, APO-METHYLDOPA, DOPAMET, NOVOMEDOPA, NU-MEDOPA

METHYLDOPA-CHLOROTHIAZIDE

SUPRES

METHYLDOPA-HYDROCHLOROTHIAZIDE

ALDORIL, APO-METHAZIDE, NOVODOPARIL, PMS DOPAZIDE

Purpose

This medicine is used to treat high blood pressure.

Allergies/Warnings

Be sure to tell your doctor and pharmacist if you are allergic to any medicine.

How to Use This Medicine

Time of Administration

Try to take the medicine at the same time(s) every day so that you have a constant level of the medicine in your body.

How to Administer

Take the medicine with food or a glass of water.

Special Instructions

Length of Therapy

High blood pressure (hypertension) is a long-term condition and it will probably be necessary for you to take the drug for a long time in spite of the fact that you feel better. If high blood pressure is not treated, it can lead to serious problems such as heart failure, strokes, blood vessel problems or kidney problems.

It is very important that you take this medicine as your doctor has directed and that you do not miss any doses. Otherwise, you cannot expect the drug to keep your blood pressure down.

Pregnancy/Breastfeeding

Women who are pregnant, breastfeeding or planning to become pregnant should tell their doctor before taking this medicine.

Drug Interactions

Some nonprescription drugs can aggravate your condition. Do not take any of the following without the approval of your doctor or pharmacist: cough, cold, or sinus products; asthma, allergy or hay fever products, since they could increase your blood pressure. Read the label of the product to see if there is a warning. If there is, check first with your doctor or pharmacist before using the product.

Alcohol

Do not drink alcoholic beverages while taking this drug without the approval of your doctor because the combination could make the possible side effect of dizziness worse.

Special Precautions

Drowsiness may occur during the first 2 or 3 days or after any increase in your dose, and then usually disappears. If you become dizzy or drowsy, you should not drive a car, pilot an airplane, operate dangerous machinery or do jobs that require you to be alert.

If this medicine causes dizziness or lightheadedness, you should be careful going up and down stairs and you should not change positions too rapidly. Lightheadedness is more likely to occur if you stand up suddenly—this is due to blood collecting in the legs and lasts for a few seconds. Therefore, get up from a sitting or lying position more slowly and tighten and relax your leg muscles or wiggle your toes to help promote circulation. In the morning, get out of bed slowly and dangle your feet over the edge of the bed for a few minutes before standing up. Sit or lie down at the first sign of dizziness. Tell your doctor if you have been dizzy. In order to help prevent dizziness or fainting, your doctor may also recommend that you avoid alcohol, strenuous exercise, standing for long periods of time (especially in hot weather), hot showers, hot baths, Jacuzzis or saunas.

This medicine sometimes causes nasal congestion (stuffy nose). Do not try to treat it yourself but check with your doctor.

Follow any special diet your doctor may have ordered. He or she may want you to limit the amount of salt in your diet.

Your doctor will want to do laboratory tests to check your liver function, especially during the first 2 to 3 months of treatment.

If you were prescribed ALDORIL, APO-METHAZIDE, NOVODOPARIL, PMS DOPAZIDE *or* SUPRES, *the following special instructions also apply*:

- This medicine normally causes your body to lose potassium. The body has warning signs to let you know if too much potassium is being lost. Call your doctor if you become unusually thirsty or if you develop leg cramps, unusual weakness, fatigue, vomiting, confusion or an irregular pulse. Since these symptoms may not be present in all patients, your doctor may wish to check your blood occasionally to see if it is low in potassium. Depending upon your dose, your doctor may prescribe some medicine to replace the potassium or he or she may recommend that you regularly eat foods that contain a lot of potassium (see Appendix A). *Do not change your diet unless your doctor tells you to.*
- This medicine may make some people more sensitive to sunlight and some tanning lamps. When you begin taking this medicine, try to avoid too much sun until you see how you are going to react. If your skin does become more sensitive to sunlight, tell your doctor and try not to stay in direct sunlight for extended periods of time. While in the sun, wear protective clothing and sunglasses. You may wish to ask your pharmacist about suitable sunscreen products. Call your doctor if you become sunburned.

For patients with diabetes who are taking ALDORIL, APO-METHAZIDE, NOVODOPARIL, PMS DOPAZIDE *or* SUPRES:

- This medicine may cause your blood sugar to rise. Carefully test your blood or urine for sugar while you are taking this medicine. Call your doctor if you think your blood sugar is higher than normal or harder to control.

When to Call Your Doctor

Most people experience few or no side effects from this drug. However, any medicine can sometimes cause unwanted effects. Call your doctor if you develop a skin rash, sore throat, fever, chills, fast heartbeats, chest pains or difficulty in breathing, unusual tiredness or weakness, swelling of the legs or ankles, sudden weight gain of 5 pounds (2.5 kg) or more, severe diarrhea (loose bowel movements), stomach upset, unusual bruising or bleeding, a yellow color to the skin or eyes, dark-colored urine, impotence or decreased sexual ability, depression or confusion.

If you were prescribed ALDORIL, APO-METHAZIDE, NOVODOPARIL, PMS DOPAZIDE *or* SUPRES:

- In addition to the previous symptoms, also call your doctor if you develop sharp stomach pain or sharp joint pain or yellow color to the skin or eyes. Call your doctor if you feel sick or develop persistent nausea, vomiting or diarrhea.

Refills

Do not stop taking this medicine without your doctor's approval and do not go without medicine between prescription refills. Call your pharmacist for a refill 2 or 3 days before you will run out of the medicine.

Discuss with your pharmacist the implications of dispensing all your refills for this medicine with the same manufacturer's product. (*See* Generic Drugs, page 13.)

Miscellaneous

Carry an identification card in your wallet or wear a medical alert bracelet indicating that you are taking this medicine, as well as the names and phone numbers of your doctors. If you do not already carry such a card, complete the Medicine Card in this book. Always tell your dentist, pharmacist and other doctors who are treating you that you are taking this medicine.

Child-Proof Caps

If you have difficulty opening child-proof caps and there are no children in your home, you may request a regular prescription vial cap from the pharmacist.

▶ METOCLOPRAMIDE (ORAL)
Apo-Metoclop, Emex, Maxeran, Reglan

Purpose
This medicine is used to treat certain types of stomach and intestinal disorders in which there is nausea, vomiting and a persistent feeling of fullness after eating.

Do Not Self-Treat with Baking Soda

Taking a dose of baking soda with a large quantity of liquid can be dangerous or even fatal, according to a report in *Annals of Internal Medicine.*

A healthy 31-year-old man with no history of peptic ulcers, abdominal injury or surgery felt uncomfortably full after eating a large dinner. He had run out of Alka-Seltzer (his usual remedy) and decided to use ordinary baking soda. The package label of the baking soda stated that ½ teaspoon in a glass of water was effective as an antacid to help relieve heartburn, sour stomach and/or acid indigestion. The man recalled adding the recommended dose of ½ teaspoon to ½ glass of water and quickly drinking the solution. One minute later, he developed severe abdominal pain and was rushed to the hospital. An exploratory laparotomy was done and it was found that the stomach wall had ruptured and the peritoneal cavity surrounding the stomach was filled with food.

It was felt that the baking soda when combined with water produced large quantities of gas that ruptured the stomach wall. This is very rare and it usually would take larger doses in larger quantities of water to release explosive amounts of carbon dioxide. There are five reported cases of stomach rupture due to this home remedy in the medical literature.

Baking soda is another name for sodium bicarbonate. The powder is high in sodium and should not be taken by people who are on sodium-restricted diets, e.g., patients with high blood pressure or heart conditions.

Allergies/Warnings

If you have ever had an allergic reaction to any medicine or if you have seizures or any other medical condition, tell your doctor and pharmacist before you take any of this medicine.

How to Use This Medicine

Time of Administration

Take this medicine 30 minutes *before* meals and at bedtime unless otherwise directed.

Relief of nausea should occur after the first few doses.

How to Administer

For liquid medicines:

• If a spoon is used to measure the dose, it is recommended that you use a medicine spoon or an oral liquid syringe, which you can obtain from your pharmacist. *See* Oral Liquid Syringe (page 17) and Medicine Spoon (page 22).

Special Instructions

Length of Therapy

Do not take this medicine more often or longer than recommended by your doctor. To do so may increase your chance of developing side effects.

Pregnancy/Breastfeeding

Women who are pregnant, breastfeeding or planning to become pregnant should tell their doctor before taking this medicine.

Drug Interactions

Check with your pharmacist before purchasing any pain relievers, nonprescription drugs, sleeping pills, tranquilizers, medicine for seizures, muscle relaxants, anesthetics, medicines for diarrhea, glaucoma, depression or allergies without the permission of your doctor. Combining this medicine with some of these drugs could cause significant drowsiness or dizziness.

There are other drug interactions that can occur. If you are taking any other medicines, be sure to check first with your pharmacist or doctor.

Alcohol

Do not drink alcoholic beverages while taking this drug or for a few days after stopping the drug, as it may make the drowsiness worse.

Special Precautions

If you become dizzy, you should be careful going up and down stairs. Do not drive a car, pilot an airplane, operate dangerous machinery or do jobs that require you to be alert until you know how you are going to react to the drug. Sit or lie down at the first sign of dizziness. Tell your doctor if the dizziness continues.

When to Call Your Doctor

Most people experience few or no side effects from this drug. However, any medicine can sometimes cause unwanted effects. Call your doctor immediately if you develop unusual movements of the face, tongue, hands or eyes, trembling, shuffling walk, unusual muscle stiffness, stiff neck, depression or severe drowsiness.

Allergic Reactions

Call your doctor immediately if you think you may be allergic to the medicine or if you develop a skin rash, hives, itching, swelling of the face or difficulty in breathing. If you cannot reach your doctor, phone a hospital emergency department.

Storage

Store the medicine at room temperature away from heat and light.

Some Patients Should Fly with Caution

Some patients should be evaluated carefully by their doctors before traveling by airplane. Most of the medical problems associated with air travel are due to changes in the cabin pressure, concentration of oxygen in the blood and the volume of trapped gas in the body. As the airplane cabin pressure decreases with increasing altitude, gas that is normally in the person's body expands. Normally this does not create a problem. For some people, however, the effects of air travel can be dangerous:

- If a patient has an obstructed bowel, trapped gas around the bowel obstruction can cause mild to severe pain, nausea, vomiting and potential rupturing of the bowel.

- Any patient who has recently had bowel surgery or a gall-bladder operation should not fly for at least 2 weeks after surgery or until normal bowel function has been restored.
- People with low vital capacity, heart conditions or severe anemia may not be able to tolerate the hypoxemia (low amounts of oxygen in the blood) caused by the changes in cabin pressure.
- Pneumothorax is a contraindication to flying. As the altitude of the plane increases, any gas trapped within the lung cavity will expand and press against healthy lung tissue. Similarly, patients with lung cysts should avoid high altitude flying because expansion of trapped air in the cyst could result in rupture of the cyst.
- Patients with a sinus or ear infection, nasal tumor or nasal polyps, deviated septum or eustachian tube stenosis have an increased risk of developing sinus or ear problems due to the air pressure changes. If these patients must fly, they should ask their doctor or pharmacist to recommend a nasal decongestant spray or drops that can be used before and during descent. Alternatively, an oral decongestant taken 1 hour before descent may help.
- A person with a dental abscess or a defective filling should have it repaired before flying. It is believed that expanding gas trapped in or near the defective tooth could press against a nerve.
- Patients who have had a myocardial infarction (heart attack) or stroke should not fly for at least 2 to 6 weeks.
- Patients who have severe angina at sea level may find that air travel precipitates angina attacks. In contrast, some people with asthma or chronic obstructive pulmonary disease breathe more easily during airplane travel. The cabin air is less dense than air at sea level and as a result passes more easily through the obstructed bronchial tissues.
- Scuba divers should be reminded not to fly for at least 12 hours after their last dive and 24 hours after deep or repeated dives. Caution is needed because this may bring on decompression sickness (the "bends").

If you have a medical condition and wonder whether it is safe for you to travel by airplane, check with your doctor. It is better to know how safe it is to travel *before* you are aboard the plane!

▶ METRONIDAZOLE (ORAL)

APO-METRONIDAZOLE, FLAGYL, NEO-METRIC, NOVONIDAZOL, PMS METRONIDAZOLE

Purpose

This medicine is used to treat certain types of infections.

Allergies/Warnings

Be sure to tell your doctor and pharmacist if you are allergic to any medicine.

How to Use This Medicine

Time of Administration

Take this medicine with food or a glass of milk to help prevent stomach upset. If stomach upset (nausea, vomiting, stomach pain or diarrhea) continues, call your doctor.

How to Administer

The tablets may be crushed if you cannot swallow them whole.

Special Instructions

Length of Therapy

It is very important that you take this medicine exactly as your doctor has prescribed. Do not miss any doses. Try to take this medicine at the same time(s) every day so that you will have a constant level of medicine in your body.

Take the medicine until it is finished even if you begin to feel better after a few days. If you stop taking the medicine too soon, the infection may return.

Pregnancy/Breastfeeding

This medicine should not be used during pregnancy, especially during the first 3 months of pregnancy.

Women who are pregnant, breastfeeding or planning to become pregnant should tell their doctor before taking this medicine.

Alcohol

Do not drink alcoholic beverages while taking this medicine because the combination could cause a very unpleasant reaction (headache, flushing, redness of the face or an upset stomach). Do not take cough syrups, cold preparations, elixirs or tonics that contain alcohol because they could cause the same problem.

Avoid alcohol for at least 1 day after you have finished the medicine.

Special Precautions

This medicine may cause your urine to turn red-brown or darker in color. This is not an unusual effect and will go away after you have finished taking the medicine.

If your mouth becomes dry, drink water, suck ice chips or a hard, sour candy (sugarless) or chew gum (sugarless). Sugarless products are recommended in order to avoid dental problems. You may wish to ask your pharmacist about special solutions, called artificial saliva, that can also be used to help restore moisture in the mouth. It is especially important to brush and floss your teeth regularly if you develop an unpleasant metallic taste in the mouth or if you develop a dry mouth, to help prevent gum problems.

If you are taking this medicine for trichomoniasis (a genital infection):

- Your doctor may want to treat your sexual partner at the same time. In order to help prevent the infection from spreading, it is best to avoid having sex until the infection is cured. If you do have sex, the male partner should wear a condom.
- Women taking this medicine should not douche unless their doctor tells them to do so.
- It is recommended that women not wear pantyhose or tight underwear while using this medicine. Wear cotton underwear until the infection is cured. Do not wear underwear made of silk, nylon, dacron or synthetic fabrics because these materials can cause increased sweating in the genital area, which can make it more difficult to cure the infection.

When to Call Your Doctor

Call your doctor if your symptoms do not improve within a few days or if they become worse.

Most people experience few or no side effects from this drug. However, any medicine can sometimes cause unwanted effects. Call your doctor if you develop a skin rash, hives, redness, itching, severe diarrhea (lasting more than 24 hours), a sore throat and fever, sore mouth or tongue, a white coating on the tongue, confusion, insomnia, headache, numbness or tingling in the hands or feet, trembling, seizures, dizziness or drowsiness.

Allergic Reactions

Call your doctor immediately if you think you may be allergic to the medicine or if you develop a skin rash, hives, itching, swelling of the face or difficulty in breathing. If you cannot reach your doctor, phone a hospital emergency department.

▶ **MEXILETINE (ORAL)**
MEXITIL

TOCAINIDE
TONOCARD

Purpose

This medicine is used to help regulate the heartbeat so that it is strong and steady.

Allergies/Warnings

If you have ever had an allergic reaction to any local anesthetic or any other medicine or have a history of epilepsy (seizures), tell your doctor and pharmacist before you take any of this medicine.

How to Use This Medicine

Time of Administration

It is very important that you take this medicine exactly as your doctor has prescribed. Do not miss any doses and take the medicine even if you feel well. Do not take extra doses without your doctor's approval.

Take the medicine at the same time(s) every day so that you have a constant level of the medicine in your body.

How to Administer

Take the medicine with food (*See* Special Precautions, below.)

Special Instructions

Pregnancy/Breastfeeding

Women who are pregnant or planning to become pregnant should tell their doctor before taking this medicine.

This medicine should not be used in women who are breastfeeding.

Drug Interactions

It is important that you obtain the advice of your doctor or pharmacist before taking any other prescription or nonprescription medicines that can excite the heart (including certain pain relievers, sleeping pills, tranquilizers or medicines for depression, cough/cold or sinus products, asthma or allergy products, or diet medicines).

There are other drug interactions which can occur. If you are taking any other medicines, be sure to check first with your pharmacist or doctor.

For MEXILETINE:

- Avoid large amounts of foods or drugs that can increase the acidity of the urine (e.g., cranberry juice, meats, fish, eggs, gelatin products, prunes, plums, ASA, vitamin C, etc.) or the alkalinity of the urine (e.g., citrus fruits and juices, milk and milk products, most vegetables, high doses of antacids, baking soda, etc.).

For TOCAINIDE:

- Avoid large amounts of food and drugs that increase the alkalinity of the urine (e.g., citrus fruits and juices, milk and milk products, most vegetables, high doses of antacids, baking soda, etc.).

Special Precautions

This medicine sometimes causes lightheadedness, dizziness, nausea, numbness and tremor. It may help to take the medicine with some food if these side effects occur. If food does not help, call your doctor. It may be necessary to change your dosing schedule.

Your doctor will want to do blood tests, especially during the first 6 months of treatment.

If your mouth becomes dry, drink water, suck ice chips or a hard, sour candy (sugarless) or chew gum (sugarless). Sugarless products are recommended in order to avoid dental problems. You may wish to ask your pharmacist about special solutions, called artificial saliva, that can also be used to help restore moisture in the mouth. It is especially important to brush and floss your teeth regularly if you develop a dry mouth, to help prevent gum problems.

In some people, this drug may cause dizziness, drowsiness or blurred vision. Do not drive a car, pilot an airplane, operate dangerous machinery or do jobs that require you to be alert if you are dizzy or drowsy. You should also be careful going up and down stairs. Sit or lie down at the first sign of dizziness. Tell your doctor if these problems continue.

When to Call Your Doctor

Call your doctor if you develop a sore throat, fever or chills, mouth sores, coughing, wheezing, difficulty breathing, tremors, fast heartbeats, unusual bruising or bleeding, a yellow color to the skin or eyes, confusion, depression, nightmares, hallucinations, changes in vision or hearing, fainting, unusual sweating, clamminess, muscle or joint pain, heartburn, stomach pain, neck pain, constipation, diarrhea, difficulty urinating, severe nausea, vomiting or sudden weight gain of 5 pounds (2.5 kg) or more.

The appearance of tremors, e.g., mild shaking of the hands, etc., may mean that the highest dose you can tolerate has almost been reached. Tell your doctor.

Allergic Reactions

Call your doctor immediately if you think you may be allergic to the medicine or if you develop a skin rash, hives, itching, swelling of the face or difficulty in breathing. If you cannot reach your doctor, phone a hospital emergency department.

Refills

Do not stop taking this medicine without your doctor's approval and do not go without medicine between prescription refills. Call your pharmacist for a refill 2 or 3 days before you will run out of the medicine.

Miscellaneous

Carry an identification card in your wallet or wear a medical alert bracelet indicating that you are taking this medicine, as well as the names and phone numbers of your doctors. If you do not already carry such a card, complete the Medicine Card in this book. Always tell your dentist, pharmacist and other doctors who are treating you that you are taking this medicine.

▶ **MICONAZOLE NITRATE (TOPICAL)**
MICATIN CREAM, MICATIN LOTION, MONISTAT DERM CREAM

TIOCONAZOLE
TROSYD

MICONAZOLE NITRATE (VAGINAL)
MONISTAT CREAM, MONISTAT 5 TAMPONS, MONISTAT 7 VAGINAL SUPPOSITORIES, MONISTAT 7 CREAM, MONISTAT 3 VAGINAL OVULES, MONISTAT 3 DUAL-PAK

TIOCONAZOLE
GYNO-TROSYD

Purpose
This medicine is used to treat fungal or yeast infections.

Allergies/Warnings
Be sure to tell your doctor and pharmacist if you are allergic to any medicine.

How to Use This Medicine

Time of Administration
For vaginal medicines:
- This medication is usually inserted into the vagina at bedtime to help prevent draining or leaking of the drug.

For topical creams and lotions:
- This medicine is usually applied to the skin twice daily, in the morning and evening.

How to Administer
For topical creams and lotions:
- *See* Creams, Ointments, Gels, Solutions and Lotions (page 36).

For vaginal cream:
- *See* Vaginal Creams, Ointments and Gels (page 42).

For vaginal suppositories or ovules:
- *See* Vaginal Suppositories (page 44) and read the instructions that come with the package.

For vaginal tampons:
- Insert the tampon into the applicator according to the package instructions.
- Insert the applicator containing the tampon into the vagina every day at bedtime. Leave in place overnight and remove the next morning. Repeat for 5 days.

For GYNO-TROSYD VAGINAL OINTMENT:
- This medication comes in a pre-filled applicator. Open just before administration in order to prevent contamination. Follow the directions in the package.

For MONISTAT DUAL-PAK:
- This package contains vaginal suppositories and skin cream.
- Follow the instructions that come with the package. Also *see* Vaginal Suppositories (page 44).
- The skin cream is to be applied to the genital area. Cleanse the genital area with warm water and soap. You may find it easiest to take a bath. Dry the area gently and apply a small amount of cream twice daily, unless otherwise directed. Wash your hands after applying the cream.

Special Instructions

Length of Therapy

It is important to use all of this medicine plus any refills that your doctor has recommended in spite of the fact that your symptoms seem to have improved. Do not stop using it earlier than your doctor has recommended or the infection may return.

Recurrences are common and at the first sign of any recurrence, call your doctor. It may be necessary to use this medicine long-term if you have frequent recurrent infections.

Do not use this medicine more frequently or in larger quantities than prescribed by your doctor. To be effective, the vaginal medicine must be used *daily* for the length of time prescribed by your doctor.

For GYNO-TROSYD:
- This medicine usually requires only one application to be effective.

Pregnancy/Breastfeeding

Women who are pregnant, breastfeeding or planning to become pregnant should tell their doctor before using this medicine.

Caution: During pregnancy, the vaginal applicator should be used *only* on the advice of a doctor.

Special Precautions

For treatment of vaginal conditions:

- During treatment, your doctor may recommend that you do not have sex. If you do have sex, your partner should use a condom.
- Tell your doctor if you are using a diaphragm for birth control. Some products containing this medicine have been reported to interact with certain rubber products used in some diaphragms and condoms to make them less effective.
- It is recommended that you wear a sanitary napkin to prevent staining of your clothing by medicine that leaks from the vagina.
- Use this medicine continuously—even during your menstrual period. Do not use a menstrual tampon because it may absorb some of the drug. Wear a sanitary napkin during the menstrual period.
- Do not douche while using this medication unless your doctor tells you to.
- It is recommended that women not wear pantyhose or tight underwear while using this medicine. Wear cotton underwear until the infection is cured. Do not wear underwear made of silk, nylon, dacron or synthetic fabrics because these materials can cause increased sweating in the genital area, which can make it more difficult to cure the infection. Also, your doctor may recommend tub baths twice a day for good hygiene.

When to Call Your Doctor

Call your doctor if the condition for which this drug is being used continues or becomes worse or the medication causes a constant irritation such as itching or burning that was not present before you started using it.

Most people experience few or no side effects from this drug. However, any medicine can sometimes cause unwanted effects. If you are taking this medicine for a vaginal infection, call your doctor if you develop pelvic or abdominal cramps, hives, a skin rash or increased frequency of urination (passing your water).

Storage

For vaginal suppositories:
- *See* Vaginal Suppositories (page 44).

Miscellaneous

This drug is for external use only. Do not swallow it. Keep away from the eyes.

Do You Know What These Words Mean?

In a recent study reported in the *Journal of Family Practice*, several patient brochures prepared by various health organizations and pharmaceutical companies were evaluated. Many patients did not understand a wide variety of medical terms used in the brochures.

Word	Patients who did not understand meaning
"Symptom"	22%
"Orally"	38%
"Hereditary"	44%
"Hypertension"	56%
"Stroke"	76%
"Atherosclerosis"	96%

To be able to manage your drug therapy at home, you must first understand your doctor's and pharmacist's instructions. Medical terms are a "second language" to these health professionals and it is easy for them to forget to translate these words for people who do not use them in their everyday language.

Whenever you do not understand a particular word, just ask your doctor or pharmacist to explain it. Do not be embarrassed to ask. Remember there are many other people who probably would not be able to understand the same word either. If you don't ask for clarification, there is the possibility that you could misinterpret an important instruction and suffer a serious consequence.

▶ **MISOPROSTOL**
CYTOTEC

Purpose

This medicine is used to help protect your stomach from ulcers caused by certain arthritis medicines known as Non-Steroidal Anti-Inflammatory Drugs (also called NSAID drugs). These arthritis medicines can weaken the body's protective mucous lining in the stomach and cause a stomach ulcer *that has no warning symptoms or pain.*

CYTOTEC helps prevent stomach ulcers from NSAID medicines. It does this by decreasing the amount of acids in the stomach and by strengthening the mucous layer on the inside of the stomach. It is also used to treat duodenal ulcers.

Allergies/Warnings

If you have ever had an allergic reaction to this medicine, have ever had epilepsy or a stomach ulcer, have ever had stomach upset in the past while taking arthritis medicines, or if there are other medicines that upset your stomach, tell your doctor before taking this medicine.

How to Use This Medicine

Time of Administration

Take this medicine *after* eating food or a snack. This will help prevent loose stools, diarrhea and abdominal cramping that may occur during the first few days of treatment.

Special Instructions

Length of Therapy

If you develop loose stools, diarrhea or abdominal cramping during the first few days of treatment, do not be concerned. This is an expected side effect. Keep taking the medicine and these symptoms should disappear within a few days.

Pregnancy/Breastfeeding

Women of childbearing age should not take this medicine. If you are pregnant or think you might be pregnant, do not take this medicine. This medicine can cause miscarriages. The effects of the medicine on the fetus (developing baby) are not known.

Do not become pregnant while taking this medicine. Use an effective form of birth control. If you think you have become pregnant, stop the medicine and call your doctor immediately.

It is generally not recommended that women breastfeed (nurse) their infants while taking this medicine. The medicine could cause diarrhea in the infant.

Drug Interactions

Do not take antacids that contain magnesium while you are taking this medicine. If you need an antacid, ask your pharmacist to recommend one that does not contain magnesium.

Special Instructions

When To Call Your Doctor
Call your doctor if the loose stools, diarrhea or abdominal cramping do not go away within one week or become bothersome.

Birth Control Pills Lower Vitamin B_6 and Folic Acid

Birth control pills are known to lower blood levels of certain vitamins, such as vitamin B_6 and folic acid. Usually the vitamin depletion is not serious enough to cause any symptoms, especially if the woman has a good diet. However, if a woman has a poor diet—if she eats primarily snack foods, or is always on a diet—there is a chance that she could develop a deficiency of folic acid and vitamin B_6.

It is important for any woman taking the "pill" to eat a well-balanced diet including green leafy vegetables, which are a good source of folic acid.

▶ **NICOTINE RESIN COMPLEX (SMOKING CESSATION AID)**
NICORETTE

Purpose
Nicorette is a sugar-free chewing gum which contains nicotine and is a temporary aid to help you stop smoking. The nicotine in the gum is released only during chewing. This replaces the nicotine from smoking and makes it easier to break the habit of smoking.

The gum should be used as part of a total stop-smoking program and is usually used for approximately 3 months or less.

Allergies/Warnings
Nicorette should never be used by non-smokers or children.

Tell your doctor if you have a history of stomach ulcers, heart problems, circulation problems or any other medical condition.

How to Use This Medicine

Time of Administration
Chew ONE piece of gum *slowly* whenever you have the urge to smoke.

Most people require about 10 pieces of gum each day during the first month of treatment. Never exceed 20 of the 2 mg or 10 of the 4 mg pieces of gum during one day.

As your desire to smoke disappears, gradually decrease the number of pieces of gum you chew each day. Unless your doctor tells you otherwise, do not attempt to stop chewing the gum until you are only using 1 or 2 pieces a day.

How to Administer

Chew the gum slowly and gently. As you chew the gum, nicotine is slowly released. If you chew too rapidly, the nicotine will be released too quickly and side effects similar to oversmoking can develop, e.g., nausea, vomiting, increased saliva, diarrhea, stomach upset (indigestion or heartburn), hiccups, lightheadedness, hearing and vision problems, throat irritation or convulsions.

To receive the full effect of this drug, you must alternate between chewing the gum and not chewing the gum using the following steps:

- Chew 1 piece of gum slowly for up to 30 minutes. The first few pieces should be placed in the side of your mouth and chewed slowly at a rate of 2 or 3 bites per minute.
- If Nicorette starts to taste "hot," you are releasing too much of the drug and should stop chewing.
- Start chewing again until it becomes uncomfortable, then stop again.
- Continue chewing this way for 30 minutes. After 30 minutes, most of the nicotine should be released from the gum and no warmth or tingling will occur during chewing.
- Then *throw away* this piece of gum and wait until you have an urge to smoke before using another piece of gum.
- Later in the treatment, you may be able to chew the gum a little more often. Follow your doctor's directions.
- Read carefully the patient instruction sheet that comes with this medicine. Ask your doctor or pharmacist for "How To Stop Smoking with Nicorette" by Merrell Pharmaceuticals.

Special Instructions

Length of Therapy

Do not stop taking this medicine suddenly without the approval of your doctor. The medicine must be slowly stopped over a period of 1 to 2 weeks after the smoking habit has been broken. However, the nicotine gum should be carried for up to 3 months after it has been stopped in case you have a desire to smoke.

Pregnancy/Breastfeeding

NICORETTE contains nicotine, which may cause fetal harm when administered to a pregnant woman. Do not chew NICORETTE if you are pregnant or nursing. Take precautions to avoid pregnancy while using NICORETTE, but if you suspect you are pregnant, stop the medication and tell your doctor at once.

Drug Interactions

Smoking can alter the response to some drugs, e.g.: THEOPHYLLINE, IMIPRAMINE, PENTAZOCINE, FUROSEMIDE, PROPRANOLOL, PROPOXYPHENE.

Therefore, when smoking is stopped, the response to these drugs can be changed. It is important to tell your pharmacist and doctor all the medications you are taking so that they can monitor your dose of these other medicines.

Special Precautions

You must have a sincere desire to quit smoking immediately before this medicine can be beneficial.

Carry the gum with you at all times.

Do not smoke while you are on this medicine. There could be a risk of a nicotine overdose.

Anyone needing the gum for longer than 3 months should be evaluated by his or her doctor because he or she may be using the gum as a substitute source of nicotine.

If the gum sticks to dentures, there is a possibility that it might damage the dentures. Check with your doctor or dentist.

If you swallow a piece of gum, you should not experience any adverse effects since the nicotine should not be released unless the gum is chewed. If you do develop side effects, however, call your doctor or a poison center immediately.

When to Call Your Doctor

Most people experience few or no side effects from this drug. However, any medicine can sometimes cause unwanted effects. Call your doctor if you develop mouth ulcers, heart palpitations, faintness, weakness, confusion, headaches, vision or hearing problems, convulsions, aching of teeth or jaw or problems with dentures.

Allergic Reactions

Call your doctor immediately if you think you may be allergic to the medicine or if you develop a skin rash, hives, itching, swelling of the face or difficulty in breathing. If you cannot reach your doctor, phone a hospital emergency department.

Storage

WARNING: Store this gum away from children. Nicotine is very toxic and children could be poisoned if they chewed only a few pieces of the gum.

► ## NITROFURANTOIN (ORAL)

APO-NITROFURANTOIN, MACRODANTIN, NEPHRONEX, NOVOFURAN

Purpose

This medicine is used to treat certain types of infections of the bladder and kidneys.

Your doctor has prescribed this antibiotic for your present infection only. Do not use it for other infections or give it to other people.

Allergies/Warnings

If you have ever had an allergic reaction to any other medicine, tell your doctor and pharmacist.

Do not give this medicine to infants under 1 month of age.

How to Use This Medicine

Time of Administration

It is best to take all forms of this medicine with food or a full glass of milk. This will help your body absorb the drug better and will also help to prevent stomach upset.

How to Administer

For tablets and capsules:

- Swallow the tablets and capsules whole. Do not crush, chew or break them into pieces.

For liquid medicines:

- If you were prescribed a *suspension*, shake the bottle well each time before pouring so that you can measure an accurate dose.
- If a spoon is used to measure the dose, it is recommended that you use a medicine spoon or an oral liquid syringe, which you can obtain from your pharmacist. *See* Oral Liquid Syringe (page 17) and Medicine Spoon (page 22).

Special Instructions

Length of Therapy

It is important to take all of this medicine plus any refills that your doctor told you to take. Do not stop taking this medicine earlier than your doctor has recommended even if you begin to feel better. If you stop taking the medicine too soon, the infection may return.

Pregnancy/Breastfeeding

Women who are pregnant, breastfeeding or planning to become pregnant should tell their doctor before taking this medicine.

Drug Interactions

Some antacids and other nonprescription products containing magnesium can make this medicine less effective if they are taken at the same time. Check with your pharmacist before you purchase any nonprescription drugs.

Special Precautions

Try to drink at least 6 to 8 8-oz (240 mL) glasses of water or other fluids a day, unless your doctor has otherwise directed. The extra intake of water will help to wash the bacteria causing the infection out into the urine.

In some people, this drug may cause dizziness or drowsiness. Do not drive a car, pilot an airplane, operate dangerous machinery or do jobs that require you to be alert if you are dizzy or drowsy. You should also be careful going up and down stairs. Sit or lie down at the first sign of dizziness. Tell your doctor if the dizziness or drowsiness continues.

In some people, this medicine may cause the urine to turn rust-yellow to brown in color. This is only temporary and will go away after you have finished the medicine.

When to Call Your Doctor

Call your doctor if your symptoms do not improve within a few days or if they become worse.

Most people experience few or no side effects from this drug. However, any medicine can sometimes cause unwanted effects. Call your doctor if you develop a skin rash, fever or chills, troublesome nausea or diarrhea, headache, unusual tiredness, cough, difficulty in breathing, chest pain, numbness or tingling in the mouth, face, fingers or toes, milky or foul-smelling urine, painful urination, unusually pale skin or a yellow color to the skin or eyes.

Allergic Reactions

Call your doctor immediately if you think you may be allergic to the medicine or if you develop a skin rash, hives, itching, swelling of the face or difficulty in breathing. If you cannot reach your doctor, phone a hospital emergency department.

Storage

Store the medicine in a cool, dark place and keep the bottle tightly closed. Do not refrigerate or freeze the liquid medicine.

If for some reason you cannot take all of the medicine, take the unused portion back to your pharmacist. You should discuss why you cannot finish the medicine with your pharmacist. Do not take any unused medicine after the discard (expiration) date on the bottle.

Refills

Do not go without medicine between prescription refills. Call your pharmacist for a refill 2 or 3 days before you will run out of the medicine.

▶ **NITROGLYCERIN (BUCCAL)**
NITROGARD-SR

NITROGLYCERIN (SUBLINGUAL)
NITROGLYCERIN, NITROSTAT

NITROGLYCERIN (TRANSLINGUAL)
NITROLINGUAL SPRAY

Purpose

This medicine is used to relieve and prevent the chest pains of angina attacks. It does this by easing the workload of the heart and decreasing the demand on the heart for oxygen.

Allergies/Warnings

Be sure to tell your doctor and pharmacist if you are allergic to any medicine.

How to Use This Medicine

Time of Administration

Carry this medicine with you all the time but do not carry it in a pocket close to the body because body heat can destroy the drug.

This medicine should be used at the *first* sign of an attack of angina (chest pains or tightness or squeezing in the chest). The pain may travel to the arms, shoulders, neck and lower jaw. Do not wait until the pain becomes severe. *Sit down* as soon as you feel an attack of angina coming on.

NITROGLYCERIN and NITROSTAT SUBLINGUAL TABLETS may also be used 5 to 10 minutes before exercise or activities that might cause chest pain.

How to Administer
For NITROGARD-SR:
- Do not chew, swallow, or place the tablet under the tongue.
- Place the tablet high up between the upper lip and the gum to either side of the front teeth or in the pouch between the cheek and the teeth. Denture wearers should place the tablet against the gum above the denture plate.
- To decrease the risk of tooth decay, it is important to change the sites of application and to brush your teeth after each dose. Be sure the tablet has completely dissolved before brushing.
- If you accidentally swallow a single NITROGARD-SR BUCCAL TABLET do not be too concerned. Ask your doctor or pharmacist when you should take your dose.
- A slight tingling sensation may be felt for a few minutes. This is normal.
- The tablet will soften and release the medicine until it dissolves completely. Do not be concerned if the tablet feels mushy before it dissolves. It takes about 3 to 5 hours for the tablet to dissolve.

For sublingual tablets:
- Place a tablet *under your tongue* and let it dissolve completely. If your mouth is very dry and the tablet will not dissolve, add 1 mL (a few drops) of water under your tongue. Do not swallow or chew the tablet since this drug works faster when it is absorbed through the lining of the mouth.
- Always sit down while you are taking this medicine and waiting for it to dissolve.
- Try not to swallow until the tablet is dissolved and do not rinse your mouth for a few minutes. Do not eat, drink or smoke while the tablet is dissolving.
- The medicine may cause a tingling or burning sensation in the mouth while it is dissolving. This is not harmful.

354

- This medicine usually has an effect in 1 to 5 minutes. If your angina is not relieved within 5 minutes, you may dissolve a second tablet under your tongue. If the angina continues for another 5 minutes, you may dissolve a third tablet. If 3 doses do not relieve your chest pains, call your doctor or local emergency medical service immediately or go to the nearest hospital emergency department.

For NITROLINGUAL SPRAY:
- Remove the plastic cap from the canister.
- DO NOT SHAKE canister before use because this will cause a smaller dose to be delivered.
- It is recommended that you sit down before using this medication.
- Hold the canister upright and place your forefinger on the top of the button.
- Open your mouth and bring the canister as close to the mouth as possible.
- Press the button firmly to release one spray—preferably onto or under the tongue.
- DO NOT INHALE THE SPRAY.
- Close your mouth. Try not to swallow and do not rinse your mouth for a few minutes. Do not eat, drink or smoke while the medicine is being absorbed.
- Replace the plastic cap on the canister.
- This medicine usually has an effect within 5 minutes. If your angina is not relieved within 5 minutes, you may use a second dose. If the chest pains continue, you may repeat the dose. Do not use more than 3 doses in 15 minutes. If 3 doses do not relieve your chest pains, call your doctor or local emergency medical service immediately or go to the nearest hospital emergency department.

Try to relax for 15 to 20 minutes after taking the drug, and remain calm since this will also help to relieve the attack sooner. If you become dizzy or feel faint, take slow, deep breaths and bend forward with your head between your knees. Always get up slowly after you have been sitting or lying down.

Special Instructions

Pregnancy/Breastfeeding
Women who are pregnant, breastfeeding or planning to become pregnant should tell their doctor before taking this medicine.

Drug Interactions

Some nonprescription drugs can aggravate your heart condition. Do not take any of the following without the approval of your doctor or pharmacist: cough, cold or sinus products; asthma or allergy products. Read the label of the product to see if there is a warning. If there is, check with your doctor or pharmacist before using the product.

Alcohol

Do not drink alcoholic beverages too soon after taking this medicine as the combination may cause a serious drop in blood pressure, dizziness and/or fainting.

Special Precautions

After using this medicine, you may get a headache or flushing of the face that will usually disappear within a few minutes. These are common side effects. If the headaches are severe or do not go away, tell your doctor.

Keep a supply of the medicine at your bedside in case you need it during the night. Be sure you know how to operate the spray in the dark. Tell other family members where you are keeping this medicine so that they will be able to help you.

Keep a record of the number of angina attacks and number of tablets or sprays needed to relieve the chest pain, and possible causes of the attacks. This information will help your physician give you the best treatment.

You may help prevent angina attacks by taking a tablet 5 or 10 minutes before situations you know are likely to trigger attacks, such as strenuous exercise, sexual activity, emotional stress, a heavy meal, high altitudes or exposure to cold. Let your doctor know what things usually cause your angina so that he or she can advise you about preventing attacks.

Cigarette smoking can aggravate angina and is a special risk for people who have heart conditions.

When to Call Your Doctor

Most people experience few or no side effects from this drug. However, any medicine can sometimes cause unwanted effects. Call your doctor if you develop a skin rash, fainting, blurred vision, dry mouth, nausea, vomiting or severe headaches, or if your chest pain is not relieved after you have taken the number of tablets that your doctor has prescribed.

Storage

For sublingual tablets:

This medicine must be fresh in order to work. It should be stored in the following way:

- Keep the tablets in the original *glass* container supplied by your pharmacist and keep the bottle tightly closed and away from moisture and light. This will help keep the tablets fresh. Do not put the tablets in containers made of metal, plastic or cardboard or mix the tablets with other medicines.
- Throw away the cotton that comes in the bottle and do not put labels, other drugs or any other material into the bottle.
- Carry the medicine with you *at all times* in the original glass container in a cool place, such as in a coat pocket or a purse. Do not carry the container close to your body because the body warmth may weaken the tablets.
- As soon as you remove a tablet, put the cap on the bottle tightly.
- Store unopened bottles of the medicine at room temperature away from direct heat or sunlight. Do *not* store it in the refrigerator or the bathroom medicine cabinet because the moisture in these areas could spoil the tablets. Do *not* store it in the glove compartment of your car.

For buccal tablets:

- Store the medicine in the original container supplied by your pharmacist. Keep the container tightly closed and away from moisture and light. This will help keep the tablets fresh.
- Store the medicine in a cool place.

For spray:

- Store the inhaler at room temperature. Do not place it in hot water or near radiators, stoves or other sources of heat. Do not puncture, burn or incinerate the container (even when it is empty).
- The spray is stable for 3 years.

Refills

If you use the spray, it is a good idea to have an extra canister at home in case of an emergency.

Discuss with your pharmacist the implications of dispensing all your refills for this medicine with the same manufacturer's product. (*See* Generic Drugs, page 13.)

Miscellaneous

Carry an identification card in your wallet or wear a medical alert bracelet indicating that you are taking this medicine, as well as the names and phone numbers of your doctors. If you do not already carry such a card, complete the Medicine Card in this book. Always tell your dentist, pharmacist and other doctors who are treating you that you are taking this medicine.

▶ NITROGLYCERIN (ORAL)
NITRONG-SR

Purpose

This medicine is used to help prevent angina attacks (chest pains). It does this by easing the workload of the heart and decreasing the demand on the heart for oxygen. It will not relieve an angina attack that has already started because the medicine starts to work too slowly. Therefore, it will probably also be necessary for you to have a prescription for a quick-acting medicine to treat any angina attacks.

Allergies/Warnings

If you have ever had an allergic reaction to any medicine, tell your doctor and pharmacist before you take any of this medicine.

How to Use This Medicine

Time of Administration

Take this medicine on an empty stomach at least 1 hour before (or 2 hours after) eating food.

How to Administer

Take the medicine with a glass of water.

This medicine must be swallowed whole. Do not crush, chew or break it into pieces.

Special Instructions

Length of Therapy

Do not take any more of this medicine than your doctor has prescribed and do not stop taking this medicine suddenly without the approval of your doctor. It may be necessary for your doctor to reduce your dose slowly since your body will need time to adjust. It could be harmful and could cause an angina attack if you suddenly stopped taking the medicine.

Pregnancy/Breastfeeding

Women who are pregnant, breastfeeding or planning to become pregnant should tell their doctor before taking this medicine.

Drug Interactions

Some nonprescription drugs can aggravate your heart condition. Do not take any of the following without the approval of your doctor or pharmacist: cough, cold or sinus products; asthma or allergy products. Read the label of the product to see if there is a warning. If there is, check with your doctor or pharmacist before using the product.

Alcohol

Do not drink alcoholic beverages too soon after taking this medicine as the combination may cause a serious drop in blood pressure, dizziness and/or fainting.

Special Precautions

The first few doses of this medicine may cause dizziness, headache or flushing of the face. This is normal and will usually disappear after you have taken the drug a few times. Sit or lie down until these effects pass. Take slow, deep breaths and bend forward with your head between your knees if you feel faint. Get up slowly after you have been sitting or lying down. However, if the dizziness or the headaches do not go away, tell your doctor. Your dose may have to be adjusted.

If you become dizzy, you should be careful going up and down stairs. Do not drive a car, pilot an airplane, operate dangerous machinery or do jobs that require you to be alert.

Keep a record of the number of angina attacks and possible causes of the attack. This information will help your physician give you the best treatment. Be sure to tell your doctor if you have an increase in number, length or severity of attacks.

Cigarette smoking can aggravate angina and is a special risk for people who have heart conditions.

When to Call Your Doctor

Most people experience few or no side effects from this drug. However, any medicine can sometimes cause unwanted effects. Call your doctor if you develop a skin rash, fainting, blurred vision, dry mouth, nausea, vomiting or severe headaches, or if you develop chest pains not relieved by quick-acting anti-anginal medicine.

Storage
Store in a cool, dry place but not in the refrigerator.

Refills
Do not stop taking this medicine without your doctor's approval and do not go without medicine between prescription refills. Call your pharmacist for a refill 2 or 3 days before you will run out of the medicine.

Miscellaneous
Carry an identification card in your wallet or wear a medical alert bracelet indicating that you are taking this medicine, as well as the names and phone numbers of your doctors. If you do not already carry such a card, complete the Medicine Card in this book. Always tell your dentist, pharmacist and other doctors who are treating you that you are taking this medicine.

▶ NITROGLYCERIN OINTMENT (TOPICAL)
NITRO-BID, NITROL, NITROL TSAR KIT, NITRONG

Purpose
This medicine is used to help prevent angina (chest pains). It does this by easing the workload of the heart and decreasing the demand on the heart for oxygen. It will not relieve an angina attack that has already started because the medicine starts to work too slowly. Therefore, it will probably also be necessary for you to have a prescription for a quick-acting medicine to treat any angina attacks.

Allergies/Warnings
Be sure to tell your doctor and pharmacist if you are allergic to any medicine.

How to Use This Medicine

How to Administer
For ointment:
- Remove any old ointment before applying a new dose. Dry the skin completely before applying the ointment.
- This ointment must be carefully measured using the special dose-measuring papers that come with it. Use these papers to measure the length of ointment which you are to use.

- Place the printed side down and squeeze the prescribed amount of ointment onto the paper. Use this paper to spread the ointment on the skin—*do not use your fingers* to apply the ointment.
- Apply the ointment in a thin, even layer to any convenient part of the body *except* below the knee or below the elbow. Most people apply the ointment to the chest, abdomen, front of the thighs or upper arm. Do not use it on excessively hairy areas.
- Do not use the same spot all the time but rotate to different areas. This will help prevent skin irritation.
- Apply the ointment lightly—*do not rub or massage* the ointment into the skin because this would interfere with the constant slow release of the drug. Just spread it in a thin, even layer approximately the size of the special dose-measuring papers, unless otherwise directed by your doctor.
- Once the ointment is applied, use the application paper as a cover to prevent clothes from being soiled. Hold the paper in place with adhesive tape.
- If your doctor wants you to cover the ointment with transparent kitchen (plastic) wrap or other suitable material, be sure you understand the correct method. This can be held in place with adhesive or transparent tape.

For NITROL TSAR KIT:
- This medicine comes with a bandage backing so you do not have to cover it with plastic wrap.
- Tear off one TSAR patch from the roll.
- Measure the correct dose of ointment using the special dose-measuring ruler on the TSAR patch. Do not use more than 5 cm (2 inches) of ointment on each patch.
- Carefully fold the TSAR patch in half to spread the ointment. Do not get the ointment on the outer dotted border or you will not get the full dose.
- Peel off and discard the outer dotted border.
- Apply to any non-hairy area of the body *except* below the knee or below the elbow. Most people apply the patch to the upper chest, abdomen, back or upper arm. Do not shave the area.
- Do not apply the patch over cuts, scrapes or areas with calluses or scars because this can change the absorption of the drug through the skin.
- Do not use the same spot all the time but rotate to different areas. This will help prevent skin irritation.

- Do not apply directly after showering, bathing or swimming. Wait until you are sure the skin is completely dry.
- Attach the patch to the skin and press firmly in place for 10 to 15 seconds. Run your finger along the outside edge and the center of the patch. Once the patch has been applied, do not test it by pulling on it.
- Remove and throw away the patch before applying the next dose. Discard patch in a garbage container.
- When you remove the patch from the skin, wash the area with soap and water.

Special Instructions

Length of Therapy

Do not use any more of this medicine than your doctor has prescribed and do not stop using this medicine suddenly without the approval of your doctor. It will be necessary for your doctor to reduce your dose slowly since your body will need time to adjust. It could be harmful and could cause an angina attack if you suddenly stopped using the medicine.

Pregnancy/Breastfeeding

Women who are pregnant, breastfeeding or planning to become pregnant should tell their doctor before taking this medicine.

Drug Interactions

Some nonprescription drugs can aggravate your heart condition. Do not take any of the following without the approval of your doctor or pharmacist: cough, cold or sinus products; asthma or allergy products. Read the label of the product to see if there is a warning. If there is, check with your doctor or pharmacist before using the product.

Alcohol

Do not drink alcoholic beverages too soon after taking this medicine as the combination may cause a serious drop in blood pressure, dizziness and/or fainting.

Special Precautions

The first few doses of this medicine may cause dizziness, headache or flushing of the face. This is normal and will usually disappear after you have taken the drug a few times. Sit or lie down until these effects pass. Breathe deeply and bend forward with your head between your knees if you feel faint. Get up slowly after you have been sitting or lying down. However, if the dizziness or the headaches do not go away, tell your doctor. Your dose may have to adjusted.

If you become dizzy, you should be careful going up and down stairs. Do not drive a car, pilot an airplane, operate dangerous machinery or do jobs that require you to be alert.

Keep a record of the number of angina attacks and possible causes of the attacks. This information will help your physician give you the best treatment. Be sure to tell your doctor if you have an increase in number, length or severity of attacks.

Cigarette smoking can aggravate angina and is a special risk for people who have heart conditions.

When to Call Your Doctor

Most people experience few or no side effects from this drug. However, any medicine can sometimes cause unwanted effects. Call your doctor if you develop a skin rash, fainting, blurred vision, dry mouth, nausea, vomiting or severe headaches, or if you develop chest pains not relieved by sublingual nitroglycerin.

Storage

Keep tube tightly closed. Store in a cool, dry place but not in the refrigerator.

Refills

Do not stop using this medicine without your doctor's approval and do not go without medicine between prescription refills. Call your pharmacist for a refill 2 or 3 days before you will run out of the medicine.

Discuss with your pharmacist the implications of dispensing all your refills for this medicine with the same manufacturer's product. (See Generic Drugs, page 13.)

Miscellaneous

Carry an identification card in your wallet or wear a medical alert bracelet indicating that you are taking this medicine, as well as the names and phone numbers of your doctors. If you do not already carry such a card, complete the Medicine Card in this book. Always tell your dentist, pharmacist and other doctors who are treating you that you are taking this medicine.

▶ **OMEPRAZOLE (ORAL)**
LOSEC

Purpose
This medicine is used in the treatment of certain types of stomach and duodenal ulcers and in conditions in which the stomach is producing too much acid.

Allergies/Warnings
If you have ever had an allergic reaction to any medicine, tell your doctor and pharmacist before you take any of this medicine.

How to Use This Medicine

How to Administer
This medicine should be swallowed whole with a full glass of water.

Time of Administration
This medicine may be taken without regard to meals. Take it either with food or on an empty stomach.

Special Instructions

Pregnancy/Breastfeeding
Women who are pregnant, breastfeeding or planning to become pregnant should tell their doctor before taking this medicine.

Drug Interactions
This medicine may interact with certain medicines. Do not start or stop taking any drugs without checking with your physician.

Alcohol
Do not drink alcoholic beverages while taking this medicine because it may make the ulcer pain worse and interfere with healing of the ulcer.

Special Precautions
People with ulcers should generally avoid medicines that can upset the stomach, such as ASA or salicylates, since they may interfere with the healing of the ulcer. Always read the label and check with your pharmacist if you have any questions. Also avoid those foods and beverages that cause your ulcer symptoms to reappear.

This medicine is for short-term use and should be taken only for the period of time prescribed by your physician.

When to Call Your Doctor

If you are being treated for an ulcer, call your doctor immediately if you develop fainting spells, unusual thirst, dizziness, sweating, vomiting of blood, passing of bloody or black stools or sudden increase in stomach pain. This may mean your condition is getting worse.

Most people experience few or no side effects from this drug. However, any medicine can sometimes cause unwanted side effects. Call your doctor if you develop severe nausea, diarrhea, headache, constipation or stomach upset.

Storage

This medicine is very sensitive to moisture. Keep the medicine in the original bottle and keep the bottle tightly capped in a dry place. A small packet may be inside the bottle. This helps to reduce the amount of moisture in the bottle. Do not remove the packet from the bottle.

▶ **PENICILLIN G POTASSIUM (ORAL)**
MEGACILLIN, NOVOPEN-G-500

PENICILLIN V
PEN-VEE, PVF

PENICILLIN V POTASSIUM
APO-PEN-VK, LEDERCILLIN-VK, NADOPEN-V, NOVOPEN-VK, NU-PEN-VK, PVF-K, VC-K 500, V-CILLIN K

Purpose

This medicine is an antibiotic used to treat certain types of infections.

Your doctor has prescribed this antibiotic for your present infection. Do not use it for other infections or give it to other people.

Allergies/Warnings

If you have ever had an allergic reaction to PENICILLIN, a cephalosporin or any other medicine (including ASA) or if you have any allergies (for example, asthma or hay fever), tell your doctor and pharmacist before you take any of this medicine.

How to Use This Medicine

Time of Administration

It is best to take this medicine on an empty stomach 1 hour before (or 2 hours after) meals or food unless otherwise directed by your doctor. Take it at the proper time even if you skip a meal.

Space your doses of the medicine around the clock (throughout the entire day of 24 hours). For example, if you are to take 4 doses each day, space the doses 6 hours apart. This will keep a constant level of the medicine in your body.

How to Administer

For tablets:

- Take the tablets with a full glass of water unless otherwise directed.
- If you were prescribed PENICILLIN G, do not drink acidic fruit juices, such as grapefruit juice, cranberry juice or orange juice, within 1 hour of the time you take the medicine. Acidic fruit juices may prevent the medicine from working as well as it should.

For liquid medicines:

- If you were prescribed a liquid medicine, shake the bottle well each time before pouring so that you can measure an accurate dose.
- If a spoon is used to measure the dose, it is recommended that you use a medicine spoon or an oral liquid syringe, which you can obtain from your pharmacist. *See* Oral Liquid Syringe (page 17) and Medicine Spoon (page 22).

Special Instructions

Length of Therapy

It is important to take all of this medicine plus any refills that your doctor told you to take. Do not stop taking this medicine earlier than your doctor has recommended even if you begin to feel better. If you stop taking the medicine too soon, the infection may return.

This is especially important if you are taking the medicine to cure a strep infection, because if the infection is not completely cleared up, serious problems could develop later. After treatment for a strep infection, your doctor may want to do a test to make sure that the infection is gone.

Pregnancy/Breastfeeding

Women who are pregnant or planning to become pregnant should tell their doctor before taking this medicine.

Women who are breastfeeding should tell their doctor before taking this medicine. PENICILLIN can pass into the breast milk and may cause unwanted side effects in the baby.

Drug Interactions

There have been some reports that oral contraceptives (birth control pills) may not work as well while you are taking this medicine. Unplanned pregnancies may occur. Ask your doctor about another form of birth control while you are taking this antibiotic. Also call your doctor if you develop spotting or breakthrough bleeding since these can be signs of decreased birth control effect.

Special Precautions

In some people, this medicine may cause the tongue to become dark-colored. This is only temporary and will go away after you have finished the medicine.

If you develop diarrhea, do not treat it yourself without first checking with your doctor or pharmacist.

When to Call Your Doctor

Call your doctor if your symptoms do not improve within a few days or if they become worse.

Most people experience few or no side effects from this drug. However, any medicine can sometimes cause unwanted effects. Call your doctor if you develop fever, chills, severe watery diarrhea, yellow-green stools, nausea or vomiting, abdominal or stomach cramps, bloating, unusual thirst, unusual weakness or unusual weight loss. These effects are rare and may occur even after the medicine has been stopped. Also call your doctor if you develop rectal itching or, in women, vaginal itching or a vaginal discharge that was not present before you started taking the medicine.

Allergic Reactions

Call your doctor immediately if you think you may be allergic to the medicine or if you develop a skin rash, hives, itching, swelling of the face or difficulty in breathing. If you cannot reach your doctor, phone a hospital emergency department.

Storage

If for some reason you cannot take all of the medicine, take the unused portion back to your pharmacist. You should discuss why you cannot finish the medicine with your pharmacist. Do not take any unused medicine after the discard (expiration) date on the bottle.

For liquid medicines:
- Some liquid PENICILLIN medicines must be stored in the refrigerator. Check with your pharmacist if you have any questions.

Refills

Do not go without medicine between prescription refills. Call your pharmacist for a refill 2 or 3 days before you will run out of the medicine.

Transdermal Patch Rubs Off on Baby

The parents of a 9-month-old infant took their baby into their bed one night after the child woke up with the symptoms of a cold and teething. The baby stayed in the bed for several hours until he was comforted.

When the father got up the following morning, he noticed that a transdermal patch (containing a high blood pressure medicine) that he had applied was missing. A search of the bedding, shower and floor failed to locate the missing patch and it was decided that the patch must have been lost in the clothing.

According to a report in *The New England Journal of Medicine*, the baby was unusually irritable the next morning, less active than usual and slept frequently. The baby refused to eat but drank more than three times the normal amount of fluids. His urine output was also three times normal. While he was being prepared for his evening bath, the missing high blood pressure patch was noticed on his back. The patch was folded over and less than $\frac{1}{10}$ of the surface of the patch containing the medicine was touching his skin. This means the baby received $\frac{1}{10}$ the dose of the medicine being released from the patch.

The patch was immediately removed and the child began returning to normal within 6 hours. By the next day he was back to normal despite his cold and teething symptoms.

Even though this was a freak occurrence, it does alert us to the possibility that transdermal patches can be transferred between two people sleeping in the same bed. It also alerts us to the need to discard patches in a place where children cannot retrieve them. Children are attracted to "bandages" and it is quite possible that they would play with them if they found them in a wastepaper basket.

▶ PENTOXIFYLLINE (ORAL)
TRENTAL

Purpose

This medicine is used in the treatment of intermittent claudication (a severe pain in calf muscles occurring during walking but subsiding with rest). The medicine improves blood flow to the legs and feet. It does this by making the red blood cells more flexible so that they can more easily carry oxygen to the tiny blood vessels called capillaries. This helps to reduce painful leg cramps that occur while walking and makes it possible to walk farther with fewer rests.

Allergies/Warnings

If you have ever had an allergic reaction to this medicine or caffeine, any other xanthine drugs such as THEOPHYLLINE, THEOBROMINE or AMINOPHYLLINE or any drugs used to treat asthma, tell your doctor and pharmacist before you take any of this medicine.

How to Use This Medicine

Time of Administration

Take this medicine with food or immediately after meals to help prevent stomach upset (indigestion, heartburn), dizziness and headache unless otherwise directed by your doctor.

How to Administer

Take the medicine with a full glass of water unless otherwise directed.

This medicine has a special formulation so the drug is slowly released. It must be swallowed whole. Do not crush, chew or break it into pieces.

Special Instructions

Length of Therapy

The full effect of the medicine may not be noticed immediately, but may take from 2 to 8 weeks. Be patient. Take the medicine regularly and try not to miss any doses.

Pregnancy/Breastfeeding

Women who are pregnant or planning to become pregnant should tell their doctor before taking this medicine.

Alcohol

Do not drink alcoholic beverages while taking this drug without the approval of your doctor. The combination could irritate your stomach and could cause drowsiness or dizziness. One drink may have the same effect that 2 or 3 drinks normally would have.

Special Precautions

The most common side effects are upset stomach (indigestion, heartburn), nausea, dizziness and headache. Taking the medicine with some food can usually help decrease these side effects.

If this medicine causes dizziness or lightheadedness, you should be careful going up and down stairs and you should not change positions too rapidly. Therefore, get up from a sitting or lying position more slowly and tighten and relax your leg muscles or wiggle your toes to help promote circulation. Sit or lie down at the first sign of dizziness. Do not drive a car, pilot a plane, operate dangerous machinery or do jobs that require you to be alert if you are dizzy. Tell your doctor if you have been dizzy.

It is recommended that you do not smoke while you are on this medicine because smoking can aggravate your condition.

You can monitor your own progress by keeping a daily record of how far you can walk without having to stop for a rest. This record will also be very useful to your doctor.

When to Call Your Doctor

Most people experience few or no side effects from this drug. However, any medicine can sometimes cause unwanted effects. Call your doctor if you develop vomiting, severe dizziness, severe headache, fainting, chest pains, flushing of the face, nosebleeds, flu-like symptoms, fever, fast or slow heartbeats, a yellow color to the skin or eyes, dark-colored urine or a skin rash.

Allergic Reactions

Call your doctor immediately if you think you may be allergic to the medicine or if you develop a skin rash, hives, itching, swelling of the face or difficulty in breathing. If you cannot reach your doctor, phone a hospital emergency department.

Storage

Store this medicine in a cool, dry place.

Refills

Do not stop taking this medicine without your doctor's approval and do not go without medicine between prescription refills. Call your pharmacist for a refill 2 or 3 days before you will run out of the medicine.

▶ POTASSIUM SUPPLEMENTS (ORAL)

APO-K, KALIUM DURULES, KAOCHLOR, KAOCHLOR-20 CONCENTRATE, KAON, KAY-CIEL, KCI 5%, K-DUR, K-LONG, K-LOR, K-LYTE, K-LYTE/C1, K-10, K-MED, K-MED 900, MICRO-K EXTENCAPS, MICRO-K-10 EXTENCAPS, MICRO-K LS, NEO-K, NOVOLENTE-K, POTASSIUM-ROUGIER, POTASSIUM SANDOZ, ROYCHLOR 10%, ROYCHLOR 20%, SLOW-K

Purpose

This medicine is a potassium supplement that is used by people who have certain medical conditions or who are taking prescription medicines that can cause the body to be low in potassium.

Allergies/Warnings

Be sure to tell your doctor or pharmacist if you are allergic to any medicine.

How to Use This Medicine

Time of Administration

It is very important that you take this medicine exactly as your doctor has prescribed. Do not miss any doses and take the medicine even if you feel well. Try to take this medicine at the same time(s) every day so that you will have a constant level of medicine in your body.

Do not take extra doses without your doctor's approval. This is very important if you are also taking both diuretics ("water pills") and digitalis medicines for your heart.

How to Administer

Always take this medicine immediately *after* food to help prevent stomach upset and diarrhea. Follow each dose with at least $1/2$ glass of water unless otherwise directed.

For liquid medicine:

- Mix each dose of the liquid with some water, root beer or orange juice. The amount of water, root beer, or orange juice used will depend on the brand of liquid medicine you were prescribed. Ask your pharmacist if you do not know how much water to use. Do not use tomato juice if you are on a low-salt diet.

For effervescent tablets (K-LYTE, POTASSIUM SANDOZ) *and for effervescent powders* (K-LOR, K-LYTE/C1, NEO-K EFFERVESCENT GRANULES):

- Dissolve each tablet or dose of the powder or granules in at least 1/2 glass of *cold* water or fruit juice. Let the bubbles disappear before drinking the solution. *Sip slowly* over a period of 5 to 10 minutes.

For MICRO-K LS POWDER:

- Pour contents of packet slowly into 1/2 glass of water or juice.
- Stir thoroughly for 30 seconds until slightly thickened.
- Drink immediately.

For APO-K, KALIUM DURULES, K-LONG, K-MED, NOVOLENTE-K, SLOW-K:

- This medicine must be swallowed whole. Do not crush, chew or break it into pieces and do not take chipped tablets. Swallow with plenty of water.
- Sit up or stand up when you take each dose in order to help prevent heartburn or irritation of the esophagus. It is also best to take any evening doses at least 1 hour before going to bed.

For MICRO-K EXTENCAPS, MICRO-K-10 EXTENCAPS:

- These capsules should be swallowed whole. Do not crush or chew.
- If you have difficulty swallowing the capsules, they may be opened and the contents sprinkled on a spoonful of soft food. The mouth should be rinsed well with water to remove any particles left in the mouth.

For K-DUR TABLETS:

- Take these tablets with a glass of water or other liquid.
- If you have trouble swallowing the tablets:
  - Break the tablet in half and swallow each half separately
    OR
  - Place the whole tablet in 4 oz (120 mL) of water and allow to stand for 2 to 3 minutes. After the tablet has disintegrated (broken

up) stir for 30 seconds and drink immediately. Add another small amount of water, stir and drink immediately. This will ensure that you receive the full dose of medicine.

Special Instructions

Pregnancy/Breastfeeding

Women who are pregnant, breastfeeding or planning to become pregnant should tell their doctor before taking this medicine.

Special Precautions

Do not use salt substitutes, low-salt milk or low-salt soups without the approval of your doctor. They may contain large amounts of potassium.

Do not take laxatives without the permission of your doctor. Incorrect use of laxatives could interfere with the potassium level in your body. Some laxatives contain extra potassium and other laxatives could cause your body to lose too much potassium.

When to Call Your Doctor

Most people experience few or no side effects from this drug. However, any medicine can sometimes cause unwanted effects. Call your doctor if you develop sharp stomach pain, black or bloody stools, an unusual feeling of heaviness or weakness in the legs, numbness or tingling of the hands or feet, confusion, shortness of breath, unusual nervousness or irregular heartbeats.

Eye Drop Timing

If you must use more than 1 kind of eye drop, it is best to wait about 5 minutes between the drops.

This permits the buildup of the first drug in the cornea of the eye while allowing for minimal loss through drainage into the nasolacrimal ducts in the corner of the eye.

▶ **PRAZOSIN (ORAL)**
MINIPRESS

TERAZOSIN
HYTRIN

Purpose

This medicine is used to treat high blood pressure.

Allergies/Warnings

Be sure to tell your doctor and pharmacist if you are allergic to any medicine.

How to Use This Medicine

Time of Administration

It is generally recommended that you lie down for approximately 1 to 2 hours after you take the first dose of this medicine or after the first dose of any dosage increases. The *first* dose of this medicine is generally taken at bedtime to help prevent dizziness or fainting, which may occur within 30 to 90 minutes after the first dose or any increase in the dosage. This is called the "first dose phenomenon" and is often decreased by starting with a low dose and gradually increasing it.

Check with your doctor if you do not know when to take the first dose. If you must get up during the night (especially after the first dose), get up very slowly (*see* Special Precautions, below).

Try to take the medicine at the same time(s) every day so that you have a constant level of the medicine in your body.

How to Administer

It is best to take this medicine (especially the first dose) in a sitting position with some food or immediately after meals. This will help prevent dizziness or fainting.

Special Instructions

Length of Therapy

High blood pressure (hypertension) is a long-term condition and it will probably be necessary for you to take the drug for a long time in spite of the fact that you feel better. If high blood pressure is not treated, it can lead to serious problems such as heart failure, strokes, blood vessel problems or kidney problems.

It may take 4 to 6 weeks for you to feel the full effect of this medicine. It is very important that you take this medicine as your doctor has directed and that you do not miss any doses. Otherwise, you cannot expect the drug to keep your blood pressure down.

Pregnancy/Breastfeeding

Women who are pregnant, breastfeeding or planning to become pregnant should tell their doctor before taking this medicine.

Drug Interactions

Some nonprescription drugs can aggravate your condition. Do not take any of the following without the approval of your doctor or pharmacist: cough, cold, or sinus products; asthma, allergy or hay fever products, since they could increase your blood pressure. Read the label of the product to see if there is a warning. If there is, check with your doctor or pharmacist before using the product.

Alcohol

Do not drink alcoholic beverages while taking this drug without the approval of your doctor because the combination could make the possible side effect of dizziness worse.

Special Precautions

In some people, this drug will cause dizziness, lightheadedness or drowsiness (especially during the first few days of therapy). Do not drive a car, pilot an airplane, operate dangerous machinery or do jobs that require you to be alert during the first 24 hours of using this drug, when the dose is increased or until you have taken several doses and you know how you are going to react to the drug.

If you become dizzy, you should be careful going up and down stairs and you should not change positions too rapidly. Lightheadedness is more likely to occur if you stand up suddenly—this is due to blood collecting in the legs and lasts for a few seconds. Therefore, get up from a sitting or lying position more slowly and tighten and relax your leg muscles or wiggle your toes to help promote circulation. In the morning, get out of bed slowly and dangle your feet over the edge of the bed for a few minutes before standing up. Sit or lie down at the first sign of dizziness. Tell your doctor you have been dizzy. You can help prevent dizziness or fainting by avoiding alcoholic beverages, strenuous exercise, standing for long periods of time (especially in hot weather), hot showers, hot baths, Jacuzzis or saunas.

Follow any special diet your doctor may have ordered. It may be necessary for you to limit the amount of salt in your diet.

If your mouth becomes dry, drink water, suck ice chips or a hard, sour candy (sugarless) or chew gum (sugarless). Sugarless products are recommended in order to avoid dental problems. You may wish to ask your pharmacist about special solutions, called artificial saliva, that can also be used to help restore moisture in the mouth. It is especially important to brush and floss your teeth regularly if you develop a dry mouth, to help prevent gum problems.

When to Call Your Doctor

Most people experience few or no side effects from this drug. However, any medicine can sometimes cause unwanted effects. Call your doctor if you develop a skin rash, fainting, fast heartbeats, swelling of the legs or ankles, sudden weight gain of 5 pounds (2.5 kg) or more, chest pains or difficulty in breathing, difficulty in controlling urination (passing your water) or numbness or tingling in the hands or feet.

Refills

Do not stop taking this medicine without your doctor's approval and do not go without medicine between prescription refills. Call your pharmacist for a refill 2 or 3 days before you will run out of the medicine.

Miscellaneous

Carry an identification card in your wallet or wear a medical alert bracelet indicating that you are taking this medicine, as well as the names and phone numbers of your doctors. If you do not already carry such a card, complete the Medicine Card in this book. Always tell your dentist, pharmacist and other doctors who are treating you that you are taking this medicine.

▶ PROCAINAMIDE (ORAL)

APO-PROCAINAMIDE, PROCAN SR, PRONESTYL, PRONESTYL SR

Purpose

This medicine is used to help regulate the heartbeat so that it is strong and steady.

Allergies/Warnings

If you have ever had an allergic reaction to any local anesthetic or any medicine, tell your doctor and pharmacist before you take any of this medicine.

Sit Up When Swallowing Medicines

People who are bedridden should *sit up* if at all possible to take their medicines.

British physicians have reported that esophageal ulceration occurred in a patient with no history of upper gastrointestinal disease who took a TETRACYCLINE tablet with no water and went to bed. He woke up during the night with severe pain that was later diagnosed as an ulceration of the wall of the esophagus (food pipe). This problem is also likely to occur if the person has a hiatal hernia, narrowed esophagus or reflux of stomach contents back up the esophagus.

There is less of a chance that a medicine will lodge in the esophagus and fail to pass into the stomach if the person sits up for a few minutes and takes the medicine with a full glass of water (unless the patient has been told to restrict fluids). The water will quickly carry the drug into the stomach so that it does not get stuck in the esophagus or upper stomach (heartburn area). This way gravity can also assist in transporting medications past the esophagus and the heartburn area. For this reason, it is also a good idea to take bedtime doses of a medicine 20 to 30 minutes before lying down.

How to Use This Medicine

Time of Administration

It is very important that you take this medicine exactly as your doctor has prescribed. Do not miss any doses and take the medicine even if you feel well. Do not take extra tablets or capsules without your doctor's approval.

Take the medicine at the same time(s) every day so that you have a constant level of the medicine in your body.

How to Administer

It is best to take this medicine with a glass of water on an empty stomach at least 1 hour before (or 2 hours after) eating food. Take it at the proper time even if you skip a dose. If you develop stomach upset after taking the drug, take it with some food. Call your doctor if you continue to have an upset stomach (indigestion or heartburn).

For PROCAN SR, PRONESTYL SR:

- This medicine has a special formulation so the drug is slowly released. It must be swallowed whole. Do not crush or chew it.

Special Instructions

Length of Therapy

Do not take any more of this medicine than your doctor has prescribed and do not stop taking this medicine suddenly without the approval of your doctor. It may be necessary for your doctor to slowly reduce your dose since your body may need time to adjust. It might be harmful if you suddenly stopped taking the medicine.

Pregnancy/Breastfeeding

Women who are pregnant, breastfeeding or planning to become pregnant should tell their doctor before taking this medicine.

Drug Interactions

It is important that you obtain the advice of your doctor or pharmacist before taking any other prescription or nonprescription medicines that can increase the heart rate (including pain relievers, sleeping pills, tranquilizers or medicines for depression, cough/cold or sinus products, asthma or allergy products).

There are other drug interactions which can occur. If you are taking any other medicines, be sure to check first with your pharmacist or doctor.

Special Precautions

If this medicine causes dizziness or lightheadedness, you should be careful going up and down stairs and you should not change positions too rapidly. Lightheadedness is more likely to occur if you stand up suddenly—this is due to blood collecting in the legs and lasts for a few seconds. Therefore, get up from a sitting or lying position more slowly and tighten and relax your leg muscles or wiggle your toes to help promote circulation. In the morning, get out of bed slowly and dangle your feet over the edge of the bed for a few minutes before standing up. Sit or lie down at the first sign of dizziness. Do not drive a car, pilot an airplane, operate dangerous machinery or do jobs that require you to be alert if you are dizzy. Tell your doctor if you have been dizzy.

In order to help prevent dizziness or fainting, your doctor may also recommend that you avoid strenuous exercise, standing for long periods of time (especially in hot weather), hot showers, hot baths, Jacuzzis or saunas.

If this medicine is taken for longer than 1 month, your doctor will want to do blood tests.

If you were prescribed PROCAN SR: Do not become alarmed if you notice something that looks like a tablet in your stool. This medicine is contained in a wax core that has been designed to release the drug slowly in your body. The empty wax core is eliminated in the stool.

When to Call Your Doctor

Most people experience few or no side effects from this drug. However, any medicine can sometimes cause unwanted effects. Call your doctor if you develop a sore throat, fever, chills, nausea or vomiting, mouth sores, flu-like symptoms, muscle aches and joint pains, chest pains, coughing, skin lesions, fast heartbeats, depression, confusion, unusual bruising or bleeding, unexplained weakness, fainting or a skin rash.

Allergic Reactions

Call your doctor immediately if you think you may be allergic to the medicine or if you develop a skin rash, hives, itching, swelling of the face or difficulty in breathing. If you cannot reach your doctor, phone a hospital emergency department.

Refills

Do not stop taking this medicine without your doctor's approval and do not go without medicine between prescription refills. Call your pharmacist for a refill 2 or 3 days before you will run out of the medicine.

Discuss with your pharmacist the implications of dispensing all your refills for this medicine with the same manufacturer's product. (*See* Generic Drugs, page 13.)

Miscellaneous

Carry an identification card in your wallet or wear a medical alert bracelet indicating that you are taking this medicine, as well as the names and phone numbers of your doctors. If you do not already carry such a card, complete the Medicine Card in this book. Always tell your dentist, pharmacist and other doctors who are treating you that you are taking this medicine.

▶ PROMETHAZINE (ORAL)
HISTANTIL, PHENERGAN, PMS PROMETHAZINE SYRUP

Purpose
This medicine is an antihistamine that is used to help relieve symptoms (such as itching) of certain types of allergic conditions. It is often used to treat nausea, vomiting and motion sickness. This drug has several other uses and the reason it was prescribed depends upon your condition. Check with your doctor if you do not understand why you are taking it.

Allergies/Warnings
If you have ever had an allergic reaction to any medicine or if you have asthma, glaucoma, an enlarged prostate or urinary retention (a type of bladder problem), high blood pressure or diabetes, tell your doctor and pharmacist before you take any of this medicine.

This medicine is not recommended for children less than 2 years of age.

How to Use This Medicine

Time of Administration
If you are taking this medicine to help prevent motion sickness, take it 30 minutes to 1 hour before travel and repeat if necessary according to your doctor's instructions.

How to Administer
This medicine may be taken without regard to meals. Take it either with food or on an empty stomach. If stomach upset occurs, take it with some food or a glass of milk.

If you were prescribed the syrup:
• See Oral Liquid Medicines (page 17).

Special Instructions

Length of Therapy
Do not take this medicine more often or longer than recommended by your doctor. To do so may increase your chance of developing side effects.

Pregnancy/Breastfeeding

Women who are pregnant, breastfeeding or planning to become pregnant should tell their doctor before taking this medicine.

Drug Interactions

It is important that you obtain the advice of your doctor or pharmacist before taking any other prescription or nonprescription medicines including pain relievers, sleeping pills, tranquilizers, medicine for seizures, muscle relaxants, anesthetics, medicines for depression or other medicines for allergies. Combining this medicine with some of these drugs could cause drowsiness or dizziness.

There are other drug interactions that can occur. If you are taking any other medicines, be sure to check first with your pharmacist or doctor.

Alcohol

Do not drink alcoholic beverages while taking this drug without the approval of your doctor because the combination could cause drowsiness. One drink may have the same effect that 2 or 3 drinks normally would have.

Special Precautions

In some people, this drug may initially cause dizziness or drowsiness. Do not drive a car, pilot an airplane, operate dangerous machinery or do jobs that require you to be alert until you know how you are going to react to the drug. If you become dizzy or drowsy, you should be careful going up and down stairs. Sit or lie down at the first sign of dizziness. Tell your doctor if the dizziness or drowsiness continues.

People over 65 years of age may be more sensitive to these side effects.

If your mouth becomes dry, drink water, suck ice chips or a hard, sour candy (sugarless) or chew gum (sugarless). Sugarless products are recommended in order to avoid dental problems. You may wish to ask your pharmacist about special solutions, called artificial saliva, that can also be used to help restore moisture in the mouth. It is especially important to brush and floss your teeth regularly if you develop a dry mouth, to help prevent gum problems.

This medicine may make some people more sensitive to sunlight and some tanning lamps. When you begin taking this medicine, try to avoid too much sun until you see how you are going to react. If your skin does become more sensitive to sunlight, tell your doctor and try not to stay in direct sunlight for extended periods of time. While in the sun, wear protective clothing and sunglasses. You may wish to ask your pharmacist about suitable sunscreen products. Call your doctor if you become sunburned.

When to Call Your Doctor

Most people experience few or no side effects from this drug. However, any medicine can sometimes cause unwanted effects. Call your doctor if you develop a skin rash, fast or irregular heartbeats, blurred vision, stomach pain, unexplained weakness or tiredness, unexplained sore throat, fever, mouth sores, unusual bruising or bleeding, unexplained nervousness, restlessness or irritability (especially in children), trouble sleeping or difficulty in urinating (passing your water).

▶ PROPAFENONE (ORAL)
RYTHMOL

Purpose

This medicine is used to help make the heart beat at a regular and normal rate.

Allergies/Warnings

If you have ever had an allergic reaction to any medication, tell your doctor and pharmacist before you take this medicine. Also tell your doctor if you have ever had asthma or diseases of the lungs, liver or kidneys.

How to Use This Medicine

Time of Administration

It is best to take this medication with food.

Space doses of medicine around the clock (throughout the entire day of 24 hours). For example, if you take 3 doses each day, space the doses 8 hours apart.

Special Instructions

Length of Therapy

It is very important that you take this medicine exactly as your doctor has prescribed. Do not miss any doses. Take the medicine even if you feel well.

Try to take this medicine at the same time(s) every day so that you will have a constant level of medicine in your body. Do not take extra tablets without the approval of your doctor.

Do not stop taking this medicine suddenly without the approval of your doctor. It will be necessary for your doctor to reduce your dose slowly since your body will need time to adjust. It could be harmful to you and make your condition worse if you suddenly stopped taking the medicine.

Too Much Vitamin A Can Be Harmful

Too much vitamin A can cause weakness; muscle cramps; soreness, cracking and scaling around the mouth and anus; diffuse loss of scalp hair, eyebrows and eyelashes; and unintentional weight loss.

These were the symptoms of a 41-year-old woman who had been taking high doses of vitamin A 3 months prior to being admitted to hospital. According to *The American Journal of Medicine*, the physicians calculated that she had ingested 22,190,000 International Units (IU) of vitamin A over the 3-month period. Seven months after she stopped the vitamin A supplement, her scalp hair, eyebrows and eyelashes returned and her weakness and muscle cramps disappeared.

The Canadian Council on Nutrition recommends 2,600 IU to 3,000 IU per day of vitamin A in a mixed diet for adult men and adult women who are not pregnant or breastfeeding.

Pregnancy/Breastfeeding
Women who are pregnant, breastfeeding or planning to become pregnant should tell their doctor before taking this medicine.

Drug Interactions
Some prescription drugs can interact with this medicine. Therefore, do not start or stop taking any drugs you are currently taking without first consulting your doctor or pharmacist.

Special Precautions
Any imbalance in the level of potassium in your blood may alter the effect of this drug. Your doctor may prescribe some medicine to

adjust your potassium level or recommend certain changes in your diet. Do NOT change your diet without your doctor's permission.

If this medicine causes dizziness or lightheadedness, you should be careful going up and down stairs and you should not change positions too quickly. This medicine may also cause drowsiness. Do not drive a car, pilot an airplane, operate dangerous machinery or do jobs that require you to be alert if you are dizzy or drowsy.

This medicine may cause you to become constipated. To help prevent constipation, try increasing the amount of bulk in your diet (for example, bran, fresh fruit and salads), exercising more often or drinking more fluids (unless otherwise directed). Call your doctor if constipation continues.

This medicine may cause an unusual taste in the mouth. This effect may disappear as your body adjusts to the medicine. If it continues to be a bothersome problem, inform your doctor.

If your mouth becomes dry, drink water, suck ice chips or a hard sour candy (sugarless) or chew gum (sugarless). Sugarless products are recommended in order to avoid dental problems. You may wish to ask your pharmacist about special solutions, called artificial saliva, that can also be used to help restore moisture in the mouth. To help prevent gum problems, it is especially important to brush and floss your teeth regularly if you develop a dry mouth.

Important Numbers to Keep in Your Wallet

It is wise to keep the phone numbers of your doctors, pharmacy and nearest emergency center next to the telephone *and* on a card that you can carry in your wallet or purse. This simple step will help you be better prepared if an emergency occurs or if you have a problem with your medications.

When to Call Your Doctor

Call your doctor immediately if you develop unusual bruising, bleeding, unusual tiredness, fever, sore throat, chills or any signs of an infection. Call your doctor if you develop shortness of breath, chest pain, swelling of the legs or ankles, muscle weakness, joint pain, nausea or vomiting, irregular or rapid heartbeat, tingling or numbness in the fingers or toes.

Allergic Reactions

Call your doctor immediately if you think you may be allergic to the medicine or if you develop skin rash, hives, itching, swelling of the face or difficulty in breathing. If you cannot reach your doctor, phone a hospital emergency department.

Refills

Do not stop taking this medicine without your doctor's approval and do not go without medicine between refills. Call your pharmacist for a refill 2 or 3 days before you will run out of medicine.

Miscellaneous

Carry an identification card in your wallet or wear a medical alert bracelet containing the names of your medicines and the names and phone numbers of your doctors. If you do not already carry such a card, complete the Medicine Card in this book. Always tell your dentist, pharmacist and other doctors who are treating you that you are taking this medicine.

▶ **QUINIDINE BISULFATE (ORAL)**
BIQUIN DURULES

QUINIDINE GLUCONATE
QUINAGLUTE DURA-TABS, QUINATE

QUINIDINE POLYGALACTURONATE
CARDIOQUIN

QUINIDINE SULFATE
APO-QUINIDINE, QUINIDEX EXTENTABS

Purpose

This medicine is used to help make the heart beat at a regular and normal rate.

Allergies/Warnings

Be sure to tell your doctor and pharmacist if you are allergic to any medicine.

How to Use This Medicine

Time of Administration

It is best to take this medicine with a glass of water on an empty stomach at least 1 hour before (or 2 hours after) eating food. Take it at the proper time even if you skip a meal. However, if you develop stomach upset after taking the drug, take it with some food. Call your doctor if you continue to have an upset stomach.

How to Administer

Take the medicine with a full glass of water unless otherwise directed.

If you were prescribed BIQUIN DURULES, QUINAGLUTE DURA-TABS *or* QUINIDEX EXTENTABS:

- These tablets have a special coating and must be swallowed whole. Do not crush, chew or break them into pieces. Do not take chipped tablets.

Special Instructions

Length of Therapy

It is very important that you take this medicine exactly as your doctor has prescribed. Do not miss any doses and take the medicine even if you feel well. Try to take this medicine at the same time(s) every day so that you will have a constant level of medicine in your body. Do not take extra tablets without your doctor's approval.

Pregnancy/Breastfeeding

Women who are pregnant, breastfeeding or planning to become pregnant should tell their doctor before taking this medicine.

Drug Interactions

Some nonprescription drugs can interfere with this medicine or aggravate your heart condition. Do not take any of the following without the approval of your doctor or pharmacist: antacids or baking soda; cough, cold or sinus products; asthma or allergy products.

Do not use salt substitutes without the approval of your doctor. They may contain potassium, which could affect the way you respond to this medicine.

Special Precautions

The effect of a prescribed dose of QUINIDINE varies with each person and is not entirely predictable. Therefore, your doctor may wish to do a blood test to check the level of QUINIDINE in your serum or do a heart tracing or other tests to assess the effect of the drug in your body more thoroughly.

Tell your doctor if you become dizzy or feel faint. If you become dizzy or feel faint, you should be careful going up and down stairs, getting out of bed or out of chairs. Sit or lie down at the first sign of dizziness. Do not drive a car, pilot an airplane, operate dangerous machinery or do jobs that require you to be alert.

Some foods can affect the way your body handles this medicine. Avoid eating or drinking *excessive* amounts of citrus juices, milk and vegetables. Check with your doctor if you have any questions about your diet or before you make any drastic changes in your diet.

In some people, this medicine may cause a bitter taste. This problem is only temporary.

When to Call Your Doctor

Most people experience few or no side effects from this drug. However, any medicine can sometimes cause unwanted effects and some people may be more sensitive to QUINIDINE and develop side effects after taking the first few doses. Call your doctor if you develop ringing or buzzing in the ears or any loss of hearing, blurred vision, a skin rash, unexplained fever, irregular heartbeats, dizziness or a feeling of faintness, severe headaches, nausea, vomiting, stomach cramps, troublesome diarrhea, shortness of breath, joint pain or unusual bruising or bleeding.

Allergic Reactions

Call your doctor immediately if you think you may be allergic to the medicine or if you develop a skin rash, hives, itching, swelling of the face or difficulty in breathing. If you cannot reach your doctor, phone a hospital emergency department.

Refills

Do not stop taking this medicine without your doctor's approval and do not go without medicine between refills. Call your pharmacist for a refill 2 or 3 days before you will run out of the medicine.

Discuss with your pharmacist the implications of dispensing all your refills for this medicine with the same manufacturer's product. (*See* Generic Drugs, page 13.)

Miscellaneous

Carry an identification card in your wallet or wear a medical alert bracelet indicating that you are taking this medicine, as well as the names and phone numbers of your doctors. If you do not already carry such a card, complete the Medicine Card in this book. Always tell your dentist, pharmacist and other doctors who are treating you that you are taking this medicine.

What to Do with the Cotton in Medicine Bottles

The cotton that is packed in many new bottles of nonprescription medicines and vitamins is meant to be discarded after the bottle is opened.

The cotton is inserted by the manufacturer to prevent the tablets or capsules from rattling around and breaking during shipment. After the bottle has been opened, the cotton should generally be discarded. With some prescription medications, such as certain brands of sublingual NITROGLYCERIN tablets, the cotton must be discarded to help ensure potency of the medicine. Ask your pharmacist if you have any questions.

▶ SODIUM SULFACETAMIDE (OPHTHALMIC)

AK-SULF EYE DROPS, BALSULPH, BLEPH-10 LIQUIFILM, CETAMIDE EYE OINTMENT, ISOPTO-CETAMIDE EYE DROPS, OPHTHO-SULF, SODIUM SULAMYD EYE DROPS, SODIUM SULAMYD EYE OINTMENT, SULFEX 10% EYE DROPS

Purpose

This medicine is an antibiotic used to treat certain types of eye infections. It is to be used *only* for the eye infection you have now and should not be used for any other eye infections.

Allergies/Warnings

Be sure to tell your doctor and pharmacist if you are allergic to sulfa or sulfonamide medicines or any antibiotic medicine.

How to Use This Medicine

How to Administer
For eye drops:
- *See* Eye Drops (page 24).

For eye ointment:
- *See* Eye Ointments (page 26).

Special Instructions

Length of Therapy
It is important to use all of this medicine, plus any refills that your doctor told you to use. Do not stop using it earlier than your doctor has recommended in spite of the fact that your symptoms seem to have improved. Otherwise, the infection may return.

Pregnancy/Breastfeeding
Women who are pregnant, breastfeeding or planning to become pregnant should tell their doctor before taking this medicine.

Drug Interactions
Do not use this medicine at the same time as any other eye medicine without the approval of your doctor. Some medicines cannot be mixed.

Special Precautions
Do not use eye drop solutions that have turned dark in color.

Your vision may be blurred for a few minutes after you use the eye medicine. Do not drive a car, pilot an airplane, operate dangerous machinery or do jobs that require you to be alert until your vision has cleared.

When to Call Your Doctor
Contact your doctor if the eye infection for which you are using this medicine does not begin to improve in 3 to 4 days, if increased eye redness or eye pain develops or if the eye becomes irritated by the medicine for more than a few minutes. Many eye medicines sting for a short time immediately after use.

Storage
Store this medicine in a cool place away from heat.

Miscellaneous
This medicine is for external use only. Do not swallow it.

Do not share this eye medication with family members or friends. The infection could be transferred.

▶ **SPIRONOLACTONE (ORAL)**
ALDACTONE, NOVOSPIROTON

SPIRONOLACTONE-HYDROCHLOROTHIAZIDE
ALDACTAZIDE, NOVOSPIROZINE

Purpose

This medicine is used to help the body get rid of excess fluids and to decrease swelling. The medicine does this by increasing the amount of urine and is commonly called a water pill or fluid pill. It is commonly used to treat high blood pressure and other medical conditions.

Allergies/Warnings

Be sure to tell your doctor or pharmacist if you are allergic to any medicine.

How to Use This Medicine

Time of Administration

Try to take this medicine at the same time(s) every day so that you have a constant level of the medicine in your body.

When you first start taking this medicine, you will probably urinate (pass your water) more often and in larger amounts than usual. Therefore, if you are to take 1 dose each day, take it in the morning after breakfast. Do not initially take a dose at bedtime or you may have to get up during the night to go to the bathroom.

If you are to take more than 1 dose each day, take the last dose approximately 6 hours before bedtime so that you will not have to get up during the night to go to the bathroom. This effect will usually decrease after you have taken the drug for a while.

How to Administer

Take this medicine with food, meals or milk to decrease stomach upset and increase the absorption of this medicine. If stomach upset occurs, call your doctor.

Special Instructions

Length of Therapy

For patients with high blood pressure:
- High blood pressure (hypertension) is a long-term condition and it will probably be necessary for you to take the drug for a long time

even if you feel better. If high blood pressure is not treated, it can lead to serious problems such as heart failure, strokes, blood vessel problems or kidney problems.

It is very important that you take this medicine as your doctor has directed and that you do not miss any doses. Otherwise, you cannot expect the drug to keep your blood pressure down or remove excess fluid.

Pregnancy/Breastfeeding
Women who are pregnant, breastfeeding or planning to become pregnant should tell their doctor before taking this medicine.

Drug Interactions
Do not take large doses of ASA or other salicylates without the approval of your doctor or pharmacist.

Some nonprescription drugs can aggravate high blood pressure. Do not take any of the following without the approval of your doctor or pharmacist: cough, cold or sinus products; asthma or allergy products, since they may increase your blood pressure. Read the label of the nonprescription drug product to see if there is a warning. If there is, check with your doctor or pharmacist before using the product.

Alcohol
Be careful drinking alcoholic beverages while taking this medicine because it could make the possible side effect of dizziness worse.

Special Precautions
If this medicine causes dizziness or lightheadedness, you should be careful going up and down stairs and you should not change positions too rapidly. Lightheadedness is more likely to occur if you stand up suddenly—this is due to blood collecting in the legs and lasts for a few seconds. Therefore, get up from a sitting or lying position more slowly and tighten and relax your leg muscles or wiggle your toes to help promote circulation. In the morning, get out of bed slowly and dangle your feet over the edge of the bed for a few minutes before standing up. Sit or lie down at the first sign of dizziness. Do not drive a car, pilot an airplane, operate dangerous machinery or do jobs that require you to be alert if you are dizzy. Tell your doctor if you have been dizzy.

In order to help prevent dizziness or fainting, your doctor may also recommend that you avoid strenuous exercise, standing for long periods of time (especially in hot weather), hot showers, hot baths, Jacuzzis or saunas.

People more than 65 years of age may be more sensitive to the side effect of dizziness.

This medicine does not cause your body to lose potassium as some other types of water pills do. Therefore, it is not usually necessary for you to eat foods rich in potassium. In fact, too much potassium while you are taking this medicine could be harmful. Call your doctor if you develop any of the warning signs of too much potassium: irregular heartbeats, numbness or tingling in the hands, feet or lips, confusion, difficulty breathing, unusual tiredness or weakness, unexplained nervousness, weakness or a feeling of heaviness in the legs. Since not all patients develop these symptoms, your doctor may want to check your blood occasionally to see if the potassium level is normal.

Do not use salt substitutes, low-salt milk or low-salt soups without the approval of your doctor. They may contain large amounts of potassium, which could affect the way you respond to this medicine.

If you were prescribed ALDACTAZIDE *or* NOVOSPIROZINE:
- This medicine may make some people more sensitive to sunlight and some tanning lamps. When you begin taking this medicine, try to avoid too much sun until you see how you are going to react. If your skin does become more sensitive to sunlight, tell your doctor and try not to stay in direct sunlight for extended periods of time. While in the sun, wear protective clothing and sunglasses. You may wish to ask your pharmacist about suitable sunscreen products. Call your doctor if you become sunburned.
- If you are a diabetic, this medicine may cause your blood sugar to rise. Carefully test your blood or urine for sugar while you are taking this medicine. Call your doctor if you think your blood sugar is higher than normal or harder to control.

When to Call Your Doctor

Most people experience few or no side effects from this drug. However, any medicine can sometimes cause unwanted effects. Call your doctor if you develop a sore throat, fever, skin rash, a dry mouth (or if you become very thirsty), nausea, tiredness, drowsiness, weakness, swelling of the legs or ankles, stomach pain, a sudden weight gain of 5 pounds (2.5 kg) or more, swelling or tenderness of the breasts (men or women), increased facial hair (in women) or menstrual problems (in women).

Also call your doctor if you feel sick or develop persistent vomiting or diarrhea.

If you were prescribed ALDACTAZIDE *or* NOVOSPIROZINE:
- Also call your doctor if you develop sharp joint pain, unusual bruising or bleeding, a yellow color to the skin or eyes or dark-colored urine.

Allergic Reactions
Call your doctor immediately if you think you may be allergic to the medicine or if you develop a skin rash, hives, itching, swelling of the face or difficulty in breathing. If you cannot reach your doctor, phone a hospital emergency department.

Refills
Do not stop taking this medicine without your doctor's approval and do not go without medicine between prescription refills. Call your pharmacist for a refill 2 or 3 days before you will run out of the medicine.

Discuss with your pharmacist the implications of dispensing all your refills for this medicine with the same manufacturer's product. (*See* Generic Drugs, page 13.)

What to Do if You Forget to Refill Your Prescription

It is important to tell your doctor if you did not have a prescription refilled.

If you forget or decide not to have a prescription refilled, tell your physician so that he or she can take this into consideration when planning your future treatment. If you stop taking a medication but do not tell your doctor, he or she may decide that the medication is not producing the expected effect and may switch you to another medication.

The best policy is to tell your doctor when you have not taken the medication correctly. Patients usually have good reasons for being unable to continue with a therapy, and it is important to tell your doctor your reasons. Once your doctor is aware of the problems the medication is causing, there are usually several things that can be done to help make the therapy more acceptable.

The most important thing to remember is that no medication—not even a "wonder drug"—can be effective if it is not taken correctly.

▶ **SUCRALFATE (ORAL)**
SULCRATE

Purpose
This medicine is used in the treatment and prevention of duodenal and stomach ulcers.

Allergies/Warnings
If you have ever had an allergic reaction to SUCRALFATE or any other medicine, tell your doctor and pharmacist before you take any of this medicine.

How to Use This Medicine

Time of Administration
Take this medicine with a glass of water on an empty stomach at least 1 hour before meals and at bedtime unless otherwise directed.

How to Administer
If you were prescribed liquid medicine:
- Shake the bottle well before pouring so that you can measure an accurate dose. It is recommended that you use a medicine spoon or oral liquid syringe, which you can obtain from your pharmacist.
- *See* Oral Liquid Syringe (page 17) and Medicine Spoon (page 22).

Special Instructions

Length of Therapy
It is very important that you take this medicine for the full length of treatment as your doctor has prescribed. Try not to miss any doses because the medicine will not be as effective. It may take several days or a few weeks before you feel the full benefit of this medicine.

Pregnancy/Breastfeeding
Women who are pregnant, breastfeeding or planning to become pregnant should tell their doctor before taking this medicine.

Drug Interactions
If you develop stomach pain between doses of this medicine, ask your doctor if you may take an antacid between doses. If you do take an antacid, do not take the antacid within $1/2$ hour before or

after this medicine. Taking the drugs too close together will keep the SUCRALFATE from producing as much benefit as it normally would.

If you are taking any other medicines, be sure to tell your doctor and pharmacist because this medicine can interact with certain prescription drugs. SUCRALFATE should not be taken within 2 hours of any other medicines.

Alcohol

Do not drink alcoholic beverages while taking this drug because it may make the ulcer pain worse and interfere with healing of the ulcer.

Special Precautions

People with ulcers should avoid ASA-containing medicines since they may interfere with healing of the ulcer. Also avoid those foods and beverages that cause your ulcer symptoms to reappear.

Rarely, this drug may cause dizziness or drowsiness. Do not drive a car, pilot an airplane, operate dangerous machinery or do jobs that require you to be alert until you know how you are going to react to the drug. If you become dizzy, you should be careful going up and down stairs. Sit or lie down at the first sign of dizziness. Tell your doctor if the dizziness or drowsiness continues.

This medicine may cause some people to become constipated. To help prevent constipation, try increasing the amount of bulk in your diet (for example, bran, fresh fruits and salads), exercising more often or drinking more fluids (unless otherwise directed). Call your doctor if the constipation continues.

If your mouth becomes dry, drink water, suck ice chips or a hard, sour candy (sugarless) or chew gum (sugarless). Sugarless products are recommended in order to avoid dental problems. You may wish to ask your pharmacist about special solutions, called artificial saliva, that can also be used to help restore moisture in the mouth. It is especially important to brush and floss your teeth regularly if you develop a dry mouth, to help prevent gum problems.

When to Call Your Doctor

Most people do not develop side effects from this medicine. If side effects do occur, they are usually mild and usually disappear when you stop taking the medicine.

Call your doctor immediately if you are being treated for an ulcer and you develop fainting spells, unusual thirst, dizziness, sweating, vomiting of blood or bloody or black stools. This may mean your condition is getting worse.

Allergic Reactions

Most people experience few or no side effects from this drug. However, any medicine can sometimes cause unwanted effects. Call your doctor if you develop a skin rash, hives, itching, back pain, stomach pain or severe constipation.

Do Not Share Medicines

Even though two drugs may look alike, this does not mean that they are the same. NEVER SHARE YOUR MEDICINES.

Even if a friend takes the same drugs as you, the drug could be a different strength and serious problems could result if your friend took one of your medicines.

▶ **SULFADIAZINE-TRIMETHOPRIM (ORAL)**
COPTIN

SULFAMETHOXAZOLE
APO-SULFAMETHOXAZOLE, GANTANOL

SULFAMETHOXAZOLE-TRIMETHOPRIM
APO-SULFATRIM, APO-SULFATRIM DS, APO-SULFATRIM PEDIATRIC, BACTRIM, BACTRIM DS, NOVOTRIMEL, NOVOTRIMEL DS, PROTRIN, PROTRIN DF, ROUBAC, SEPTRA, SEPTRA DS

SULFAPYRIDINE
DAGENAN

SULFISOXAZOLE
NOVOSOXAZOLE

SULFONAMIDE-PHENAZOPYRIDINE PREPARATIONS
AZO-GANTRISIN, URO GANTANOL

Purpose

This medicine is an anti-infective used to treat certain types of infections.

Allergies/Warnings

If you have ever had an allergic reaction to sulfa drugs, thiazide diuretics (water pills), diabetes medicine that you take by mouth or glaucoma medicine that you take by mouth, tell your doctor and pharmacist before you take any of this medicine.

This medicine should *not* be given to infants under 2 months of age.

How to Use This Medicine

Time of Administration

It is best (but not necessary) to take this medicine on an empty stomach 1 hour before (or 2 hours after) eating food, unless otherwise directed. Take the medicine at the proper time even if you skip a meal. If stomach upset occurs, call your doctor.

Space your doses of the medicine around the clock (throughout the entire day of 24 hours). For example, if you are to take 4 doses each day, space the doses 6 hours apart. This will keep a constant level of the medicine in your body.

How to Administer

Take this medicine with a full glass (8 oz or 240 mL) of water and try to drink at least 6 to 8 additional glasses of water or other liquids every day unless otherwise directed by your doctor. This will help prevent unwanted side effects on the kidneys and, if the medicine was prescribed to treat an infection of the bladder, the extra intake of water will help to wash the bacteria causing the infection out in the urine.

For tablets and capsules:
• Take the medicine with a full glass of water unless otherwise directed.

For liquid medicines:
• If you were prescribed a *suspension*, shake the bottle well each time before pouring so that you can measure an accurate dose.
• If a spoon is used to measure the dose, it is recommended that you use a medicine spoon or an oral liquid syringe, which you can obtain from your pharmacist. *See* Oral Liquid Syringe (page 17) and Medicine Spoon (page 22).

Special Instructions

Length of Therapy

It is important to take all of this medicine plus any refills that your doctor told you to take. Do not stop taking this medicine earlier than your doctor has recommended even if you begin to feel better. If you stop taking the medicine too soon, the infection may return.

Pregnancy/Breastfeeding

Women who are pregnant or planning to become pregnant should tell their doctor before taking this medicine. This medicine should generally not be taken during the last month of pregnancy.

Women who are breastfeeding should tell their doctor before taking this medicine.

Special Precautions

This medicine may make some people more sensitive to sunlight and some tanning lamps. When you begin taking this medicine, try to avoid too much sun until you see how you are going to react. If your skin does become more sensitive to sunlight, tell your doctor and try not to stay in direct sunlight for extended periods of time. While in the sun, wear protective clothing and sunglasses. You may wish to ask your pharmacist about suitable sunscreen products. Call your doctor if you become sunburned.

If you become dizzy, you should be careful going up and down stairs. Sit or lie down at the first sign of dizziness. Do not drive a car, pilot an airplane, operate dangerous machinery or do jobs that require you to be alert until you know how you are going to react to the drug. Tell your doctor if the dizziness continues.

If you were prescribed AZO-GANTRISIN or URO GANTANOL:

• Your urine may turn orange-red in color. This is a temporary effect and will go away after you have finished the medicine. Protect your undergarments while you are taking this medicine as your urine could cause staining of clothing.

When to Call Your Doctor

Call your doctor if your symptoms do not improve within a few days or if they become worse.

Most people experience few or no side effects from this drug. However, any medicine can sometimes cause unwanted effects. Call your doctor if you develop a sore throat, fever, mouth sores, nausea or vomiting, unusually pale skin, unusual bruising or bleeding, swelling of the front part of the neck, difficulty in swallowing, unusual tiredness or weakness, unusual joint or lower back pain, blood in the urine, pain while urinating (passing your water), redness, blistering, peeling or loosening of the skin or a yellow color to the skin or eyes.

Allergic Reactions

Call your doctor immediately if you think you may be allergic to the medicine or if you develop a skin rash, hives, itching, swelling of the face or difficulty in breathing. If you cannot reach your doctor, phone a hospital emergency department.

Storage

Store the medicine in a cool, dark place and keep the bottle tightly closed. Do not freeze the liquid preparation.

If for some reason you cannot take all of the medicine, take the unused portion back to your pharmacist. You should discuss why you cannot finish the medicine with your pharmacist. Do not take any unused medicine after the discard (expiration) date on the bottle.

Refills

Do not go without medicine between prescription refills. Call your pharmacist for a refill 2 or 3 days before you will run out of the medicine.

▶ SULFASALAZINE (ORAL)

PMS SULFASALAZINE, PMS SULFASALAZINE E.C., SALAZOPYRIN, SALAZOPYRIN EN-TABS, S.A.S.-500, S.A.S. ENTERIC-500

Purpose

This medicine is used to treat certain conditions of the intestines such as ulcerative colitis and Crohn's disease.

SALAZOPYRIN EN-TABS are also used to treat rheumatoid arthritis.

Allergies/Warnings

If you have ever had an allergic reaction to sulfa drugs, salicylates or ASA, thiazide water pills, diabetes medicine that you take by mouth or glaucoma medicine that you take by mouth, tell your doctor and pharmacist before you take any of this medicine. Also tell your doctor if you have a condition known as porphyria or any other medical problems.

This medicine should *not* be given to children under 2 years of age.

Expensive Drug Interactions

A 32-year-old woman who wore a gas-permeable (hard) contact lens in one eye and a soft contact lens in the other eye developed an acute attack of colitis. She was treated with SULFASALAZINE. During the first 2 days of drug therapy, she did not wear the contact lenses. On the third day she started wearing the lenses again, and within 12 hours, the soft contact lens became stained a yellow color and the blue color of the iris in the eye appeared green when the lens was in place. The hard lens was not stained and the iris was normal blue in color.

SULFASALAZINE predictably stains the urine an orange color and has also been reported to color tears yellow to orange. The staining of the soft contact lens in this patient was attributed to the ability of the drug to stain tears, which in turn stained the lens.

This was an expensive drug interaction since extended-wear contact lenses cost approximately $250.

Other drugs which have been reported to discolor soft contact lenses are RIFAMPIN (orange staining), EPINEPHRINE HYDROCHLORIDE 2% and EPINEPHRYL BORATE 1% (dense brown staining). During treatment with any of these medicines, soft contact lenses should not be worn. Most eye drops are labeled to indicate whether they can be used with soft contact lenses, but it is always a good idea to check with the pharmacist before using any eye drops if soft contact lenses are worn.

How to Use This Medicine

Time of Administration

Space your doses of the medicine around the clock (throughout the entire day of 24 hours). For example, if you are to take 4 doses each day, space the doses 6 hours apart. This will keep a constant level of the medicine in your body.

The interval between the nighttime dose and the next morning dose should generally not be greater than 8 hours unless otherwise directed by your doctor.

How to Administer

It is best to take this medicine with food or immediately after meals to help prevent stomach upset. Call your doctor if you continue to have stomach upset.

Take each dose of medicine with a full glass (8 oz or 240 mL) of water and try to drink 8 glasses of water or other fluids every day unless otherwise directed by your doctor. This will help prevent some unwanted side effects.

For PMS SULFASALAZINE E.C., SALAZOPYRIN EN-TABS, S.A.S. ENTERIC-500, SULFASALAZINE (Kenral):

- These tablets have a special coating and must be swallowed whole. Do not crush, chew or break them into pieces. Do not take chipped tablets.

Special Instructions

Length of Therapy

It is important to take all of this medicine plus any refills that your doctor told you to take. Do not stop taking this medicine earlier than your doctor has recommended even if you begin to feel better. Otherwise, you cannot expect the drug to work for you.

Pregnancy/Breastfeeding

Women who are pregnant or planning to become pregnant should tell their doctor before taking this medicine.

Women who are breastfeeding should tell their doctor before taking this medicine. This medicine can pass into the breast milk.

Special Precautions

Be sure to keep your doctor's appointments so that he or she can check your progress and make sure that you are getting the most benefit from this medicine.

This medicine may make some people more sensitive to sunlight and some tanning lamps. When you begin taking this medicine, try to avoid too much sun until you see how you are going to react. If your skin does become more sensitive to sunlight, tell your doctor and try not to stay in direct sunlight for extended periods of time. While in the sun, wear protective clothing and sunglasses. You may wish to ask your pharmacist about suitable sunscreen products. Call your doctor if you become sunburned.

In some people, this drug may cause dizziness or drowsiness. Do not drive a car, pilot an airplane, operate dangerous machinery or do jobs that require you to be alert until you know how you are going to react to this drug. You should also be careful going up and down stairs. Sit or lie down at the first sign of dizziness. Tell your doctor if the dizziness continues.

This medicine may cause the urine to turn orange-yellow in color. This is not an unusual effect and is not harmful. It will go away after you have finished the medicine.

This medicine has also been reported to stain soft contact lenses yellow. (*See* Expensive Drug Interactions, page 400.)

When to Call Your Doctor

Call your doctor if your symptoms (including diarrhea) do not improve within 1 month or if they become worse.

Most people experience few or no side effects from this drug. However, any medicine can sometimes cause unwanted effects. Call your doctor if you develop a sore throat, fever, mouth sores, unusual bruising or bleeding, skin blisters or peeling or loosening of the skin, a yellow color to the skin and eyes, unusual tiredness or weakness, constant headache, unusual joint or low back pain, pain while urinating (passing your water), blood in the urine, difficulty swallowing, swelling of the throat or neck, itching or unusually pale skin.

Allergic Reactions

Call your doctor immediately if you think you may be allergic to the medicine or if you develop a skin rash, hives, itching, swelling of the face or difficulty in breathing. If you cannot reach your doctor, phone a hospital emergency department.

Storage

If for some reason you cannot take all of the medicine, take the unused portion back to your pharmacist. You should discuss why you cannot finish the medicine with your pharmacist. Do not take any unused medicine after the discard (expiration) date on the bottle.

Miscellaneous

Carry an identification card in your wallet or wear a medical alert bracelet indicating that you are taking this medicine, as well as the names and phone numbers of your doctors. If you do not already carry such a card, complete the Medicine Card in this book. Always tell your dentist, pharmacist and other doctors who are treating you that you are taking this medicine.

Bacteria on Toothbrushes

Medical World News reports that lingering throat and mouth infections may be aggravated by the transfer of the bacteria to toothbrushes and subsequent multiplication of the bacteria.

A professor of oral pathology compared the toothbrushes of 10 healthy people and 10 people with mouth and throat infections. He discovered that it takes only 17 to 35 days for a toothbrush to become heavily infected. This is not surprising since bacteria in toothbrushes find moisture, warmth (from a warm bathroom) and food (from the mouth) to grow.

When the oral pathologist suggested that those people with mouth and throat infections start using new toothbrushes every few weeks, they quickly recovered. It may be advisable for people with mouth infections to change their toothbrushes frequently. Depending on the toothbrush, it may be possible to thoroughly clean toothbrushes frequently by putting them through a dishwasher cycle and allowing them to dry completely.

▶ TETRACYCLINE HCl (ORAL)
ACHROMYCIN V, APO-TETRA, NOVOTETRA, NU-TETRA, TETRACYN

Purpose
This medicine is an antibiotic used to treat certain types of infections and help control acne.

Your doctor has prescribed this antibiotic for your present infection only. Do not use it for other infections or give it to other people.

Allergies/Warnings
If you have ever had an allergic reaction to TETRACYCLINE or any other medicine or if you have any allergies (for example, asthma, hay fever or hives), tell your doctor or pharmacist before you take any of this medicine.

This medicine should not be given to children under 12 years of age unless directed by your doctor. TETRACYCLINE may permanently discolor the child's teeth and slow down the growth of the teeth and bones.

How to Use This Medicine

Time of Administration

It is best to take this medicine on an empty stomach 1 hour before (or 2 hours after) meals or food unless otherwise directed. Take the medicine at the proper time even if you skip a meal.

If you develop stomach upset after taking the drug, take it with some crackers (not with dairy products). Call your doctor if you continue to have stomach upset.

Space your doses of the medicine around the clock (throughout the entire day of 24 hours). For example, if you are to take 4 doses each day, space the doses 6 hours apart. This will keep a constant level of the medicine in your body.

How to Administer

For capsules:

- Take the capsules with a full glass (8 oz or 240 mL) of water. This will help prevent irritation of the stomach and esophagus.

For liquid medicines:

- If you were prescribed a *suspension*, shake the bottle well each time before pouring so that you can measure an accurate dose.
- If a spoon is used to measure the dose, it is recommended that you use a medicine spoon or an oral liquid syringe, which you can obtain from your pharmacist. *See* Oral Liquid Syringe (page 17) and Medicine Spoon (page 22).

Do not drink milk or eat cheese, cottage cheese, ice cream or other dairy products 1 hour before or 2 hours after you have taken a dose of this medicine. If taken too close to this medicine, these foods can interfere with the absorption of the medicine and make it less effective.

Special Instructions

Length of Therapy

It is important to take all of this medicine plus any refills that your doctor told you to take. Do not stop taking this medicine earlier than your doctor has recommended even if you begin to feel better. If you stop taking the medicine too soon, the infection may return.

Pregnancy/Breastfeeding

Women who are pregnant or planning to become pregnant should not take this medicine. This medicine could cause permanent discoloration of the infant's teeth and may slow down the normal growth and development of the infant's teeth and bones.

Women who are breastfeeding should tell their doctor before taking this medicine. This medicine may pass into the breast milk and cause discoloration of the infant's teeth and may slow down the normal growth and development of the infant's teeth and bones.

Drug Interactions

Some antacids and laxatives can make this medicine less effective if they are taken at the same time. This includes products that contain aluminum, bismuth, calcium, magnesium, Epsom salt or sodium bicarbonate (baking soda). Check with your pharmacist before you purchase any antacids or laxatives. If you must take certain antacids or laxatives, they should be taken at least 2 hours before or after this medicine.

Iron or zinc pills or vitamins containing minerals can also make this medicine less effective. If you must take iron, zinc or vitamins containing minerals, take them 3 hours before (or 2 hours after) the TETRACYCLINE.

There have been some reports that oral contraceptives (birth control pills) may not work as well while you are taking this medicine. Unplanned pregnancies may occur. Ask your doctor about using another form of birth control while you are taking this antibiotic. Also call your doctor if you develop spotting or breakthrough bleeding since these can be signs of decreased birth control effect.

Special Precautions

This medicine may make some people more sensitive to sunlight and some tanning lamps. When you begin taking this medicine, try to avoid too much sun until you see how you are going to react. If your skin does become more sensitive to sunlight, tell your doctor and try not to stay in direct sunlight for extended periods of time. While in the sun, wear protective clothing and sunglasses. You may wish to ask your pharmacist about suitable sunscreen products. Call your doctor if you become sunburned.

When to Call Your Doctor

Call your doctor if your symptoms do not improve within a few days (or a few weeks or months if you are taking the medicine for acne) or if they become worse.

Most people experience few or no side effects from this drug. However, any medicine can sometimes cause unwanted effects. Call your doctor immediately if you develop severe cramps or burning of the stomach, vomiting, severe watery diarrhea, skin rash, dark-colored tongue, sore mouth or tongue, itching of the rectal or genital areas or, in women, a vaginal discharge that was not present before you started the medicine.

Allergic Reactions

Call your doctor immediately if you think you may be allergic to the medicine or if you develop a skin rash, hives, itching, swelling of the face or difficulty in breathing. If you cannot reach your doctor, phone a hospital emergency department.

Drug Affects Bones and Teeth

TETRACYCLINES should not be taken by pregnant women, infants or children up to 12 years of age.

TETRACYCLINES can stain the teeth of the child if they are given during the time that the baby teeth or permanent teeth are forming. The drugs combine with calcium in the teeth and stain the dentin (the part of the tooth that lies directly beneath the white enamel). The stained dentin shows through the white enamel of the tooth and gives a yellow-gray appearance to the tooth.

If a TETRACYCLINE drug is given to a woman during the last 3 months of pregnancy or to a baby during the first 3 months of life, staining of the teeth can occur.

If a TETRACYCLINE drug is given to a child between the ages of 3 months and 8 years, staining of the permanent teeth can occur. The severity of the stain appears to depend on the dose of the antibiotic and the stage of tooth development.

At the present time, there is no treatment which will remove the stain permanently. Some dentists have reported limited success with bleaching techniques and others have placed artificial crowns or plastic materials over the teeth.

The best treatment is prevention.

Storage

Store the tablets and capsules in a cool, dark place and keep the bottle tightly closed. Do not freeze the liquid preparation.

If for some reason you cannot take all of the medicine, take the unused portion back to your pharmacist. You should discuss why you cannot finish the medicine with your pharmacist. Do not take any unused medicine after the discard (expiration) date on the bottle. Outdated TETRACYCLINE can cause serious problems.

Refills

Do not go without medicine between prescription refills. Call your pharmacist for a refill 2 or 3 days before you will run out of the medicine.

▶ **TRETINOIN (TOPICAL)**
RETIN-A, STIEVA-A, STIEVA-A FORTE, VITAMIN A ACID

Purpose

This medicine is used to treat mild to moderate acne. Its use is presently being investigated in the treatment of sun-damaged skin.

Allergies/Warnings

Tell your doctor and pharmacist if you are allergic to TRETINOIN or any vitamin A medicine.

How to Use This Medicine

Time of Administration

The medicine is usually applied once a day before going to bed.

How to Administer

For cream and gel:
- Each time you apply the medicine, wash your hands and gently cleanse the skin area well with a mild soap and water unless otherwise directed by your doctor. Pat the skin gently with a clean towel until dry. *Wait about 20 to 30 minutes to be sure that the skin is completely dry.*
- Apply a small amount of the drug to the area under treatment and gently massage into the skin. Only the medicine that is actually touching the skin will work. A thick layer is not more effective than

a thin layer. Do not bandage unless directed by your doctor. After applying this medication, you may notice a slight stinging sensation or feeling of warmth. This is normal.

- Do not use the drug more frequently or in larger quantities than prescribed by your doctor. Overuse of this medicine may cause increased skin irritation and bleeding.
- Wash your hands thoroughly after applying the cream or gel.

For solution:

- Cleanse the skin area well with water unless otherwise directed. Pat the skin with a clean towel until the skin is completely dry. *Wait about 20 to 30 minutes to be sure that the skin is completely dry.*
- Apply the solution using the applicator that comes with the bottle. After applying this medication to the area under treatment, you may notice a slight stinging sensation or feeling of warmth. This is normal.
- Do not use the drug more frequently or in larger quantities than prescribed by your doctor. Overuse of this medicine may cause increased skin irritation and bleeding.
- Wash your hands thoroughly if you applied the solution with your fingertips.

Special Instructions

Length of Therapy

It may take up to 6 to 10 weeks before you receive the full benefit of this medicine.

For Those with Glaucoma, Timing Is Everything

The absorption of TIMOLOL eye drops, a medication prescribed for treating glaucoma, is greatly affected by the time of day it is used.

A recent study found that twice as much TIMOLOL is absorbed when administered at noon as when administered at 6:00 A.M. This is good news because proper timing may not only improve the drug's effectiveness, but make it possible for doctors to prescribe a lower dosage. With a lower dose, patients may have a lower risk of developing side effects.

The reason for this link between the time of administration and the effectiveness of the medicine is still unknown.

Pregnancy/Breastfeeding

Women who are pregnant, breastfeeding or planning to become pregnant should tell their doctor before using this medicine.

Drug Interactions

Do not use this medicine at the same time as any other acne product, or any product that is abrasive, causes peeling of the skin or contains alcohol, unless directed by your doctor. Examples of such products include abrasive soaps and cleansers, soaps and cosmetics that are drying, astringents or products with spices or lime in them.

Usually it is all right to continue using cosmetics (as long as they are not too drying), but it is a good idea to check with your doctor first. Some cosmetics can be extremely drying and this could cause problems. Always remove cosmetics before a new dose of the medicine is applied.

Special Precautions

While you are using this medicine, your skin may become more sensitive to sunlight. Do not use sunlamps, and wear protective clothing. Check with your doctor if you must work outside in the sunlight. It may be wise to use sunscreens with an SPF of 15 or higher. Also call your doctor if you get sunburned.

When you apply this medicine, you may have a mild stinging sensation or redness. This is not unusual. At first, your acne may even seem to get worse. This is due to the effect of the medicine on deep acne lesions that could not be seen previously. After a few days, you can expect some peeling to occur.

Your skin may become more sensitive to wind or cold temperatures. Dress warmly.

Do not apply this medicine to chapped, windburned or sunburned skin or to open cuts or wounds.

Keep this preparation away from the eyes, eyelids, mouth and inside of the nose. If you should accidentally get some in your eyes, wash it away with water immediately.

When to Call Your Doctor

Call your doctor if the condition for which you are using this medicine becomes worse or if the medicine causes itching or severe burning or redness for more than a few minutes after application. When you first start using the medicine, be prepared for some redness, dryness and scaling of the skin at the place the medicine was applied.

Also call your doctor if you develop blistering or crusting, swelling of the skin or darkening or lightening of treated areas.

Miscellaneous
This medicine is for external use only. Do not swallow it.

▶ **TRIAMTERENE (ORAL)**
DYRENIUM

TRIAMTERENE-HYDROCHLOROTHIAZIDE
APO-TRIAZIDE, DYAZIDE, NOVOTRIAMZIDE

Purpose
This medicine is used to help the body get rid of excess fluids and to decrease swelling. The medicine does this by increasing the amount of urine and is commonly called a *water pill* or *fluid pill*. It is commonly used to treat high blood pressure and other medical conditions.

Allergies/Warnings
Be sure to tell your doctor or pharmacist if you are allergic to any medicine.

How to Use This Medicine

Time of Administration
Try to take this medicine at the same time(s) every day so that you have a constant level of the medicine in your body.

When you first start taking this medicine, you will probably urinate (pass your water) more often and in larger amounts than usual. Therefore, if you are to take 1 dose each day, take it in the morning after breakfast. Do not initially take a dose at bedtime or you may have to get up during the night to go to the bathroom.

If you are to take more than 1 dose each day, take the last dose approximately 6 hours before bedtime so that you will not have to get up during the night to go to the bathroom. This effect will usually decrease after you have taken the drug for a while.

How to Administer
Take this medicine with food, meals or milk if it upsets your stomach. If stomach upset continues, call your doctor.

Special Instructions

Length of Therapy

For patients with high blood pressure:

- High blood pressure (hypertension) is a long-term condition and it will probably be necessary for you to take the drug for a long time even if you feel better. If high blood pressure is not treated, it can lead to serious problems such as heart failure, strokes, blood vessel problems or kidney problems.

It is very important that you take this medicine as your doctor has directed and that you do not miss any doses. Otherwise, you cannot expect the drug to keep your blood pressure down or remove excess fluid.

Pregnancy/Breastfeeding

Women who are pregnant or planning to become pregnant should tell their doctor before taking this medicine.

This medicine can pass into the breast milk and women should not breastfeed while they are on this drug.

Drug Interactions

Some nonprescription drugs can aggravate high blood pressure. Do not take any of the following without the approval of your doctor or pharmacist: cough, cold, or sinus products; asthma or allergy products, since they may increase your blood pressure. Read the label of the nonprescription drug product to see if there is a warning. If there is, check with your doctor or pharmacist before using the product.

Alcohol

Be careful drinking alcoholic beverages while taking this medicine because it could make the possible side effect of dizziness worse.

Special Precautions

If this medicine causes dizziness or lightheadedness, you should be careful going up and down stairs and you should not change positions too rapidly. Lightheadedness is more likely to occur if you stand up suddenly—this is due to blood collecting in the legs and lasts for a few seconds. Therefore, get up from a sitting or lying position more slowly and tighten and relax your leg muscles or wiggle your toes to help promote circulation. In the morning, get out of bed slowly and dangle your feet over the edge of the bed for a few minutes before standing up. Sit or lie down at the first sign of dizziness. Do not drive a car, pilot an airplane, operate dangerous machinery or do jobs that require you to be alert if you are dizzy. Tell your doctor if you have been dizzy.

In order to help prevent dizziness or fainting, your doctor may also recommend that you avoid strenuous exercise, standing for long periods of time (especially in hot weather), hot showers, hot baths, Jacuzzis or saunas. People more than 65 years of age may be more sensitive to the side effect of dizziness.

This medicine does not cause your body to lose potassium as some other types of water pills do. Therefore, it is not usually necessary for you to eat foods rich in potassium. In fact, too much potassium while you are taking this medicine could be harmful. Call your doctor if you develop any of the warning signs of too much potassium: irregular heartbeats, numbness or tingling in the hands, feet or lips, confusion, difficulty breathing, unusual tiredness or weakness, unexplained nervousness, weakness or a feeling of heaviness in the legs. Since not all patients develop these symptoms, your doctor may want to check your blood occasionally to see if the potassium level is normal.

Do not use salt substitutes, low-salt milk or low-salt soups without the approval of your doctor. They may contain large amounts of potassium, which could affect the way you respond to this medicine.

This medicine may make some people more sensitive to sunlight and some tanning lamps. When you begin taking this medicine, try to avoid too much sun until you see how you are going to react. If your skin does become more sensitive to sunlight, tell your doctor and try not to stay in direct sunlight for extended periods of time. While in the sun, wear protective clothing and sunglasses. You may wish to ask your pharmacist about suitable sunscreen products. Call your doctor if you become sunburned.

This medicine may cause your urine to turn pale blue in color.

If you are a diabetic and were prescribed APO-TRIAZIDE, DYAZIDE *or* NOVOTRIAMZIDE:
• This medicine may cause your blood sugar to rise. Carefully test your blood or urine for sugar while you are taking this medicine. Call your doctor if you think your blood sugar is higher than normal or harder to control.

When to Call Your Doctor
Most people experience few or no side effects from this drug. However, any medicine can sometimes cause unwanted effects. Call your

doctor if you develop sore throat, fever, skin rash, mouth sores, nausea or vomiting, dry mouth (or if you become very thirsty), bright red tongue, cracked corners of the mouth, weakness, irregular pulse, shortness of breath, stomach pain, headaches, swelling of the legs or ankles or a sudden weight gain of 5 pounds (2.5 kg).

Also call your doctor if you feel sick or develop persistent vomiting or diarrhea.

If you were prescribed APO-TRIAZIDE, DYAZIDE *or* NOVOTRIAMZIDE:
- Also call your doctor if you develop sharp joint pain, muscle weakness, unusual bruising or bleeding, a yellow color to the skin or eyes or dark-yellow-colored urine.

Taking the Birth Control Pill?

Certain medicines, if taken at the same time as birth control pills, may reduce the reliability and effectiveness of the contraceptive or increase the incidence of breakthrough bleeding.

If you are prescribed any of the following medications while you are taking the birth control pill, check with your doctor or pharmacist about using an additional method of contraception for the remainder of your cycle:

- AMPICILLIN
- Antimigraine preparations
- ISONIAZID
- NITROFURANTOIN
- PHENYLBUTAZONE
- TETRACYCLINE
- Analgesics (pain killers)
- CHORAMPHENICOL
- NEOMYCIN
- PENICILLIN V
- SULFONAMIDES

If you must take any of these medicines for a long period of time, the efficacy of the birth control pills could be decreased throughout the entire period of time. Discuss an alternative method of birth control with your doctor.

Allergic Reactions

Call your doctor immediately if you think you may be allergic to the medicine or if you develop a skin rash, hives, itching, swelling of the face or difficulty in breathing. If you cannot reach your doctor, phone a hospital emergency department.

Refills

Do not stop taking this medicine without your doctor's approval and do not go without medicine between prescription refills. Call your pharmacist for a refill 2 or 3 days before you will run out of the medicine.

▶ WARFARIN SODIUM (ORAL)
COUMADIN, WARFILONE

Purpose

This medicine is used to treat or help prevent harmful blood clots from forming in the blood vessels. It is commonly called a blood thinner.

Allergies/Warnings

If you have ever had an allergic reaction to any blood thinner, tell your doctor and pharmacist before you take any of this medicine.

How to Use This Medicine

Time of Administration

Take this medicine exactly as your doctor has prescribed. Try to take the medicine at the same time(s) every day and do not miss any doses. If you miss a dose, do not take extra tablets without your doctor's approval because overtreatment may cause serious bleeding problems.

How to Administer

It is best to take this medicine with a glass of water. Do not take it with food or other drugs unless otherwise directed because there are many possible interactions that could occur.

Special Instructions

Length of Therapy

Do not take any more of this medicine than your doctor has prescribed and do not stop taking this medicine suddenly without the approval of your doctor.

After you stop taking the medicine, it will take your body some time to eliminate the drug and return to normal. Your doctor or pharmacist will tell you how long you must follow these instructions after you have stopped taking this medicine.

Pregnancy/Breastfeeding

Women who are pregnant or planning to become pregnant should tell their doctor before taking this medicine. This medicine should not be taken during certain stages of pregnancy.

Women who are breastfeeding should tell their doctor before taking this medicine. This medicine can pass into the breast milk.

Drug Interactions

Do not start or stop taking any drugs you are currently taking without first consulting with your doctor. Many medicines can increase or decrease the effect of this drug. This includes both prescription and nonprescription medicines, especially pain relievers, sleeping pills, tranquilizers, medicine for seizures, muscle relaxants, anesthetics, medicines for depression or medicines for allergies. Always check with your pharmacist before you take or buy *any* nonprescription products.

Do not treat yourself with any product containing ASA or salicylate. This includes many pain killers, drugs for fever, cold medicines and antacids. ASA may interact with this medicine and cause serious bleeding problems.

Do not take any vitamin or health food supplements, especially those containing vitamin K, without the approval of your doctor or pharmacist.

Alcohol

It is best to avoid alcoholic beverages while you are taking this medicine. However, your doctor may feel it is safe for you to have an occasional drink. Small amounts of wine or beer may be safe. Brandy, cognac, whiskey or gin could be dangerous.

Broccoli Interacts with "Blood Thinners"

Large amounts of broccoli have been reported to interfere with the action of WARFARIN, an anticoagulant (blood thinner).

WARFARIN is used to help prevent clots from forming in the blood vessels. The dose of WARFARIN must be carefully adjusted so that the person has just the right amount in the bloodstream. If the dose is too low, clots could form. If the dose is too high, the person could start bleeding and hemorrhage.

Some foods (turnip greens, broccoli, lettuce, and cabbage) contain high amounts of vitamin K and should not be eaten in large quantities if the person is taking WARFARIN. Vitamin K is used in hospitals as an antidote if the patient has too high a blood level of WARFARIN. If a patient receiving WARFARIN ate unusually large amounts of any foods high in vitamin K, the effect of the medicine could be cancelled.

For example, one patient who was not responding to WARFARIN had been having both broccoli soup and raw broccoli salad for lunch almost every day. Now she is undergoing treatment on a broccoli-free diet. Another patient had been eating at least 1 pound of broccoli daily for several years. Once broccoli was eliminated from her diet, she responded to the drug treatment.

For this reason, patients are warned not to eat unusually large amounts of leafy green vegetables or change their diets without checking with their doctor. Small amounts are not likely to cause problems.

Special Precautions

Regular blood tests, called prothrombin times or PTs, are necessary in order for your doctor to prescribe the correct dose for you. Your dose may change from time to time depending on these tests.

Do not change your normal diet and do not eat unusually large amounts of foods high in vitamin K, such as fish, fish oils and leafy green vegetables (broccoli, turnip greens, cauliflower, alfalfa sprouts, carrot tops, cabbage, lettuce, watercress, asparagus), or change your diet without telling your doctor. Certain foods can affect the way you will respond to this medicine and your dose may have to be adjusted.

If you have a tendency to cut yourself while shaving, you may wish to use an electric razor to avoid possible bleeding.

You may wish to use a soft-bristled toothbrush to help prevent bleeding of the gums while brushing the teeth.

Do not donate blood because the presence of this medicine in the blood could cause problems in the recipient.

Try to avoid contact sports or activities in which you could become injured because this could result in internal bleeding or severe bruises.

When to Call Your Doctor

If your body gets more medicine than it needs, bleeding may occur. Call your doctor if you notice any unusual signs of bleeding that you cannot explain, for example, nosebleeds, unusual bruising without any obvious cause, heavy menstrual bleeding (in women), bleeding from the gums after brushing the teeth, eye hemorrhage, heavy bleeding from cuts, red or black stools, red or dark brown urine or blood in the urine, stomach cramps, back pain, vomiting or coughing up of blood or material that looks like coffee grounds.

Call your doctor if you develop stomach or back pain, joint pain, chest pain, unusual headaches, changes in vision, constipation or diarrhea, loss of appetite, unusual weight gain, swelling of the feet or ankles, loss of hair, dizziness, a skin rash, unexplained sore throat, fever or mouth sores, chills, a yellow color to the skin or eyes, difficulty urinating (passing your water) or unusual tiredness. Also call your doctor if you fall or hit your head.

Allergic Reactions

Call your doctor immediately if you think you may be allergic to the medicine or if you develop a skin rash, hives, itching, swelling of the face or difficulty in breathing. If you cannot reach your doctor, phone a hospital emergency department or emergency medical service.

Refills

Do not stop taking this medicine without your doctor's approval and do not go without medicine between prescription refills. Call your pharmacist for a refill 2 or 3 days before you will run out of the medicine.

Do not change brands of this medicine without your doctor's approval. The dose you need could be different with different brands.

Miscellaneous

Carry an identification card in your wallet or wear a medical alert bracelet indicating that you are taking this medicine, as well as the

names and phone numbers of your doctors. If you do not already carry such a card, complete the Medicine Card in this book. Always tell your dentist, pharmacist and other doctors who are treating you that you are taking this medicine.

▶ **ZOPICLONE (ORAL)**
IMOVANE

Purpose

This medicine is used to treat certain types of insomnia, such as difficulty falling asleep, frequent wakings during the night, and/or waking up too early.

Allergies/Warnings

If you have ever had an allergic reaction to any medicine or if you have depression or any medical problem (especially a lung or liver problem), tell your doctor and pharmacist before you take any of this medicine.

How to Use This Medicine

Time of Administration

Take this medicine at least 20 to 30 minutes before you want to fall asleep. Go to bed after you have taken the medicine. Do not smoke in bed after you have taken it because you could fall asleep and cause a fire.

Carry a Medicine Card

If you go to more than one doctor or pharmacy, you should tell each one what medicines you are taking.

This should include both prescription and nonprescription drugs, as both types of drugs could interfere with a new medicine that the doctor may prescribe for you.

The Medicine Card in this book is an excellent way to keep a record of all your medicines. Simply show it to every doctor and pharmacist you visit.

How to Administer

This medicine may be taken either with food or on an empty stomach.

Special Instructions

Length of Therapy

Sleeping medicines are only useful for a short time and should not be used longer than 4 weeks. If used for too long, they lose their effectiveness. Do not take any more of this medicine than your doctor has prescribed.

Pregnancy/Breastfeeding

It is not recommended that women who are pregnant, breastfeeding or planning to become pregnant use this medicine.

Drug Interactions

It is important that you obtain the advice of your doctor or pharmacist before taking any other prescription or nonprescription medicines, including pain relievers, muscle relaxants, sleeping pills, tranquilizers or medicines for depression, or cough, cold or allergy medicines. Excessive drowsiness or confusion may occur when some of these drugs are taken together.

There are other drug interactions that can occur. If you are taking other medicines, be sure to check first with your pharmacist or doctor.

Alcohol

Do not drink alcoholic beverages while taking this drug or for a few days after you have stopped taking the drug without the approval of your doctor. The combination could cause drowsiness. One drink (even during the day) may have the same effect that 2 or 3 drinks normally would have.

Special Precautions

If you do not fall asleep after taking the prescribed amount, do not take an additional dose unless advised by your doctor.

Be careful if you have to get up during the night while taking this medicine. You may not feel as alert as usual.

If you have problems sleeping, you should avoid caffeinated beverages, certain cold decongestants and strenuous exercise in the evenings, as they make it more difficult to fall asleep.

If this medicine causes dizziness or drowsiness the next day after you take it, do not drive a car, pilot an airplane, operate dangerous machinery or do jobs that require you to be alert. You should be careful going up and down stairs. Sit or lie down at the first sign of dizziness. If this hangover drowsiness becomes bothersome, call your doctor.

You may experience a sleep problem (insomnia) on the first night or 2 after stopping the drug. This is not a reason for restarting the medicine and your sleep should gradually return to normal.

This medicine may cause some people to become constipated. To help prevent constipation, try increasing the amount of bulk in your diet (for example, bran, fresh fruits, salads), exercising more often or drinking more fluids (unless otherwise directed). Call your doctor if the constipation continues.

This medicine may cause a bitter taste. This is normal and will usually disappear after you have taken the drug for a while. If it continues and is bothersome, contact your doctor.

When to Call Your Doctor

Most people experience few or no side effects from this drug. However, any medicine can sometimes cause unwanted effects. Call your doctor if you develop severe daytime drowsiness, impaired coordination, weakness, confusion, forgetfulness, anxiety or nervousness, heart palpitations, trouble sleeping, shakiness or changes in appetite.

Allergic Reactions

Call your doctor immediately if you think you may be allergic to the medicine or if you develop a skin rash or hives. If you cannot reach your doctor, phone a hospital emergency department.

APPENDIX A

Foods Rich in Potassium

If you have been instructed by your doctor to eat foods rich in potassium, this chart may be helpful. In most cases, you will want to select a food that is also *low* in calories and *low* in sodium.

Foods	Average Portion	Potassium (in mg)	Calories	Sodium (in mg)
FRUITS				
Orange	1 medium	360 mg	95	0.8
Grapefruit	1 cup	380 mg	75	1.0
Banana	1 medium	630 mg	130	0.8
Strawberries	1 cup	270 mg	55	1.2
Avocado	½	380 mg	275	3.4
Apricots	3 medium	500 mg	55	0.7
Dates	1 cup	1390 mg	500	1.8
Watermelon	½ slice	380 mg	95	1.0
Cantaloupe	½ melon	880 mg	75	46.0
Raisins	1 cup	1150 mg	425	34.0
Prunes	4 large	240 mg	90	2.4
JUICES				
Orange	8-oz glass	440 mg	105	9.0
Grapefruit	8-oz glass	370 mg	130	1.0
Prune	8-oz glass	620 mg	170	5.0
Pineapple	8-oz glass	340 mg	120	1.2
MEAT				
Hamburger	3 oz	290 mg	310	92.0
Beef (chuck)	3 oz	310 mg	260	44.0
Beef (round)	3 oz	340 mg	200	58.0
Rib roast	3 oz	290 mg	270	92.0
Turkey	4 oz	350 mg	300	46.0
VEGETABLES				
Tomato	1 medium	340 mg	30	4.5
Artichoke	1 medium	210 mg	30	22.0
Brussels sprouts	1 cup	300 mg	35	11.0

Reference: Merck Sharp & Dohme Canada Limited, Dorothy L. Smith, *Medication Guide for Patient Counseling*, second edition, page 815, 1982.

APPENDIX B

General Instructions for Patients with Diabetes

Keep a regular schedule of daily activities. Eat, exercise and take your medicine at approximately the same times every day.

Diet

The diet that your doctor has prescribed has been carefully planned especially for you. It is to your advantage to follow it very closely. Your medicines will not work effectively if you do not follow your diet. This is especially important if you are overweight.

Feet

Take special care of your feet. Some people with diabetes are prone to foot infections that can lead to serious problems.

- Wash your feet daily and dry them well.
- Check your feet daily for minor injuries and athlete's foot. Tell your doctor immediately if these develop.
- Wear clean shoes and stockings and choose shoes that fit well.
- If you develop corns or calluses, soak your feet in lukewarm water for about 10 minutes. Then rub them off gently with a pumice stone. Never use a knife to cut corns or calluses on your feet. Do *not* use commercial corn removers or commercial arch supports.
- Soften dry skin by rubbing with oil or lotion.
- Trim your toenails straight across with a file or a nail cutter. Do not cut your own toenails if your eyesight is poor.
- Do not wear garters or socks with tight elastic tops. Do *not* sit with your knees crossed.
- Do not warm your feet with a hot water bottle or a heating pad. Use loose bedsocks instead. If your feet are cold, numb or tingling under normal conditions, tell your doctor. Your circulation may be poor and your doctor can offer advice.
- Test bath water temperature with your hands and not your feet since your feet may not be sensitive to heat.
- Call your doctor if you injure your toes or feet. Cuts and scratches in the diabetic person can become infected easily and take longer to heal. Do not apply iodine or strong antiseptics to the feet at any time.

Low Blood Sugar

Know the signs of *hypoglycemia* (low blood sugar). When this happens, your urine or blood sugar will be negative. Hypoglycemia may occur if you delay or skip a meal, exercise too much, feel sick or emotionally upset, take too much insulin, drink alcohol or take certain drugs.

If you develop sweating, shaking, drowsiness, headache, excessive hunger, nausea, nervousness, chills, cold sweats, cool pale skin, confusion or unusual tiredness or weakness, eat or drink any of the following *immediately*:

- A commercial sugar product (e.g., Monoject Insulin Reaction Gel) for insulin reactions.
- 2 sugar cubes or 2 teaspoons of sugar dissolved in water.
- 4 ounces orange juice.
- 4 ounces regular ginger ale, cola beverage or any other sweetened carbonated beverage. Do *not* use low-calorie or diet beverages.
- 2 to 3 teaspoons honey or corn syrup.
- 4 Lifesaver candies.

Artificial sweeteners are of no use.

Call your doctor if this does not relieve your symptoms in about 15 minutes. If you cannot locate your doctor, call a neighbor, a friend or an emergency medical service and tell them your concern.

Always carry sugar cubes or hard candy in case you have a hypoglycemic (low blood sugar) reaction.

High Blood Sugar

Call your doctor immediately if you develop any of the following symptoms of *hyperglycemia* (high blood sugar): high urine sugar, acetone in the urine, drowsiness, loss of appetite, unusual thirst, fast breathing, nausea, vomiting, confusion, a flushed dry skin, increase in urination (passing your water more often than usual) or a fruity odor to the breath. These symptoms may occur if you miss a dose of medicine or overeat, or if you have a fever or an infection.

Carry a supply of glucagon with you if your doctor has prescribed it for you.

For More Information

If you would like more information about diabetes, contact your local chapter of the Canadian Diabetes Association.

APPENDIX C

Tips to Detect Tampering

As a result of the tampering scares, several pharmaceutical manufacturers are using different types of sealing techniques so that the consumer can detect any tampering with the capsules. Lilly has developed a double-banded gelatin seal so that it is next to impossible to separate the two parts of the capsule. Warner-Lambert is using a thermal sealing technique and a flattened capsule shape which reduces the surface area that can be gripped and makes it nearly impossible to pull the 2 sections apart. R.P. Scherer and Sterling are using a special machine that seals capsules by sonic waves.

Not every company is using special sealing techniques on its capsules. As a safety measure, it is always a good idea to inspect all nonprescription drug products before using them. Things to look for include:

- Are there any breaks in the outer covering of the container, or indications of it being unwrapped or opened?
- Is the cap on the container tight?
- Do the lot numbers on the outer and inner packages match?
- Is the protective seal on the bottle in place?
- Is the container full?
- Do all the tablets or capsules have the same appearance? Are they all the same color?
- Are any of the capsules dented?
- Are the 2 halves of the capsules lined up correctly so that any imprint matches perfectly? Many capsules have half an imprint on each half of the capsule, so that when the sections are put together the imprint matches perfectly.
- Is there any unusual or disturbing odor coming from the medicines?

If there is anything unusual about the package or the medication inside it, take the product to the pharmacist and have it checked.

APPENDIX D

Avoiding Food Triggers of Migraine

Substances in many foods can act to trigger a migraine attack. The following chart lists foods which are common migraine triggers. If food is triggering your headaches, eliminating these foods from your diet will help to control your migraines.

Beverages
- beverages containing caffeine, including coffee, tea and cola-type sodas. Do not drink more than 2 cups per day of caffeine-containing beverages.
- chocolate or cocoa
- alcoholic beverages
- food or beverages containing aspartame

Meat, Fish, Poultry
- aged, canned, cured or processed meats
- canned or aged ham
- pickled herring
- salted dried fish
- chicken liver
- aged game
- hot dogs
- fermented sausage
- bologna
- salami
- pepperoni
- summer sausage
- peanuts
- peanut butter
- any meat prepared with meat tenderizer, soy sauce, or yeast extracts

Dairy Products
- cultured dairy products:
- buttermilk
- sour cream
- chocolate milk
- aged cheeses:
- blue
- Boursault
- Brie types
- Camembert types
- Cheddar
- Swiss
- Gouda
- Roquefort
- Stilton
- Mozzarella
- Parmesan
- Provolone
- Romano
- Limit intake of yogurt to ½ cup per day

Breads and Cereals
- homemade or bakery yeast breads
- breads and crackers with cheese
- yeast coffee cake
- yeast doughnuts
- sourdough breads
- any breads or cereals containing chocolate or nuts

Vegetables
- pole or broad beans
- lima or Italian beans
- pea pods
- snow peas
- fava beans
- navy beans
- pinto beans
- garbanzo beans (chick peas)
- raw onions except for flavoring
- olives
- pickles
- sauerkraut

Fruits
- Limit intake to ½ cup per day of:
  - oranges
  - grapefruit
  - tangerines
  - pineapple
  - lemon
  - lime
  - bananas
- avocados
- figs
- raisins
- papaya
- passion fruit
- red plums
- seeds:
  - sunflower
  - sesame
  - pumpkin

Soups
- canned soups
- soup cubes
- bouillon cubes
- soup bases with yeast or monosodium glutamate (MSG)

Desserts
- chocolate flavored:
  - ice cream
  - pudding
  - cookies
  - cakes
- mincemeat pies

Sweets
- chocolate candies
- chocolate syrup
- carob
- aspartame

Miscellaneous
- pizza
- cheese sauce
- soy sauce
- monosodium glutamate (MSG)
- yeast
- meat tenderizers
- seasoned salts
- mixed dishes:
  - macaroni and cheese
  - beef stroganoff
  - cheese blintzes
  - lasagna
  - frozen dinners
- any pickled, preserved or marinated foods.

Source: American Council for Headache Education (ACHE), 875 Kings Highway, Suite 200, West Deptford, New Jersey, U.S.A. 08096.

APPENDIX E

Helpful Tips to Reduce Nausea and Vomiting from Chemotherapy

Patients who are receiving chemotherapy may find the following dietary suggestions helpful in reducing nausea and vomiting:

- Eat small meals frequently throughout the day to keep your stomach from feeling too full.

- Chew your food well so that it will be easier for your body to digest it.

- Eat slowly so that only small amounts of food enter your stomach at a time.

- Avoid drinking liquids at mealtime to prevent filling up your stomach. Instead, drink liquids 1 hour before or after eating.

- Try to drink clear, cool, unsweetened beverages, such as apple juice.

- Before you go for your chemotherapy treatment, eat a light meal, such as soup and crackers.

- Try not to lie down flat for at least 2 hours after eating. However, it may be helpful to rest after eating since this will help your body digest the food.

- If the smell of food causes nausea, try to stay out of the kitchen.

APPENDIX F

First Aid for Epileptic Seizures

Many patients with grand mal epilepsy may experience a warning "aura" before the onset of seizures. This aura may be in the form of unusual colors, smells or sounds, numbness, tingling or other disturbances. Some people will utter a short cry.

- If a patient experiences a seizure, place the patient where he or she cannot fall or be hurt. Sometimes the floor is the safest area. Clear the area of any furniture and hard, sharp or hot objects.

- Check the person's wrist or neck for an emergency medical information bracelet or necklace.

- Stay calm yourself! You cannot stop a seizure once it starts, so let the seizure run its course. Do not try to revive the person.

- Loosen tight clothing (especially around the neck) to make it easier for the person to breathe.

- Do not force anything between the patient's teeth since this could result in damage to the teeth or gums, aspiration of the material or bite injuries to the person administering the first aid. Remember it is physically impossible for a person to swallow his or her tongue during a seizure.

- Try to gently turn the patient on the side to allow mucous and often large amounts of saliva to drain from the mouth.

- Do not be alarmed if the person seems to stop breathing momentarily, but if the patient passes from one seizure to another without regaining consciousness, call an ambulance or seek medical assistance.

- After the seizure is over, the patient may be confused and/or incontinent (loss of bladder control). Allow him or her to sleep or rest. If the person remains groggy, weak or confused, he or she should not be allowed to go home alone. A relative should always be contacted if the patient is a child.

- The patient should inform his or her physician of the seizure.

APPENDIX G

Poison Control Centers in Canada

NEWFOUNDLAND AND
LABRADOR

St. John's
Provincial Poison Control Centre
The Dr. Charles A. Janeway
  Child Health Centre
(709) 722-1110

Corner Brook
Western Memorial Hospital
(709) 637-5263
(709) 637-5264

Gander
James Paton Memorial Hospital
(709) 258-5552
(709) 651-2500 (Switchboard)

Grand Falls
Central Newfoundland Hospital
(709) 292-2134

Labrador City
Capt. Wm. Jackman Memorial
  Hospital
(709) 944-2632

St. Anthony Charles S. Curtis
  Memorial Hospital
Grenfell Regional Health Services
(709) 454-3333, ext. 364

PRINCE EDWARD ISLAND

Charlottetown
Queen Elizabeth Hospital
Emergency Department
(902) 566-6250

Summerside
Prince County Hospital
(902) 436-9131, ext. 175

NOVA SCOTIA

Main Center:

Halifax
The Izaak Walton Killam Hospital
  for Children
(902) 428-8161

Satellite Centers:

Amherst
Highland View Regional Hospital
(902) 667-3361, ext. 145

Antigonish St. Martha's Hospital
(902) 863-2830, ext. 122

Bridgewater
Dawson Memorial Hospital
(902) 543-4603

Dartmouth
Dartmouth General Hospital
(902) 465-8333
(902) 465-8300 (Emergency Dept.)

Halifax
Victoria General Hospital
Emergency Department
(902) 428-2043

Kentville
Blanchard-Fraser Memorial
  Hospital
(902) 678-7381, ext. 215

New Glasgow
Aberdeen Hospital
(902) 752-8311

Sydney
Sydney City Hospital
(902) 539-6400, ext. 118

Yarmouth
Yarmouth Regional Hospital
(902) 742-3541, ext. 111

NEW BRUNSWICK
There is a poison treatment
center in the Emergency Service
of most of the active treatment
hospitals in New Brunswick.

Bathurst
Chaleur General Hospital
(506) 546-4666

Campbellton
Hotel-Dieu St. Joseph
(506) 753-5212

Edmundston
Hotel-Dieu St. Joseph
(506) 735-7384

Fredericton
Dr. Everett Chalmers Hospital
(506) 452-5400
911 (Fredericton area only)

Moncton
Moncton Hospital
(506) 857-5555
911 (Moncton area only)

Saint John
Saint John Regional Hospital
Central Division
(506) 648-7111
911 (Saint John area only)

QUEBEC
There is a poison treatment
center in the Emergency Service
of every active treatment hospital
or Centre Local de Santé
Communautaire in the Province
of Quebec. There is one Poison
Control Centre in the Province
of Quebec.

Quebec City
Poison Control Centre of Quebec
Centre anti-poison du Québec
656-8090 (for Quebec City only)
1-800-463-5060 (for Quebec
  Province only)
(418) 656-8090 (for all other
  areas)

The Centre de Toxicologie du Québec is in charge of the provincial Poison Control Program.

Centre de Toxicologie du Québec
Centre Hospitalier de l'Université Laval
(418) 654-2254

ONTARIO

Main Poison Control Information Centres:

Toronto
Hospital for Sick Children
(416) 598-5900 (for area 416 and outside of Ontario)
1-800-268-9017 (for the rest of Ontario)

Ottawa
Children's Hospital of Eastern Ontario
(613) 737-1100
1-800-267-1373 (most of Ontario)

Other Centres:

Brantford
Brantford General Hospital
(519) 752-7871

Kingston
Kingston General Hospital
1-800-267-1373 (Children's Hospital of Eastern Ontario)

Kirkland Lake
Kirkland and District Hospital
(705) 567-5251

Kitchener
Kitchener-Waterloo Hospital
(519) 749-4220

St. Mary's General Hospital
(519) 744-4121

London
Victoria Hospital
(519) 667-6565

St. Catharines
St. Catharines General Hospital
Poison Control Centre
(416) 684-7271, ext. 461

Sarnia
Sarnia General Hospital
(519) 336-6311

St. Joseph's Hospital
(519) 336-3111

Sault Ste Marie
Plummer Memorial Public Hospital
(705) 759-3800

Simcoe
Norfolk General Hospital
(519) 426-0750, ext. 212

Thunder Bay
McKellar General Hospital
(807) 623-5561

Port Arthur General Hospital
911 (Thunder Bay area only)
(807) 344-6621 (outside Thunder
  Bay area)
(416) 598-5900

Toronto
East General and Orthopaedic
  Hospital
(416) 469-6245

Windsor
Hotel-Dieu de St. Joseph
(519) 973-4400

MANITOBA
Poison treatment is available in
every active emergency hospital
in Manitoba.

There is one provincial Poison
Information Centre in the
Province of Manitoba.

Winnipeg
Provincial Poison Information
  Centre
Children's Hospital Health
  Sciences Centre
(204) 787-2591

SASKATCHEWAN
There is a poison treatment
center in the Emergency Service
of most of the active treatment
hospitals in Saskatchewan.

Main Centres:

Regina
Regina General Hospital
Poison Control Centre
(306) 359-4545

Saskatoon
Saskatoon University Hospital
Poison Control Centre
(306) 966-1010

ALBERTA

Provincial Center:

Calgary
Poison and Drug Information
  Service
Foothills General Hospital
1-800-332-1414 (within Alberta
  only)
(403) 270-1414 (Calgary area
  and outside of Alberta)

Treatment Centres: All active
treatment hospitals in Alberta.

BRITISH COLUMBIA

Poison treatment is available in every active hospital emergency department in British Columbia.

Vancouver
B.C. Drug and Poison
  Information Centre (DPIC)
St. Paul's Hospital
(604) 682-5050

Victoria
Royal Jubilee Hospital
Emergency Department
(604) 595-9211

NORTHWEST TERRITORIES

Fort Smith
Fort Smith Health Centre
(403) 872-2713, ext. 211 (24 hr.
  service)
(Ask for Poison Control)

Hay River
H.H. Williams Memorial
  Hospital
(403) 874-6512

Inuvik
Inuvik General Hospital
(403) 979-2955

Iqaluit (Frobisher Bay)
Baffin Regional Hospital
(819) 979-5231, ext. 268

Yellowknife
Stanton Yellowknife Hospital
(403) 920-4111

YUKON TERRITORY

Whitehorse
Whitehorse General Hospital
Emergency Department
(403) 668-9444, ext. 226

Available information on telephones and personnel as supplied by Children's Hospital of Eastern Ontario, Ottawa, January 1991.

Credit: Canadian Pharmaceutical Association

APPENDIX H

Canadian Drug Information Centers

Regional Drug Information Centers

BRITISH COLUMBIA

B.C. Drug and Poison
  Information Centre (DPIC)
St. Paul's Hospital
1081 Burrard Street
Vancouver, B.C. V6Z 1Y6
(604) 682-2344

ALBERTA

Provincial Poison and Drug
  Information Centre (PADIS)
Foothills Hospital
1403-29th Street NW
Calgary, Alberta T2N 2T9
(403) 270-1414 (Poison
  Information)
1-800-332-1414 (Alberta only—
  Drug Information)

SASKATCHEWAN

Dial Access Drug Information
  Service
University of Saskatchewan
Saskatoon, Saskatchewan
S7N 0W0
(306) 652-1160

ONTARIO

London
Drug Information Centre
(UH-LONDIS)
Pharmacy Department
University Hospital
339 Windermere Road
Box 5339
London, Ontario N6A 5A5
(519) 663-3172

Ottawa
Ottawa Valley Regional Drug
  Information Service
Pharmacy Department
Ottawa General Hospital
501 Smyth Road
Ottawa, Ontario K1H 8L6
(613) 737-8347

QUEBEC

Centre D'Information
  Pharmaceutique (CIP)
Hôpital du Sacre-Coeur de
  Montréal
5400, Boul. Gouin Ouest
Montreal, Quebec H4J 1C5
(514) 338-2161

NOVA SCOTIA

Provincial Drug Information
  Centre
Pharmacy Department
Camp Hill Hospital
1763 Robie Street
Halifax, Nova Scotia B3H 3G2
(902) 420-2222

Other Major Hospital-Based
Drug Information Centers
For all hospitals listed direct
inquiries to:
Drug Information Center
Pharmacy Department

BRITISH COLUMBIA

Victoria
Royal Jubilee Hospital
1900 Fort Street
Victoria, B.C. V8R 1J8
(604) 595-9200

Vancouver
Vancouver General Hospital
855 West 12th Avenue
Vancouver, B.C. V5Z 1M9
(604) 875-4111

MANITOBA

Winnipeg
Health Sciences Centre
820 Sherbrook Street
Winnipeg, Manitoba R3A 1R9
(204) 787-3097

Misericordia General Hospital
99 Cornish Avenue
Winnipeg, Manitoba R3C 1A2
(204) 788-8242

St. Boniface General Hospital
409 Tache Avenue
Winnipeg, Manitoba R2H 2A6
(204) 237-2630

ONTARIO

Hamilton
McMaster University Medical
  Centre
P.O. Box 2000, Station "A"
Hamilton, Ontario L8N 3Z5
(416) 521-2100, ext. 6019

St. Joseph's Hospital
50 Charlton Avenue East
Hamilton, Ontario L8N 1Y4
(416) 522-4941

Kingston
Kingston General Hospital
76 Stuart Street
Kingston, Ontario K7L 2V7
(613) 548-3232

Kitchener
Kitchener-Waterloo Hospital
835 King Street West
Kitchener, Ontario N2G 1G3
(519) 742-3611

London
St. Joseph's Health Centre
268 Grosvenor Street
London, Ontario N5A 4V2
(519) 439-3271, ext. 4376

Victoria Hospital
South Street Campus
375 South Street
London, Ontario N6A 4G5
(519) 432-5241

Ottawa
Ottawa Civic Hospital
1053 Carling Avenue
Ottawa, Ontario K1Y 4E9
(613) 725-4115

Ottawa General Hospital
501 Smyth Road
Ottawa, Ontario K1H 8L6
(613) 737-8344

Toronto
Addiction Research Foundation
33 Russell Street
Toronto, Ontario M5S 2S1
(416) 595-6014

Princess Margaret Hospital
500 Sherbourne Street
Toronto, Ontario M4X 1K9
(416) 924-0671

St. Joseph's Health Centre
30 The Queensway
Toronto, Ontario M6R 1B5
(416) 530-6299

St. Michael's Hospital
30 Bond Street
Toronto, Ontario M5B 1W8
(416) 864-5130

Sunnybrook Medical Centre
2075 Bayview Avenue
Toronto, Ontario M4N 3M5
(416) 480-4513

The Hospital for Sick Children
555 University Avenue
Toronto, Ontario M5G 1X8
(416) 598-6703

The Wellesley Hospital
160 Wellesley Street East
Toronto, Ontario M4Y 1J3
(416) 480-4513

Toronto General Hospital
101 College Street
Toronto, Ontario M5G 1L7
(416) 595-3611

Toronto Western Hospital
399 Bathurst Street
Toronto, Ontario M5T 2S8
(416) 369-5943

QUEBEC

Montreal
Centre Hospitalier
  Maisonneuve-Rosemont
5415 Boulevard de l'Assomption
Montreal, Quebec H1T 2M4
(514) 252-3530

Mortimer B. Davis—Jewish
  General Hospital
3755 Chemin de la Côté de St.
  Catharine
Montreal, Quebec H3T 1E2
(514) 340-8222, ext. 5025

Royal Victoria Hospital
687 Avenue des Pins
Montreal, Quebec H3A 1A1
(514) 842-1231

NOVA SCOTIA

Halifax
Victoria General Hospital
1278 Tower Road
Halifax, Nova Scotia B3H 2Y9
(902) 428-3575

INDEX